HOLISTIC
HERBAL

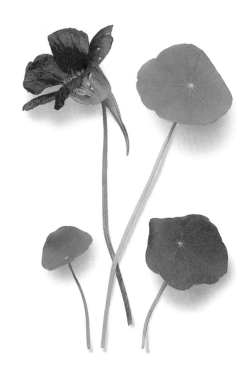

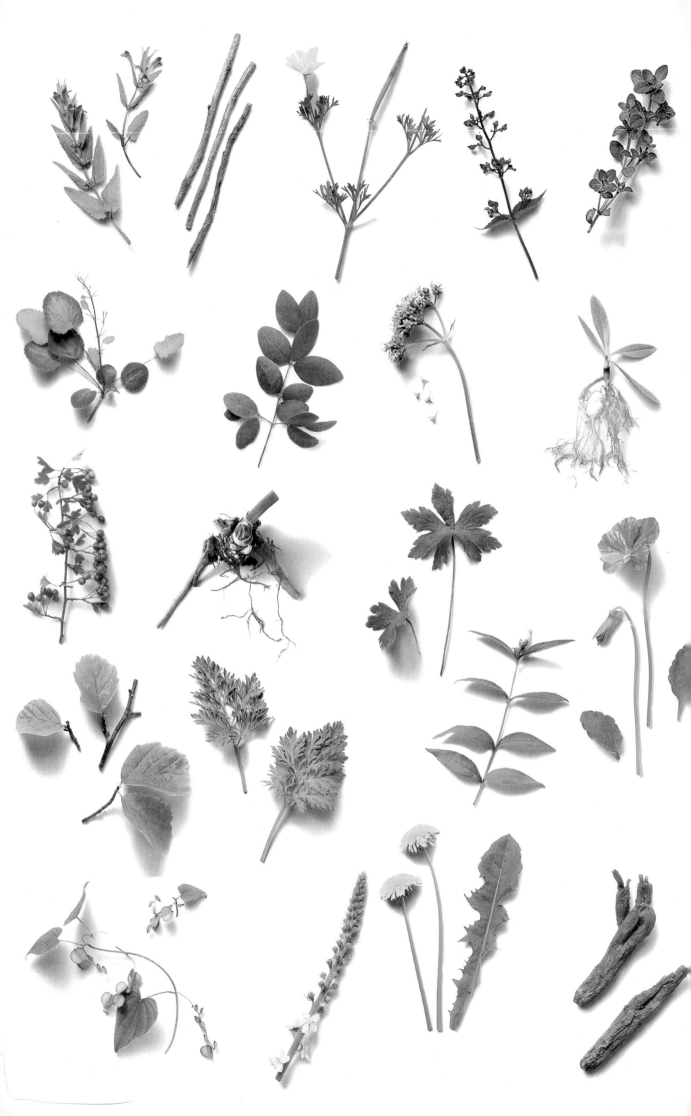

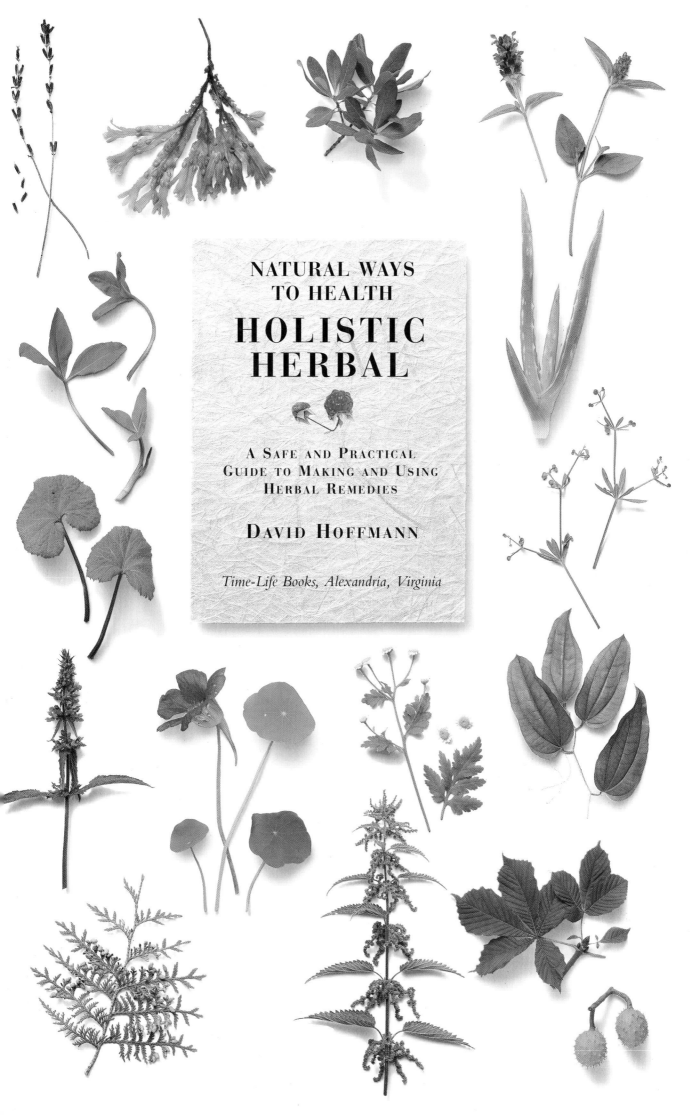

NATURAL WAYS TO HEALTH

HOLISTIC HERBAL

A Safe and Practical Guide to Making and Using Herbal Remedies

David Hoffmann

Time-Life Books, Alexandria, Virginia

Time-Life Books is a division of Time Life Inc.

TIME LIFE INC. PRESIDENT and CEO: George Artandi
TIME-LIFE BOOKS PRESIDENT: Stephen R. Frary
PUBLISHER/MANAGING EDITOR: Neil Kagan

ELEMENT BOOKS LIMITED
Shaftesbury, Dorset SP7 8BP
Reprinted 1996, 1997 and 1998

Published in USA in 1996 by
ELEMENT BOOKS LIMITED
160 North Washington Street, Boston, MA 02114

Published in Australia in 1996 by
ELEMENT BOOKS LIMITED
and distributed by Penguin Australia Ltd
487 Maroondah Highway, Ringwood, Victoria 3134

Designed and created with
The Bridgewater Book Company Limited

ELEMENT BOOKS LIMITED
Creative Director: **Ed Day**
Managing Editor: **Miranda Spicer**
Senior Comissioning Editor: **Caro Ness**
Production Manager: **Susan Sutterby**
Production Controller: **Fiona Harrison**

BRIDGEWATER BOOK CO.
Art Director: **Peter Bridgewater**
Layout/Page make-up: **Ed White**
Managing Editor: **Anne Townley**
Editor: **Viv Croot**
Plant research: **Sarah Mellish**
Picture research: **Vanessa Fletcher**
Studio photography: **Guy Ryecart**
Medical illustrator: **Michael Courtney**
Plaster models: **Mark Jamieson**
Illustrator: **Paul Allen**

Printed and bound in Singapore

British Library Cataloguing in Publication data available.

ACKNOWLEDGMENTS

The publishers wish to thank the following for the use of pictures:

A-Z Botanical Collection:
pp.21 (Derek Gould), 78R
(K. Jarayam), 81R (Geoff Kidd), 84R (Bjorn Svensson),
135L & 138L (Ron Bass), 149L, 150L (K. Jarayam),
155L (Dr Thomas Hagen)

e.t. archive: Royal Academy p.28T

Garden & Wildlife Matters Photo Library: p.176B

Hutchison Library:
pp.12 (Brian Mose), 130R (P.E.Parker),
189T (C.R. Overseas), 212B (Robert Francis),
230T (Nancy Durrell McKenna)

The Image Bank: p.183 (Grant Faint)

Images Colour Library:
pp.16B, 169T, 177T & B, 212T, 218B

Andrew Lawson: pp.142R, 160R

Oxford Scientific Films:
pp.101L (James Nash Alford/Patrick Morris), 109R & 122L
(Deni Brown), 157R (Ben Osborne), 161R (Jack Dermio)

Science Photo Library:
pp.10B (Simon Fraser), 16L & R (NIBSC), 41B (David Scharf)

Harry Smith Collection: pp.100R, 111L, 117R

Smith/Polunin Collection: p.69R

Elizabeth Whiting Associates: p.20T

Special thanks to:

Darren Webster,
Royal Botanic Gardens,
Kew, London, England

Geoff Peacock,
YSJ Seeds,
Kingsfield Conservation Nursery,
Somerset, England

Duncan Ross,
Poyntzfield Herb Nursery,
Ross-shire, Scotland

Anthony Lyman-Dixon,
Arne Herbs,
Bristol, England

Dave Masters,
Nymans Gardens,
Sussex, England

David Squire

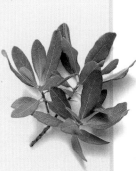

CONTENTS

How to Use This Book _____ 6

PART ONE:
THE HOLISTIC APPROACH ___ 9

Herbs and Health _____ 10

Herbs in the Holistic Context _____ 10

Healing the Whole Self _____ 11

Herbs and the Environment _____ 11

Wholeness and Prevention _____ 12

Herbs to Prevent Disease _____ 12

Tonics for the Systems of the Body _____ 12

Helping the Body Cleanse Itself _____ 14

Herbs and the Body's Defence System _____ 16

PART TWO: PRACTICAL HERBALISM ___ 19

Gathering Herbs _____ 20

The Preparation of Herbs _____ 22

Internal Remedies _____ 22

External Remedies _____ 28

The Chemistry of Herbs _____ 32

The Action of Herbs _____ 36

Fighting Off Invaders _____ 40

Herbs for Infections and Infestations _____ 42

Anti-Microbials _____ 42

Diaphoretics (Febrifuges) _____ 42

Anthelmintics (Vermifuges) _____ 43

Treating Infections _____ 44

Treating Infestations _____ 44

A Therapeutic Index _____ 46

Herbal Remedies in the Home _____ 49

PART THREE: THE HERBAL _____ 51

Introducing The Herbal _____ 52

The Herbal _____ 53

PART FOUR:
SYSTEMS OF THE BODY _____ 167

The Circulatory System _____ 168

Prevention of Circulatory Disease _____ 168

Herbs for the Heart and Circulation _____ 170

Patterns of Circulatory Disease _____ 172

The Lymphatic System _____ 175

The Respiratory System _____ 176

Prevention of Respiratory Disease _____ 176

Herbs for the Respiratory System _____ 178

Patterns of Respiratory Disease _____ 179

Ears, Nose, Throat and Eyes _____ 182

Herbs for Ears, Nose, Throat and Eyes _____ 184

Patterns of Disease _____ 184

The Digestive System _____ 188

Prevention of Digestive Disease _____ 189

Herbs for the Digestive System _____ 190

Patterns of Digestive Disease _____ 192

The Nervous System _____ 202

Herbs for the Nervous System _____ 203

Patterns of Nervous Disease _____ 204

The Skin _____ 212

Herbs for the Skin _____ 213

Patterns of Skin Disease _____ 214

The Musculo/Skeletal System _____ 218

Herbs for the Musculo/Skeletal System _____ 220

Patterns of Muscle and Bone Disease _____ 222

The Glandular System _____ 226

Herbs for the Glands _____ 227

Patterns of Glandular Disease _____ 228

The Reproductive System _____ 230

Herbs for the Female Reproductive System _____ 232

Patterns of Reproductive
Disease _____ 234

**The Urinary
System** _____ 240

Herbs for the Urinary
System _____ 241

Patterns of Urinary
Disease _____ 242

PART FIVE:
USEFUL INFORMATION _____ 245

When to Gather Herbs _____ 246

Glossary _____ 248

Further Reading and Useful Addresses _____ 251

Index _____ 252

HOW TO USE THIS BOOK

Holistic Herbal can be used in several ways: it can be read from cover to cover as an introduction to herbalism; it can be used as a textbook; it can be used as a source for finding out about the holistic treatment of specific conditions and problems; or it can be used as a traditional herbal.

There are four main sections. The introductory section, **The Holistic Approach,** places herbalism in a wider context and shows plants in their relationship to healing and humanity. The second part, **Practical Herbalism**, offers advice on how to harvest and store herbs and gives easy-to-follow instructions showing how to prepare herbal tinctures, creams, capsules and pills; it explains the underlying chemistry of herbs and describes the actions they have on the body. A therapeutic index indicates which herbs might be useful for particular diseases and suggestions are made for a practical herbal medicine chest for the home.

The third part of the book is a traditional **Herbal** which lists over 200 commonly used herbs, describes their properties and explains when and how to use them.

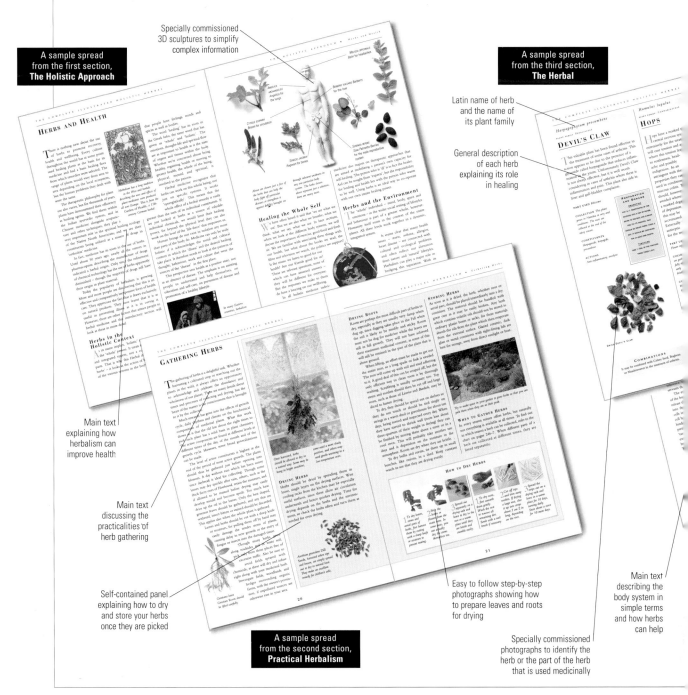

A sample spread from the first section, **The Holistic Approach**

Specially commissioned 3D sculptures to simplify complex information

A sample spread from the third section, **The Herbal**

Latin name of herb and the name of its plant family

General description of each herb explaining its role in healing

Main text explaining how herbalism can improve health

Main text discussing the practicalities of herb gathering

Self-contained panel explaining how to dry and store your herbs once they are picked

A sample spread from the second section, **Practical Herbalism**

Easy to follow step-by-step photographs showing how to prepare leaves and roots for drying

Main text describing the body system in simple terms and how herbs can help

Specially commissioned photographs to identify the herb or the part of the herb that is used medicinally

The fourth part, **Systems of the Body**, looks in detail at each system of the body in turn and the patterns of disease to which they are susceptible, and suggests the herbs or combination of herbs which can help restore and heal the body to its proper wholeness.

Finally, the fifth section contains useful information, a seasonal chart indicating when to gather herbs for maximum effectiveness, a glossary of medical and therapeutic terms, suggested further reading, a list of suppliers and organizations, and a general index.

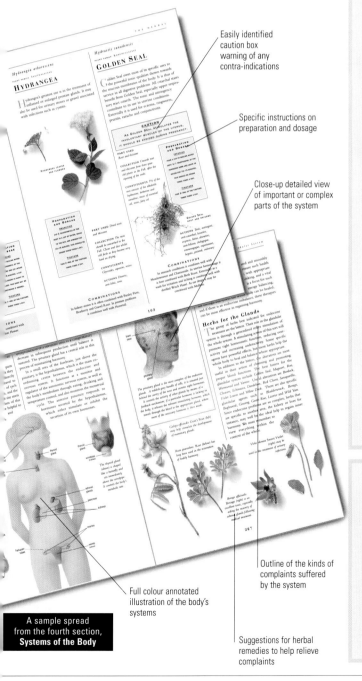

Easily identified caution box warning of any contra-indications

Specific instructions on preparation and dosage

Close-up detailed view of important or complex parts of the system

Full colour annotated illustration of the body's systems

A sample spread from the fourth section, **Systems of the Body**

Outline of the kinds of complaints suffered by the system

Suggestions for herbal remedies to help relieve complaints

WEIGHTS AND MEASURES

Measurements in this book are metric with US equivalents. Pints are US pints which contain 16 fluid ounces.

The metric system is the most widely used dosage measurement today. Many of the books used by American herbalists, however, refer to the old system of apothecaries' ounces, grains and drams (drachms). These conversion charts may be useful if you are consulting such sources.

APOTHECARIES – METRIC VOLUME CONVERSION

MINIMS	MILLILITRES	FLUID DRAMS	MILLILITRES	FLUID OUNCES	MILLILITRES
1	0.06				
2	0.12	1	3.7	1	29.57
5	0.31	2	7.39	2	59.57
10	0.62	3	11.09	5	147.87
15	0.92	4	14.79	7	207.01
20	1.23	5	18.48	10	295.73
30	1.85	6	22.18	12	354.88
40	2.46	7	25.88	14	414.02
50	3.08	8 (1fl. oz.)	29.57	16 (1pt)	473.17
60 (1fl. dr.)	3.70			32 (1qt)	946.33
				128 (1gal.)	3785.32

APOTHECARIES – METRIC WEIGHT CONVERSION

GRAINS	GRAMS	DRAMS	GRAMS	OUNCES	GRAMS
$1/2$	0.032	1	3.888	1	31.103
1	0.065	2	7.776	2	62.207
$1^1/2$	0.097(0.1)	3	11.664	3	93.310
2	0.12	4	15.552	4	124.414
5	0.30	5	19.440	5	155.517
10	0.65	6	23.328	6	186.621
15	1.00	7	27.216	7	217.724
20	1.30	8 (1oz.)	31.103	8	248.828
30	2.00			9	279.931
				10	311.035
				12	373.242

An unfortunate trend is to use drops or dropperfuls as a way of measuring dosage. The 'drop' is a totally variable quantity that depends on (for example):
● the size of the hole in the dropper
● the viscosity or density of the liquid
● the pressure applied to the bulb of the dropper
A review of modern herbals shows a range from 60 to 100 drops equalling 1 ml. Drops are only of value for measuring volatile oils not taken internally.

SYMBOLS

Recipes throughout this book use symbols for clarity.

◪ a spoon indicates the amount of herb mixture used per cup of water
▣ a cup means an infusion should be made
▣ a pan means a decoction should be made
◉ a clock indicates how many minutes the mixture should infuse or simmer
So ◪ ▣ ◉ means that 1 teaspoonful of the mixture per cup of water should be simmered for 10 minutes to make a decoction.

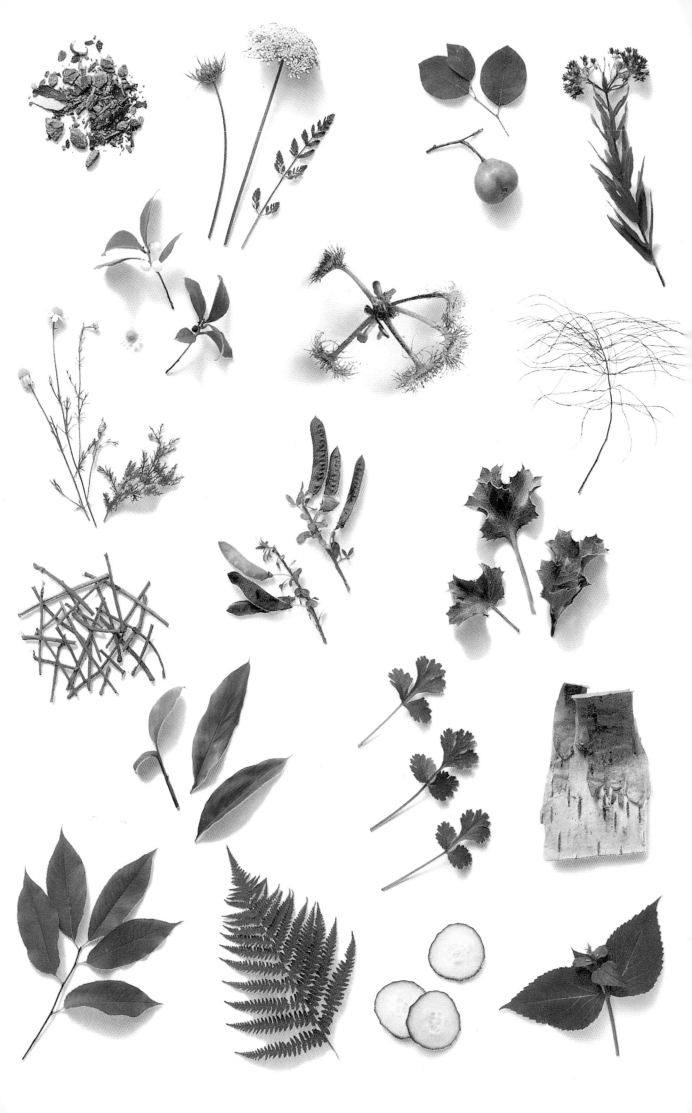

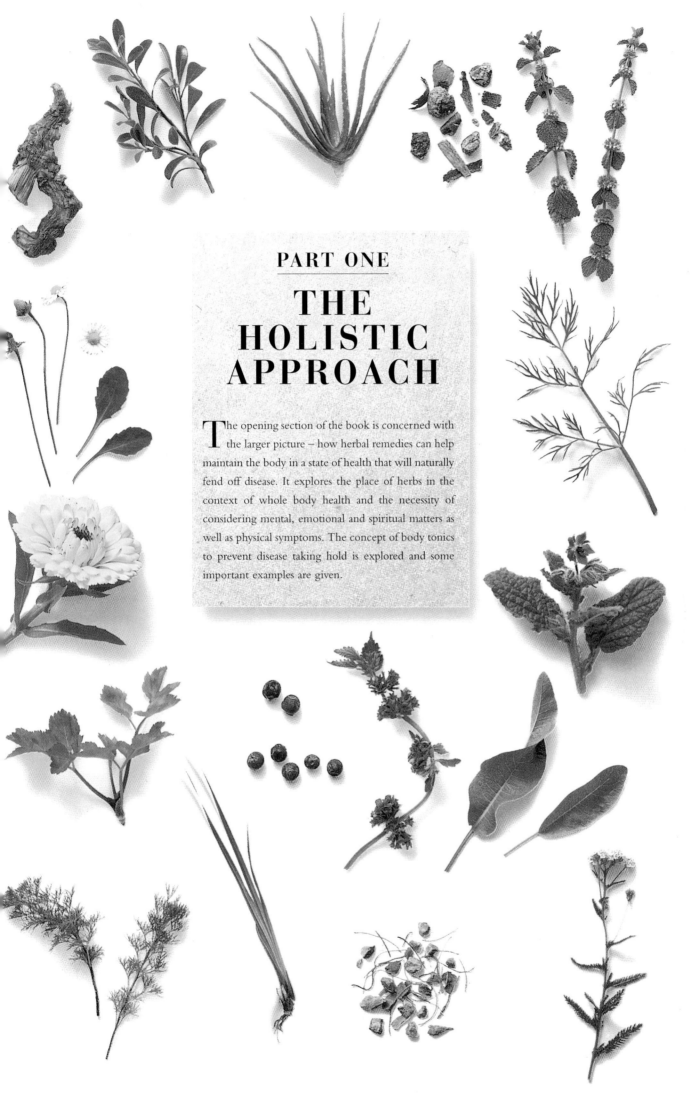

PART ONE

THE HOLISTIC APPROACH

The opening section of the book is concerned with the larger picture – how herbal remedies can help maintain the body in a state of health that will naturally fend off disease. It explores the place of herbs in the context of whole body health and the necessity of considering mental, emotional and spiritual matters as well as physical symptoms. The concept of body tonics to prevent disease taking hold is explored and some important examples are given.

HERBS AND HEALTH

There is nothing new about the use of herbs to promote recovery, health and wellbeing. Every culture throughout the world has at some point used healing plants as the basis for its medicine and had a basic healing flora from which remedies were selected. The range of plants would vary from area to area depending on the local ecosystem, but the human problems they dealt with were the same.

The therapeutic philosophy for plant use also varies, but for thousands of years plants have demonstrated their efficiency as healing agents. We find them within the Indian ayurvedic system, and in Chinese medicine alongside acupuncture and other techniques; they play a very important role in the spiritual healing ecology of the Native North Americans; and we see their constituents being utilized as a source of drugs in 'orthodox' medicine.

In fact, medicine has its roots in the use of herbs. Until about 50 years ago, nearly all the entries in pharmacopeias describing the manufacture of drugs indicated a herbal origin. Only since the refinement of chemical technology has the use of herbs apparently diminished – though the majority of drugs still have their origin in plant material.

Today the popularity of herbalism is growing. More and more people are discovering that this is an effective and comparatively inexpensive form of health care. They appreciate the fact that it draws exclusively on natural products. They have learnt that it is as useful in preventing illness as it is in curing it. However, there are other factors that attract people to herbal medicine and this introductory section will look at these in more detail.

Herbs in the Holistic Context

As its name implies, 'holistic' medicine deals with the 'whole' person. It treats the body as a whole and integrated system, not a collection of isolated parts. That is why this Herbal does not merely 'list herbs' – it looks at the action of herbs in the context of the various systems in the body and acknowledges

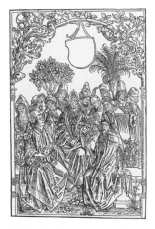

Herbalism has a long tradition in the West and herbals describing the uses and effects of plant medicines were produced all over Europe. This is from the Garden of Health, a 15th-century German herbal.

that people have feelings, minds and spirits as well as bodies.

The word 'healing' has its roots in the Greek *holos,* the same word that has given us 'whole' and 'holistic'. The emotions, thought-life and spiritual flow are as important to health as is the state of organs and tissues within the body. Whether we're concerned about being healthy, regaining health or moving to greater health, the whole of the being, physical, mental and spiritual, is involved in the process.

Herbal medicine recognizes that herbs can work on this whole being, not just on specific systems. It works 'synergistically'. This means that the whole effect of a herbal remedy is vastly greater than the sum of its individual constituents. If we just looked at herbs as a source of valuable individual chemicals, we would limit their healing power, for beyond the physical level they can also work on the level of the 'life-force' that empowers us.

Human beings do not exist in isolation any more than parts of the body do. Medicine can only be truly holistic if it acknowledges the social and cultural context in which the 'illness' and the desired healing take place. It therefore needs to look at the patterns of thought, behaviour, work and culture that were the sources of the 'disease' in the first place.

This perspective sees health as a positive state, not as an absence of disease. The emphasis is on assisting people to understand and help themselves, on education and self-care, on prevention of disease and promotion of a healthy lifestyle.

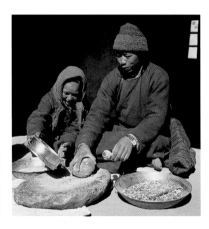

In many Eastern countries, herbalism is part of mainstream living. This is a traditional village doctor, working at his roadside pharmacy in northern India.

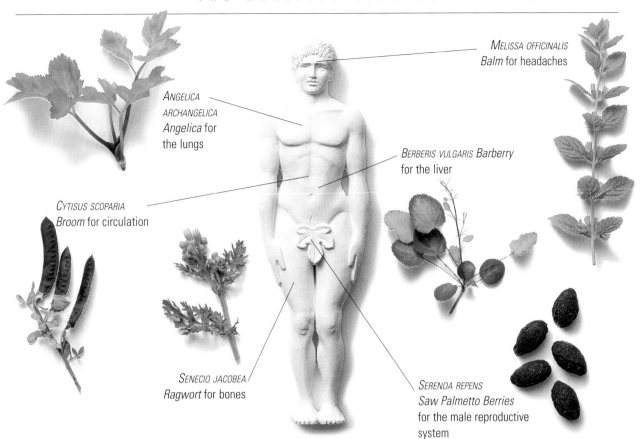

MELISSA OFFICINALIS
Balm for headaches

ANGELICA ARCHANGELICA
Angelica for the lungs

BERBERIS VULGARIS Barberry
for the liver

CYTISUS SCOPARIA
Broom for circulation

SENECIO JACOBEA
Ragwort for bones

SERENOA REPENS
Saw Palmetto Berries
for the male reproductive
system

Above are shown just a few of the herbs that can help the body fight off particular diseases or strengthen it against debility brought on through inherent weakness in any one particular body system. The herbs shown above represent just a selection; there are many more.

Healing the Whole Self

We have often heard it said that 'we are what we eat'. But we are also what we breathe, what we think, what we say, what we see. In later sections, when we look at the different body systems, we will discuss the importance of exercise, good food and fresh air. We are familiar with associating these things with our health, but what about the books we read, the films and television we watch, the politics we support? Is the music we listen to good for our health? Are our friends good for us? These are relevant questions, none of which can have assumed answers – they will be different for everyone. But the responses we make to them do have a bearing on our wellbeing.

In all holistic medicine individuality and responsibility are crucial factors. There is an emphasis on the uniqueness of the individual and the importance of tailoring treatment to meet each person's very different needs and circumstances. Holistic

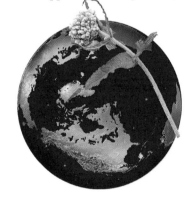

Herbalism is the natural therapy choice for people concerned with the preservation of the whole planet.

medicine also majors on therapeutic approaches that are aimed at mobilizing a person's own capacity for self-healing. The person who is 'ill' is in fact the healer. Aid can be sought from 'experts', but the responsibility for healing and health lies with the person who wants to be well. Using herbs is an ideal way to co-operate with our own innate healing power.

Herbs and the Environment

The 'whole' individual – mind, body, spirit and emotions – in the wider social setting of lifestyles and behaviour is part of a greater whole, however. Humanity itself exists in the context of the entire planet. All these levels work together in a dynamic, integrated system.

It seems clear that many health issues – stress, asthma, allergies, heart disease – are connected with cultural and ecological problems and often reflect our alienation from nature and 'natural' lifestyles. Herbalism can play a major role in bridging this separation. With its reverence for life and the relationship it establishes between plants and people, herbalism is close to the heart of the greener vision that is slowly but surely changing our cultural worldview.

1 1

WHOLENESS AND PREVENTION

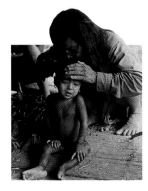

The shamanic healer is still part of daily life in many non-Westernized countries.

Herbal remedies can be used for the safe alleviation of illness, but as we shall see, this is not the only way to use these plants. Herbs can be used to support people's health and wholeness, helping them to stay at their personal peak of vitality and prevent disease development. There is food that supplies nutritional needs (calories, proteins and vitamins) and also delicious tastes and smells, and there are herbal 'foods' that nurture our wholeness, integration and wellbeing. These tonic remedies play a fundamental role in the maintenance of health and prevention of disease. In this section three aspects of this vast field will be considered: prevention; detoxification and elimination; and support for the body's immune system.

Herbs to Prevent Disease

The plant kingdom is an abundant and rich resource for anyone interested in prevention. The key is not so much in specific remedies but in an understanding of the role of herbal actions in maintaining health and correct physiological activity. With the insights that modern physiology provides about homeostasis, the body's own process of maintaining a stable environment, it is clear that herbs used in the right way will support this balancing process.

Artemisia vulgaris Mugwort, a tonic remedy for nervous complaints.

Tonics for the Systems of the Body

Tonics are herbs that strengthen and enliven either a specific organ or system, or the whole body. The concept of system tonics highlights the possibility of nourishing and toning the whole of a body system. This will aid the structural form of the tissues and organs as well as their functional activity, without eliciting a specific physiological or biochemical response.

BODY TONICS

Each system of the body has plants that are particularly suited to it, some of which are tonics. Below are listed some of the remedies which act as tonics for the major systems of the body.

Infection	*Garlic, Echinacea,* and system-specific anti-microbials such as *Bearberry* for the urinary system.
Cardiovascular System	*Hawthorn* and *Garlic.* The bioflavonoid containing herbs such as *Buckwheat* and *Lime Blossom* are especially useful for strengthening blood vessels.
Respiratory System	*Mullein, Elecampane* and *Coltsfoot.*
Digestive System	The bitter tonics will often be helpful in preventative approaches in health. Examples are *Gentian, Agrimony* and *Dandelion Root.*
The Liver	Bitter tonics, especially *Milk Thistle,* are hepatics (work on the liver).
Urinary System	*Buchu, Bearberry* and *Corn Silk* are very useful.
Reproductive System	For women use *Raspberry, False Unicorn Root* and other uterine tonics, while for men use *Saw Palmetto, Damiana* or *Sarsaparilla.*
Nervous System	*Oats, Skullcap, St John's Wort, Vervain* and *Mugwort* are all excellent tonic remedies. *Ginseng* has a toning effect when the person is under stress, because of its effect upon the adrenal glands.
Musculo/ Skeletal System	*Celery Seed, Bogbean* and *Nettles* will help prevent problems from other systems of the body manifest as disease in this system. *Comfrey* and *Horsetail* will help strengthen the bones and connective tissue.
The Skin	*Cleavers, Nettles, Red Clover* and most alterative remedies will help.

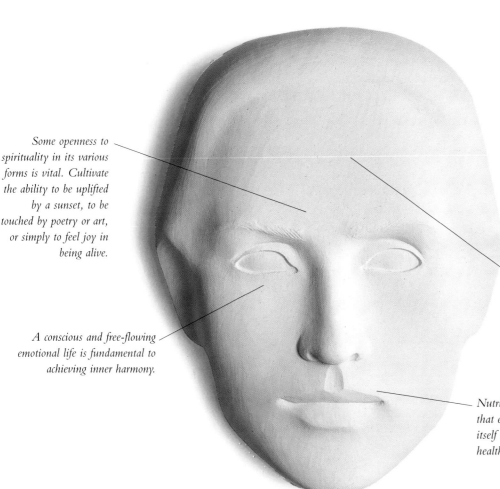

A healthy mind in a healthy body. The vigour of our mental and emotional life is just as important in the well-being of the whole person as the physical state of the body. Some factors for health annotate this illustration of a calm, balanced character.

Some openness to spirituality in its various forms is vital. Cultivate the ability to be uplifted by a sunset, to be touched by poetry or art, or simply to feel joy in being alive.

Mental factors are crucial, as we are what we think. Without a personal vision, life becomes a slow process of degeneration and decay.

A conscious and free-flowing emotional life is fundamental to achieving inner harmony.

Nutrition must be of a quality that enables the body to renew itself in a way that ensures health and wholeness.

Tonics truly are gifts of Nature to a suffering humanity – whole plants that enliven whole human beings, gifts of the Mother Earth to her children.

A characteristic of tonic herbs is that they are all gentle remedies that have a mild yet profound effect upon the body. Not all herbal remedies are tonics, of course; many have a powerful impact upon human physiology. These must be used with the greatest respect, their use being reserved for those times of illness where strong medicine is called for. The value of tonic herbs lies in their normalizing, nurturing effects. Whenever possible, the herbalist will focus on the use of such remedies, and will use an effector – a remedy that has an observable impact upon the body – only if absolutely necessary. The chemically-based effectors are hardly used at all. They are, however, the foundation of modern allopathic (orthodox) medicine.

The tonics can play a specific role in ensuring that individuals are at their own particular peak of health and vitality. The quality of such a state of wellbeing will vary from person to person, but everyone will sense an improvement in their general experience of life. Tonics may also be used specifically to ward off a known health problem or a family weakness.

By the very nature of tonics we can only talk in the most general terms when applying them to a specific system. They are usually interchangeable when it comes to their tonic action. However, always take into account the broader picture of a specific herb's range of actions, as it needs this breadth of vision to enable a coherent choice to be made.

Valeriana officinalis Valerian is a sedative herb whose properties are recognized in the orthodox pharmacy. It encourages the calming of the mind and the relaxing of unwanted tension.

Helping the Body Cleanse Itself

The herbal approach to detoxification is based upon the perception that the human body is a self-healing and homeostatic organism, and that the therapist simply has to support normal processes. The body has a wonderfully effective and astoundingly complex mechanism for ridding the body of waste and poisons.

Using simple and safe herbs will support this natural process, as long as the eliminative processes are addressed as a whole, and not just the colon, as is often the case. This means that whenever such a programme is undertaken, you must ensure that all organs of elimination are being helped at the same time. In addition always help the specific area of the body that has been under most toxic pressure. Examples would be the lungs in a tobacco smoker or the liver in someone with alcohol-related problems. The herbal approach to detoxification can thus be summarized:

- **Support** for the whole process of elimination
- **Specific support** for overly taxed organs
- **Alleviation of symptoms** and addressing any pathologies that may also be present

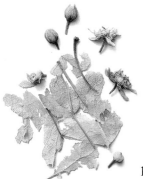

Tilea x *vulgaris* Lime Blossom *is an excellent diaphoretic, diuretic and astringent.*

HERBAL ACTIONS AND ELIMINATION

There are herbal actions whose physiological impact makes them especially indicated for the support of the different pathways of elimination in the body:

- **For the digestive system and colon** – laxative
- **For the kidneys and urinary system** – diuretic
- **For the liver and blood** – hepatic, alterative
- **For the lymphatic system** – alterative, lymphatic, tonic
- **For skin** – diaphoretic, alterative
- **For the respiratory system** – expectorant, anti-catarrhal
- **For systemic support in general** – tonic, alterative, adaptogen, anti-microbial

This does not specify which herb or even mention any remedy. There are potentially many appropriate plants that might be chosen. This diversity and abundance of healing plants is at once both the gift of herbalism and the frustration of every student of herbs!

GENTLE CLEANSERS

There are many ways in which the medical herbalist would go about the task of selecting the appropriate remedy for any particular individual. However, there is a simple basic guideline to follow. Always use gentle remedies when stimulating elimination. If overly active plants are used, then the effect may be one of intense elimination. This can be unpleasant and uncomfortable and of no therapeutic benefit. Here are some suggestions for herbs that effectively supply the relevant actions while also being safe and mild. This is not a comprehensive list but simply gives examples to point the way.

Laxative An aid to opening the bowels.	*Yellow Dock, Dandelion Root*
Diuretic An aid to promoting the flow of urine.	*Dandelion Leaf*
Hepatic Used in the treatment of disorders of the liver.	*Dandelion Root,* beetroot (as an example of a vegetable that will fulfil the same role)
Alterative Promotes the restoration of the general well-being of the body.	*Nettles, Cleavers*
Lymphatic tonic Promotes the health of the lymphatic system carrying tissue fluid.	*Cleavers, Echinacea, Marigold*
Diaphoretic Used to treat the skin and promote perspiration.	*Yellow Dock, Lime Blossom*
Expectorant Aids the removal of excess mucus from the lungs and facilitates coughing.	*Mullein, Coltsfoot*
Tonic Used to promote the health of the whole body.	any tonic remedy that has an affinity for the parts of the body under pressure from toxic build-up *(see pages 12–13).*
Adaptogen A substance that regulates the production of hormones.	*Siberian Ginseng*
Anti-microbial Helps the body fight off the organisms that cause disease.	*Echinacea, Garlic.*

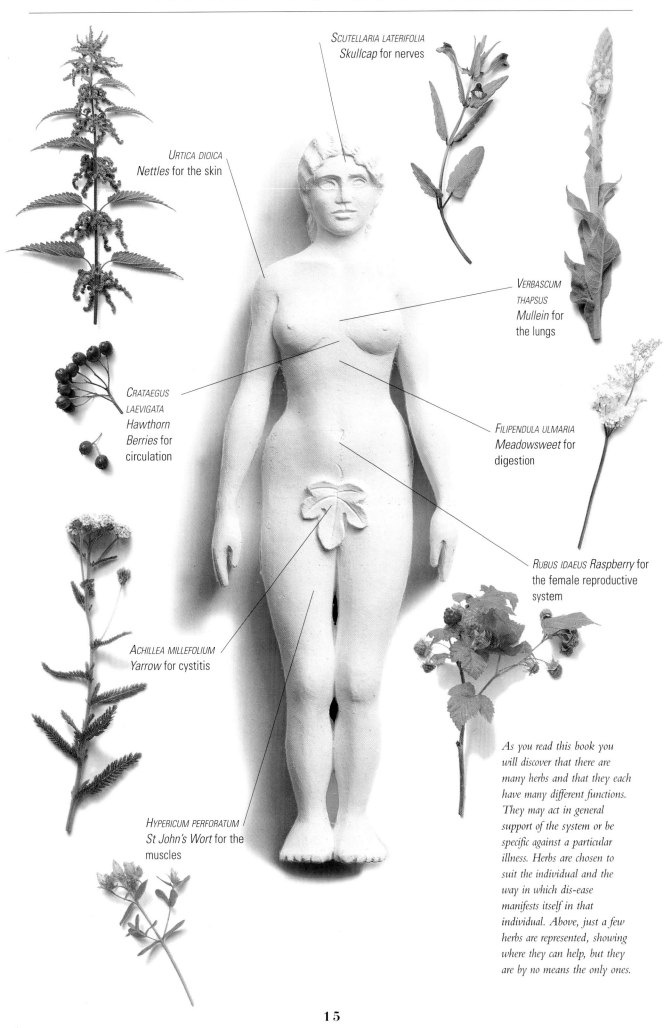

SCUTELLARIA LATERIFOLIA
Skullcap for nerves

URTICA DIOICA
Nettles for the skin

VERBASCUM THAPSUS
Mullein for the lungs

CRATAEGUS LAEVIGATA
Hawthorn Berries for circulation

FILIPENDULA ULMARIA
Meadowsweet for digestion

RUBUS IDAEUS Raspberry for the female reproductive system

ACHILLEA MILLEFOLIUM
Yarrow for cystitis

HYPERICUM PERFORATUM
St John's Wort for the muscles

As you read this book you will discover that there are many herbs and that they each have many different functions. They may act in general support of the system or be specific against a particular illness. Herbs are chosen to suit the individual and the way in which dis-ease manifests itself in that individual. Above, just a few herbs are represented, showing where they can help, but they are by no means the only ones.

15

Herbs and the Body's Defence System

One of the ways the body defends itself is to make itself resistant to disease, to become immune to attack by virus or bacterium. The human immune system has become an increasingly crucial issue in recent years. Not only in medicine but in many aspects of our lives, to have a sound grasp of the new concepts whicn concern human immunity has become essential in understanding our world and making personal choices.

This is not only due to the AIDS epidemic but also the statistical explosion of a whole range of auto-immune diseases. To understand the possibilities of the holistic approach, it is important both to have a grasp of the biological basis of immunity and to comprehend the role it plays in human life. Important insights arise when our immunity is placed in an ecological perspective. It becomes evident that human immunity is a vital component of the interface between individuals and their world.

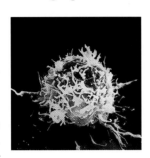

A healthy T-cell lymphocyte, one of the army of white cells that patrol the bloodstream to defend the body from invasion and infection.

WHAT IS HUMAN IMMUNITY?

Human immunity is ecology in action: there is a relationship phenomenon in play. Not only must both sides of this relationship be identified and understood but also the nature of their relationship with each other must be clarified. This can prove extremely challenging as it will be in dynamic flux at all times.

Immunity can be seen as an ecological interface between inner and outer environments where a complex of procedures and processes allows flow both inwards and outwards, resistance and embrace at the same time. To focus on one side only of this profound dialogue is to miss the point and compromise the whole thing.

Immunity is also an expression of homeostasis, the umbrella concept that describes the ability of the human body's physiological processes to maintain a stable internal environment.

It is also an expression of relationship. The very nature of relationship plays a role in the wellbeing of the immune system and so the practitioner must explore patients' relationship with their world on all levels – from the food they eat, the people they love (or hate), to the way they relate to nature.

THE HERBAL POSSIBILITIES

There are many ways of using herbs to enhance immunological vitality. All the many diverse herbal traditions, with their unique cultural roots and expressions, have valuable insights into treatments and specific herbs for the system. Herbal medicine is ecological medicine. It is based on an ecological relationship that has gradually evolved through geological time, and so of course there will be remedies that directly address the ecological process of human immunity.

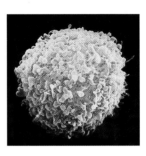

A T-cell lymphocyte attacked by the Human Immuno-deficiency Virus. The small green lumps are virus particles budding in the stricken cell.

Traditional knowledge is being confirmed by modern pharmacology. A growing number of remedies are being shown to have marked immunological effects in both the laboratory and the clinic. Some are stimulants to immunity but most can be described as modulators, that is they enable the body's natural responses to be more flexible in the face of disease. One approach is that based upon the work of the American herbalist Christopher Hobbs. His synthesis of Chinese and Western herbal modes has been an inspiration to many herbalists. It identifies three levels of herbal activity: deep immune activation; surface immune activation; and 'adaptogens' or hormonal modulators.

• **Deep immune activation** 'Deep immune activators' is the term that is used to describe plants that impact the immunological process within the tissue that mediates its work. They are also known as immunomodulators, or adjuvants.

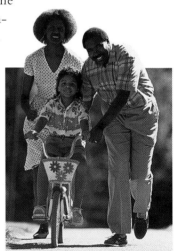

Just as in a happy, healthy family, individual members support and value each other, so the various systems of the body work together.

Chemical research points to constituents such as saponins and complex polysaccharides as key components in the immunological role played by such plants. However, it must be remembered that herbs act as biological wholes, not simply vehicles for active ingredients. These plants have an effect upon the cellular foundations of the human immune response. They do not necessarily act as stimulants or inhibitors to the vastly complex process of immunity, but rather 'feed' the whole process in some way as yet unknown.

In addition to specific remedies for immuno-modulation, the encouragement of bodily wellbeing through the support of each of the body systems will help the immune system. Bitter tonics, alteratives, hepatics, diuretics, diaphoretics and pulmonaries are all useful. *(See Actions of Herbs pages 36–9 for more information.)*

• **Surface immune activation** This level of activity focuses on the resistance aspect of immunity. Surface immune activation addresses the need to help resist pathogenic micro-organisms. There are many remedies known as anti-microbials. These are often plants that stimulate the activity and generation of white blood cells. Important examples include *Echinacea, Wild Indigo, Myrrh, Thuja, Marigold* and

---

FOUR ASPECTS OF COMPLETE HEALTH

• **Bodily health and wholeness** to ensure that the physical body has the correct nutrition and appropriate healing support for any ills it may be experiencing

• **Emotional wellbeing** to ensure a well-rounded life in which you can nurture and be nurtured and fully appreciate the human condition

• **Mental vision and perspective** to help create a frame of mind in which you can find your centre, enabling you to make choices from that centre, not from the stance of a victim

• **Spiritual openness** and vitality in whatever form that takes for the person involved

---

Garlic. More information is given in the section on Fighting off Invaders *(pages 40–5).*

• **Adaptogens or hormonal modulators** Remedies in this group work through a hormonal modulation of immune response. True adaptogens, such as *Ginseng,* work via the adrenal glands. Herbs that affect the other endocrine glands are described in the section on The Glandular System *(pages 226–9).*

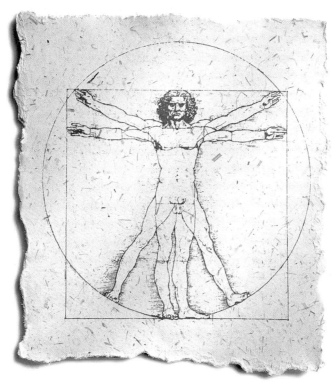

Leonardo da Vinci's celebrated figure of humanity symbolizes the balance, proportion and symmetry that define perfect health.

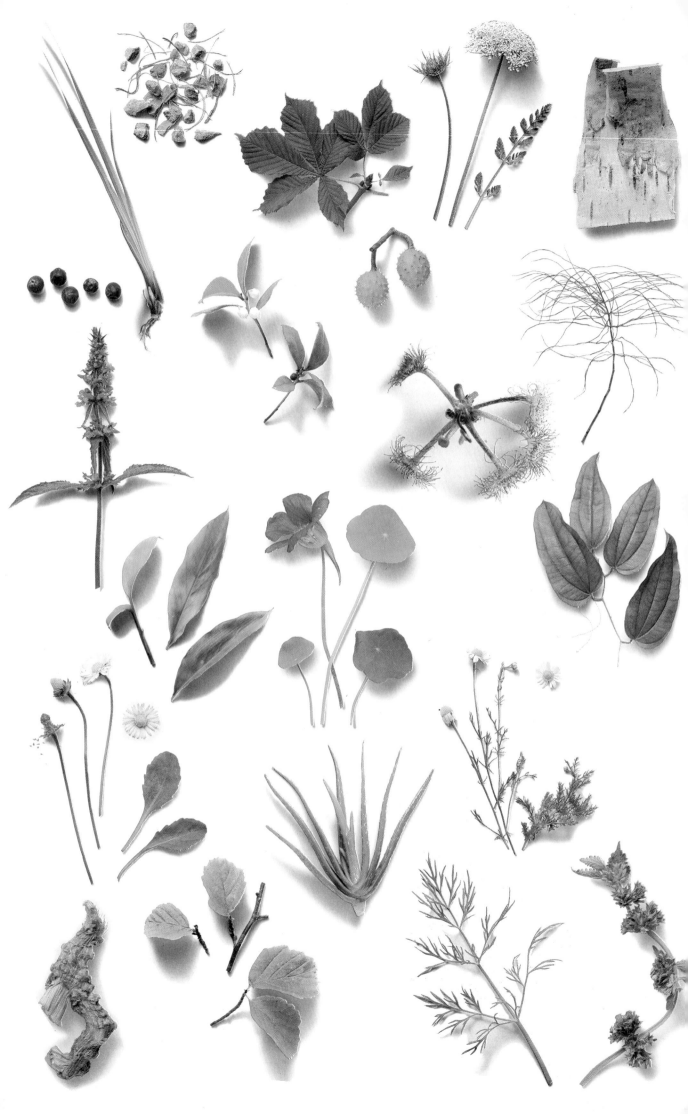

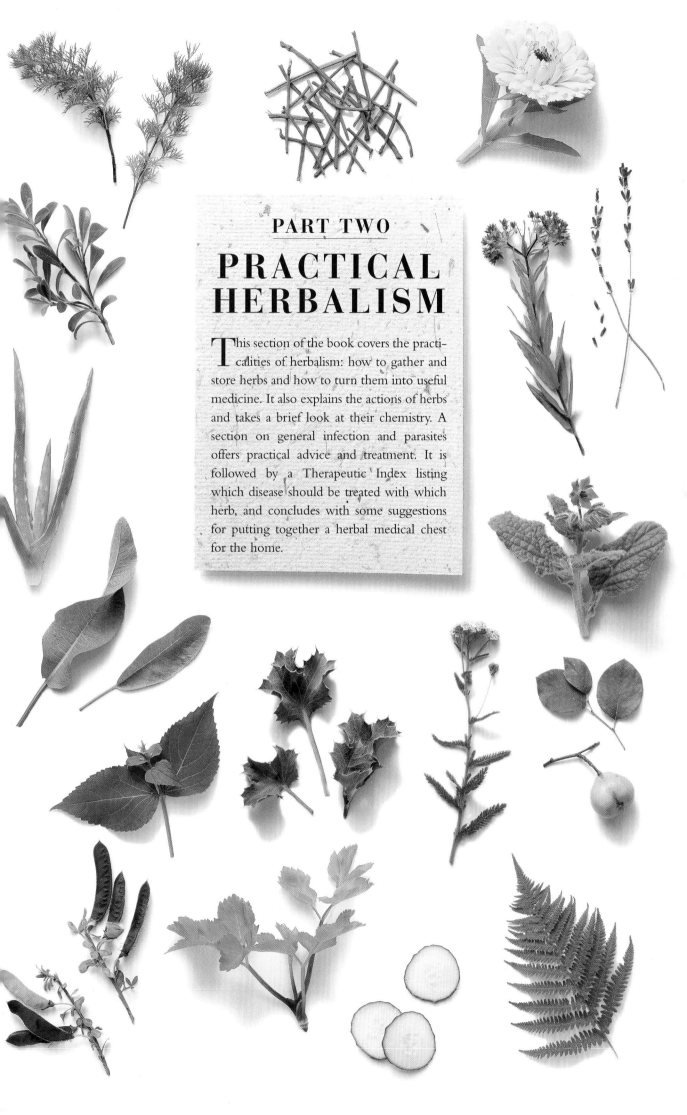

PART TWO
PRACTICAL HERBALISM

This section of the book covers the practicalities of herbalism: how to gather and store herbs and how to turn them into useful medicine. It also explains the actions of herbs and takes a brief look at their chemistry. A section on general infection and parasites offers practical advice and treatment. It is followed by a Therapeutic Index listing which disease should be treated with which herb, and concludes with some suggestions for putting together a herbal medical chest for the home.

GATHERING HERBS

The gathering of herbs is a delightful task. Whether harvesting a cultivated crop or searching out the plants in the wild, it always offers an opportunity to acknowledge and celebrate the abundance and wholeness of our planet. There are many details about times and processes of collecting and drying, but the heart of the matter is the consciousness that is brought to it by the collector.

Much research has gone into the effects of growth cycle, daily rhythms and climate on the biochemical composition of medicinal plants. What this work shows us is that the old law about the right times to pick each plant has a solid basis in plant chemistry. The active components are found at different levels at different times of the day, of the month and of the growth cycle. However, some broad generalizations can be made.

The level of active constituents is highest at the end of the period of most active growth. The plants should thus be gathered just before opening into blossom. A day without rain which has been sunny since daybreak is ideal for collecting. Though some leaves may dry quickly after rain, others, such as the thick furry ones of *Horehound,* retain the moisture, and if allowed to be massed before drying may easily develop mould and become spoilt. Too much heat dries up the oil in the leaves. Only the best shaped, greenest leaves should be gathered, and any that are withered, insect-bitten or stained should be discarded. This applies also when the whole plant is gathered.

Leaves and herbs should be cut with a sharp knife or secateurs, for pulling them off by hand may easily damage the tender stems of plants, causing delay in new growth or the entry of fungus or insects into the damaged tissue.

Though many herbs grow along roadsides and in waste soil, pick only from those places free of excessive traffic. Also be sure to avoid fields sprayed with chemicals, as these will dry and infuse right along with your medicinal herb. Investigate fields, woodlands and hedges surrounding organic farms, with the owner's permission, if unpolluted sources are otherwise rare in your area.

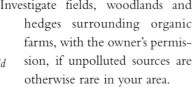

Gentiana lutea Gentian Root *should be lifted carefully.*

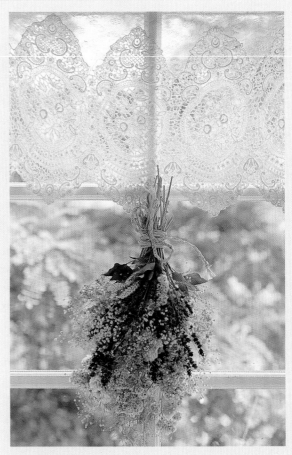

Once harvested, herbs should be allowed to dry in a natural way. Some may be hung in bright sunshine, some need a more shady position, and others may need gentle warming in a low-temperature oven.

DRYING HERBS

Herbs should be dried by spreading them in loose, single layers on flat drying surfaces. Wire cooling racks from the kitchen may be especially useful surfaces, since these allow air circulation underneath and hence quicker drying. Time for drying depends on the herbs and the environment, so check the herbs often and turn them as needed for even drying.

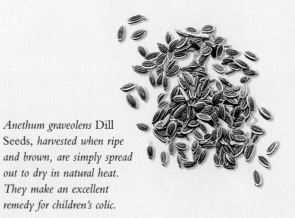

Anethum graveolens Dill Seeds, *harvested when ripe and brown, are simply spread out to dry in natural heat. They make an excellent remedy for children's colic.*

DRYING ROOTS

Roots are perhaps the most difficult part of herbs to dry, especially as they are usually very damp when dug up, since digging takes place in the Fall when the soil is likely to be muddy and sticky. Roots must not be dug for medicine while the leaves are still in full growth. They will not have achieved their maximum medicinal content, as some of this will still be retained in the part of the plant that is above ground.

When lifting, an effort must be made to get out the entire root, so a long spade or fork is needed. The root will come up with soil and mud adhering to it. A good deal of this can be scraped off, but the only efficient way to clean roots is by thorough washing. Scrubbing is usually necessary too. Top stems and rootlets should then be cut off and large roots, such as those of *Licorice* and *Burdock,* may be sliced to hasten drying.

To dry, they should be spread out on shelves so they do not touch or should be tied singly on strings in a warm shed or greenhouse for about ten days, being turned and inspected every day. When they have started to shrink well (roots lose about three-quarters of their weight in drying) they can be finished by storing them above a stove or in a cool oven. This will probably take another ten days and is dependent on the moisture in the atmosphere. Roots are dry when they are brittle.

To dry bulbs and corms, tie them up in small bunches, like onions, in a shed. Keep constant watch to see that they are drying evenly.

STORING HERBS

As soon as it is dried, the herb, whether root or aerial part, should be placed immediately into a dry container. The material should be handled with great care as it may be easily broken. Any herb which contains volatile oils should not be stored in ordinary plastic boxes or sacks, for these materials absorb the oils from the plant which then evaporate from the external surface. Glazed ceramic, dark glass or metal containers with tight-fitting lids are best for storage, away from direct sunlight or heat.

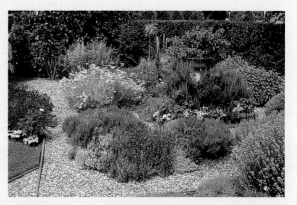

Try to make space in your garden to grow herbs so that you can pick them when they are at their peak.

WHEN TO GATHER HERBS

In every season nature offers herbs, but naturally not everything is available at all times. To find out in which season a herb can be collected, refer to the chart on pages 246–7. When different parts of a herb are collected at different times, they are listed separately.

HOW TO DRY HERBS

1 To dry leaves, stems and aerial parts of herbs, first harvest them by cutting with a sharp knife or secateurs to prevent tearing.

2 Strip the leaves or flowers from the main stem. In some cases, you can actually dry the stems themselves too.

3 Spread out separately on a drying rack and leave to dry in the sun or a warm place until they are brittle and crumble easily.

1 To dry roots, first unearth them gently. Wash the root to remove all remaining dirt. Scrub with a nail brush if necessary.

2 Cut off tops and trim away rootlets. If drying a large root, slice it up into strips about 5 cm/2 in long, depending on the root.

3 Spread the strips out on a drying rack and leave in a warm place for 10 days, turning daily. Store above a stove for 10 more days.

THE PREPARATION OF HERBS

Part of the art of herbal medicine is knowing what technique to use in preparing the remedies. Various methods of using plants have developed over the centuries to enable their healing properties to be released and become active. After the right choice of herbs has been made, the best way to prepare them must be selected.

Methods of preparation are mentioned throughout the book, but they are not described in detail each time. In this section a thorough explanation of methods is given. For clarity the methods are divided into those that are for use inside the body and those for external use.

Internal Remedies

From a holistic perspective, the best way of using herbs is to take them internally, since it is from within that healing takes place. The ways of preparing internal remedies are numerous, but with all of them it is essential to take care with the process to ensure you end up with what you want.

TO MAKE AN INFUSION

Infusions may be drunk hot – which is normally best for a medicinal herb tea – or cold, or have ice in them. They may be sweetened with *Licorice Root,* honey or even brown sugar.

Herbal teabags can be made by filling little muslin bags with herbal mixtures, taking care to remember how many teaspoonfuls have been put into each bag.

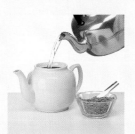 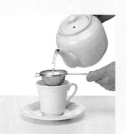

1 *Take a china or glass teapot which has been warmed and put one teaspoonful of the dried herb or herb mixture into it for each cup of tea that you intend to brew.*

2 *Pour a cup of boiling water in for each teaspoonful of herb that is already in the pot and then put the lid on. Leave to steep for ten to fifteen minutes.*

There are three basic kinds of preparations that can be taken internally: *water-based, alcohol-based,* and *fresh or dried herbs.*

WATER-BASED PREPARATIONS

There are two ways to prepare water-based extracts: *infusions* and *decoctions.* When the herbs to be used contain any hard, woody material, decoctions are used; otherwise infusions are used.

• **Infusion** If you know how to make tea, you know how to make an infusion. It is perhaps the most simple and common method of taking a herb and fresh or dried herbs can be used to prepare it. However, where one part of dried herb is prescribed, it can be replaced by three parts of the fresh herb, the difference being due to the higher water content of the fresh herb. Therefore, if the instructions call for one teaspoonful of dried herb, it can be substituted by three teaspoonfuls of fresh herb.

To make larger quantities to last for a while, the proportion should be 30g/1oz of herb to 500ml/1pt of water. The best way to store it is in a well-stoppered bottle in the refrigerator. However, the shelf life of such an infusion is not very long, as it is so full of life-force that any micro-organism that enters the infusion will multiply and thrive in it. If there is any sign of fermentation or spoiling, the infusion should be discarded. Whenever possible, infusions should be prepared when needed.

Infusions are most appropriate for plant parts such as leaves, flowers or green stems, where the substances wanted are easily accessible. If you also want to infuse bark, root, seeds or resin, it is best to powder them first, to break down some of their cell walls and make them more accessible to the water. Seeds, for instance, such as *Fennel* and *Aniseed,* should be slightly bruised before being used in an infusion to release the volatile oils from the cells. Any aromatic herb should be infused in a pot that has a well-sealing lid, to ensure that only a minimum of the volatile oil is lost through the process of evaporation.

When you are working with herbs that are very sensitive to heat, either because they contain highly volatile oils or because their constituents break down at high temperature, you can also make a cold infusion. The proportion of herb to water is the same

TO MAKE A DECOCTION

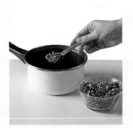

1 Put one teaspoonful of dried herb or three teaspoonfuls of fresh material for each cup of water into a pot or saucepan. Dried herbs should be powdered or broken into small pieces, while fresh material should be cut into small pieces. If large quantities are made, use 30g/1oz of dried herb for each 500ml/1pt of

water. (These are general guidelines, more specific dosages for each herb are given in The Herbal section.) The container should be glass, ceramic or earthenware. If using metal it should be enamelled. Never use aluminium.

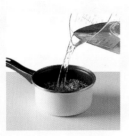

2 Add the appropriate amount of water to the herbs in the pan.

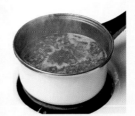

3 Bring to the boil and simmer for the time given for the mixture or specific herb, usually ten to fifteen minutes. If the herb contains volatile oils, put a lid on to the saucepan.

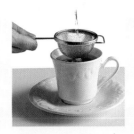

4 Strain the tea while it is still hot.

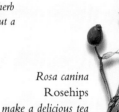

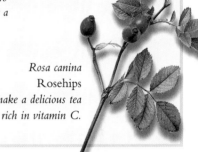

Rosa canina
Rosehips
make a delicious tea
rich in vitamin C.

but in this case the infusion should be left for six to twelve hours in a well-sealed earthenware pot. When the liquid is ready, strain and use it.

As an alternative, cold milk can also be used as a base for a cold infusion. Milk contains fats and oils which aid the dissolution of the oily constituents of plants. These milk infusions can also be used for compresses and poultices, adding the soothing action of milk to that of the herbs. There is however one contra-indication for the use of milk in an infusion: if there is any evidence of an internal reaction to milk in the form of over-sensitivity or allergy, or if the skin becomes irritated when it is applied externally, then avoid such infusions.

The infusions made as directed will be the base for many other preparations described later.

• **Decoction** Whenever the herb to be used is hard and woody, it is better to make a decoction rather than an infusion to ensure that the soluble contents of the herbs actually reach the water. Roots, rhizomes, wood, bark, nuts and some seeds are hard and their cell walls are very strong, so to ensure that the active constituents are transferred to the water, more heat is needed than for infusions and the herb has to be boiled in the water.

A decoction can be used in the same way as an infusion. General instructions for making decoctions are given above.

When preparing a mixture containing soft and woody herbs, it is best to prepare an infusion and a decoction separately to ensure that the more sensitive herbs are treated accordingly. When using a woody herb which contains a lot of volatile oils, it is best to make sure that it is powdered as finely as possible and then used in an infusion rather than a decoction, to ensure that the oils do not boil away.

DELICIOUS HERB TEAS

Herbs can make a delicious addition to everyday life and can open up a whole world of subtle delights and pleasures. They are not only medicines or alternatives to coffee, but can in their own right make excellent teas. Whilst each person will have favourite herbs, here is a list of some suggested herbs, each of which makes delicious teas, either singly or in combination. From this list you can select those which you like the taste of most, or those that also augment your health.

Flowers	Chamomile, Elder Flower, Lime Blossom, Red Clover
Leaves	Peppermint, Spearmint, Lemon Balm, Rosemary, Sage, Thyme, Hyssop, Vervain
Berries	Hawthorn, Rosehips
Seeds	Aniseed, Caraway, Celery, Dill, Fennel
Roots	Licorice

ALCOHOL-BASED PREPARATIONS

In general, alcohol is a better solvent than water for the plant constituents. Mixtures of alcohol and water dissolve nearly all the relevant ingredients of a herb and at the same time act as a preservative. Alcohol preparations are called tinctures, an expression that is occasionally also used for preparations based on glycerine or vinegar, as described below.

The methods given here for the preparation of tinctures show a simple and general approach; when tinctures are prepared professionally according to descriptions in a pharmacopeia, specific water/alcohol proportions are used for each herb, but for general use such details are unnecessary.

For home use it is best to take an alcohol of at least 30% (60 proof), vodka for instance, as this is about the weakest alcohol/water mixture with a long-term preservative action.

We can use tinctures in a variety of ways. They can be taken straight or mixed with a little water, or they can be added to

a cup of hot water. If this is done, the alcohol will partly evaporate and leave most of the extract in the water, which with some herbs will make the water cloudy, as resins and other constituents not soluble in water will precipitate. Some drops of the tincture can be added to a bath or footbath, or used in a compressor mixed with oil and fat to make an ointment. Suppositories and lozenges can be made this way too.

Another most pleasant way of making a kind of alcohol infusion is to infuse herbs in wine. Even though these wine-based preparations do not have the shelf life of tinctures and are not as concentrated, they can be very pleasant to take and most effective in some conditions. There is a long history of using wine in this way, and in fact most aperitifs and liqueurs were originally herbal remedies, based on herbs such as *Wormwood, Mugwort* and *Aniseed*, to aid the digestive process.

You can also ferment the herbs themselves; after all, even grapes are herbs. All the aromatic herbs make

---

TONIC WINE

500ml / 1pt Madeira
1 sprig of Wormwood
1 sprig of Rosemary
1 small bruised Nutmeg
2.5cm / 1in of bruised Ginger
2.5cm / 1in of bruised Cinnamon Bark
12 large organic Raisins

This is Dian Dincin Buchanan's recipe from her book *Herbal Medicine.* 'Pour off about an ounce of the wine. Place herbs in the wine. Cork the bottle tightly. Place the bottle in a dark, cool place for a week or two. Strain off the herbs. Combine this medicated wine with a fresh bottle of Madeira and mix thoroughly. Sip a small amount whenever needed. It helps settle the stomach, gives energy and makes you feel better.'

TO MAKE AN ALCOHOLIC TINCTURE

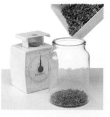

1 Put 120g/4oz of finely chopped or ground dried herbs into a container that can be tightly closed. If fresh herbs are used, twice the amount should be taken.

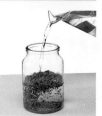

2 Pour 500ml/1pt of 30% (60 proof) vodka on the herbs and then close the container tightly.

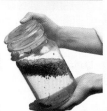

3 Keep the container in a warm place for two weeks and shake it well twice every day.

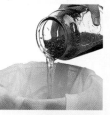

4 After decanting the bulk of the liquid, pour the residue into a muslin cloth suspended in a bowl.

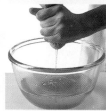

5 Wring out all the liquid. The residue makes excellent garden compost.

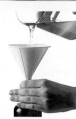

6 Pour the tincture into a dark bottle. Keep it well stoppered. Tinctures are much stronger, volume for volume, than infusions or decoctions, so check in The Herbal section for dosage details.

exquisite wines, and *Elderberry* and *Dandelion* are especially useful – and delicious – as medicinal wines.

VINEGAR-BASED TINCTURE

Tinctures can also be made using vinegar, which contains acetic acid that acts as a solvent and preservative in a way similar to alcohol. Whenever you make a vinegar tincture, it is best to use apple cider vinegar, as it has in itself excellent health-augmenting properties. Synthetic chemical vinegar should not be used. The method is the same as for alcoholic tinctures and if you steep spices or aromatic herbs in vinegar, the resulting fragrant vinegar will be excellent for culinary use.

GLYCERINE-BASED TINCTURE

Tinctures based on glycerine have the advantage of being milder on the digestive tract than alcoholic tinctures, but they have the disadvantage of not dissolving resinous or oily materials quite as well. As a solvent, glycerine is generally better than water but not as good as alcohol.

To make a glycerine tincture, make up 500ml/1pt of a mixture consisting of one part glycerine and one part water, add 120g/4oz of the dried, ground herb and leave it in a well-stoppered container for two weeks, shaking it daily. After two weeks, strain and press or wring the residue as with alcoholic tinctures. For fresh herbs, due to their greater water content, put 240g/8oz into a mixture of 75% glycerine/25% water.

• **Syrup** In the case of fluid medicine – be it infusion, decoction or tincture – that has a particularly unpleasant taste, it is sometimes advisable to mask the taste by combining the fluid with a sweetener. You could simply add a teaspoonful or two of your favourite honey, but another way to do this is to use a syrup. This is the traditional way to make cough mixtures more palatable for children, or any herbal preparation more 'toothsome', as the great herbalist Nicholas Culpeper (1616–54) used to call it.

DANDELION WINE

2l/4pts cold Water
Dandelion Flowers
15ml/1tbsp bruised
Ginger root
peel of 1 Orange, finely cut
peel of 1 Lemon, finely cut
700g/1½lb Demerara sugar
juice of 1 Lemon
5ml/1tsp Wine yeast

Bring water to the boil and leave to cool. Separate the Dandelion Flowers from their bitter stalks and calyces and put them in a large bowl. Pour the water over the flowers and leave for a day, stirring occasionally. Pour into a large pan and rinse out the bowl. Add the ginger and the orange and lemon rinds then boil for 30 minutes. Strain the liquid, pour it back into the bowl. Mix in the sugar and the lemon juice and allow to cool. Cream the wine yeast with some of the liquid and add to the mixture in the bowl. Cover the bowl with a cloth and leave the mixture to ferment in a warm place for two days. Pour the liquid into a cask. Seal the cask with a cotton wool bung, to allow gas to escape (or use a jug with an airlock available from home-brew suppliers). Leave the mixture in the cask or jug until all the fermentation has ceased and gas bubbles no longer form. Then close the cask or jug tightly for about two months. Finally, siphon the clear liquid into clean, dry bottles and seal. Keep the wine for six months before drinking.

A simple syrup base is made as follows. Pour 500ml/1pt of boiling water onto 1.1kg/2½ lb of sugar, place over heat and stir until the sugar dissolves and the liquid begins to boil. Remove from the heat.

This simple syrup can best be used together with a tincture: mix one part of the tincture with three parts of syrup and store for future use.

For use with an infusion or decoction, it is simpler to add the sugar directly to the liquid: for every 500ml/1pt of liquid add 350g/12oz of sugar and heat gently until the sugar is dissolved. This again can be stored for future use and will keep in a refrigerator.

Since too much sugar is not very healthy, syrups are best used for gargles and cough medicines only.

OXYMEL

When you have to take a particularly powerful tasting herb, such as *Garlic, Squill* or *Balm of Gilead,* the taste can best be covered by making an oxymel, which is made from five parts honey with one part vinegar. To make an oxymel base, put 500ml/1pt of vinegar and 1kg/2¼lb of honey into a pot and boil until the liquid has the consistency of syrup.

This is an established herbalist's recipe for the preparation of oxymel of *Garlic:* put 250ml/¹/₂pt of vinegar into a vessel, boil in it 7.5g/¹/₄oz of *Caraway Seeds* and the same quantity of *Fennel Seeds.* Add 45g/1¹/₂oz of fresh *Garlic Root* sliced, then press out the liquid and add 300g/10oz of honey. Boil until it has the consistency of syrup.

This oxymel can either be used as a gargle or you can take a dose of about two tablespoons internally.

Taraxacum officinale Dandelion, *a powerful diuretic herb, also has culinary uses; its leaves make a refreshing salad and its flowers make a delicious wine.*

DRY-BASED PREPARATIONS

Sometimes it is more appropriate to take herbs in a dry form, with the advantage that you do not taste the herb and also that you can take in the whole herb, including the woody material. The main drawback lies in the fact that the dry herbs are unprocessed, and therefore the plant constituents are not always as readily available for easy absorption. In a process like infusion, heat and water help to break down the walls of the plant cells and to dissolve the constituents, something which is not always guaranteed during the digestive process in the stomach and the small intestines. Also, when the constituents are already dissolved in liquid form, they are available a lot faster and begin their actions sooner.

A second drawback to taking some of the herbs dry, as in capsules, lies in the very fact that you do not taste the herb. For various reasons – even though they taste unpleasant – the bitter herbs work much better when they are tasted, as their effectiveness depends on the neurological sensation of bitterness. When you put bitters into a capsule or a pill, their action may well be lost or diminished.

Taking all these considerations into account, there are still a number of ways to use herbs in dry form. The main thing you have to pay attention to is that the herbs be powdered as finely as possible. This guarantees that the cell walls are largely broken down, and helps in the digestion and absorption of the herb.

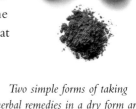

- **Capsules** The easiest way to take dry powdered herbs internally is to use gelatine capsules. (These come in various sizes and can be obtained from most chemists. Capsules not made of animal products are also available; ask in your area for suppliers.) The size you need depends on the amount of herbs prescribed per dose and on the volume of the material. A capsule size 00 for instance will hold about 0.5g/^{1}/$_{60}$oz of finely powdered herb.

- **Pills** There are a number of ways in which to make pills, depending on the degree of technical skill that you possess.

The simplest way to take an unpleasant remedy is to roll the powder into a small pill with fresh bread, which works most effectively with herbs such as *Golden Seal* or *Cayenne*. Instead of using bread, the powder can be combined with cream cheese.

Two simple forms of taking herbal remedies in a dry form are capsules and bread pills.

If necessary, you can make a more storable pill by making lozenges.

TO FILL A CAPSULE

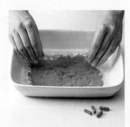

1 Place the powdered herbs in a flat dish and take the halves of the capsule apart.

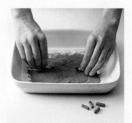

2 Move the halves of the capsules through the powder, filling them in the process.

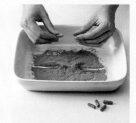

3 Push the two halves together.

Capsules are a useful option if you do not want to drink too much liquid in the forms of infusion or decoction. However, capsules are not recommended if you have been prescribed bitter herbs, as the action will be lost if you do not taste them on the tongue. You can buy ready-made capsules from a herbal pharmacy but, by making your own, you can produce customized remedies and only make as many as you need at the time.

LOZENGES

Lozenges are the ideal preparation for remedies to help the mouth, throat and upper respiratory tract, as taken in this way they can work where they are most needed. Lozenges containing the most used herbal remedies for the respiratory tract are easily available in herbal pharmacies, but it is very simple and economical to make your own. Stored in an airtight container, they will keep for months.

Herbal lozenges can easily be bought at herbal pharmacies, but making your own is more satisfactory as you can then specify a remedy you find particularly helpful.

The method of making lozenges is based on combining a powdered herb with sugar and a mucilage (thick, viscous jelly) to produce the characteristic texture.

The mucilage may be obtained from *Marshmallow Root, Slippery Elm Bark, Comfrey Root* or from one of the edible gums such as Tragacanth or Acacia.

A simple recipe and method showing how to make lozenges is given in the step-by-step illustration below. Prepare your dried herb first. A good selection for respiratory tract complaints includes anti-microbial herbs such as *Red Sage* for tonsillitis or mouth ulcers, demulcents such as *Coltsfoot, Licorice* or *Lungwort* for sore throats, expectorants such as *Angelica, Aniseed* and *Thyme* to clear mucus and specifics such as *White Horehound* for coughs.

Instead of using dry herbs, you can also use essential oils. A good example would be *Peppermint* oil. Mix 12 drops of pure *Peppermint* oil with 60g/2oz of sugar and then combine this with enough of the mucilage of Tragacanth to make a paste. Then proceed as shown in the step-by-step illustration and store the product in an airtight container for later use.

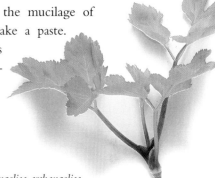

Angelica archangelica
Angelica *is a useful respiratory herb.*

TO MAKE A LOZENGE

Lozenges are easy to make using edible gum such as Tragacanth or Acacia to make a basic mucilage. Tragacanth is available at herbal pharmacies and some specialist food stores, but you can also get it from artist's material suppliers.

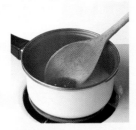

1 *Soak 30g/1oz Tragacanth in water for 24 hours, stirring as often as possible. Boil 500ml/1pt of water. Mix in the Tragacanth.*

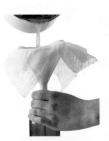

2 *Using a wooden spoon, beat the mixture to a uniform consistency. Force it through a muslin strainer to make a mucilage.*

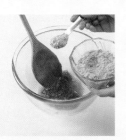

3 *Mix enough of your chosen herb (in dried, powdered form) into the mucilage to make a paste. Add unrefined brown sugar if you like.*

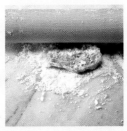

4 *Dust a pastry board and rolling pin with icing sugar or cornflour to prevent sticking and roll out the paste to a layer about 1.25cm/½in thick.*

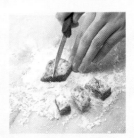

5 *When the paste has cooled slightly, cut the paste into lozenges, in any shape and size you like. Leave to dry. Store in an airtight tin.*

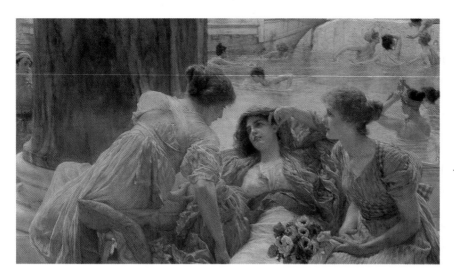

The therapeutic effects of bathing, especially in baths rich in mineral or herbal properties, have been known since ancient times. Taking a revitalizing or medicinal bath was often a social occasion rather than an individual therapy. The French-born Roman emperor Caracalla (AD176–217) constructed some famous baths in Rome. Here they are shown glowing in the sumptuous, romantic light in which the late 19th-century artist Sir Lawrence Alma-Tadema (1836–1912) customarily bathed his view of the ancient world of Greece and Rome.

External Remedies

As the body can absorb herbal compounds through the skin, a wide range of methods and formulations have been developed that take advantage of this fact. Douches and suppositories, though they might appear to be internal remedies, have traditionally been categorized as external remedies.

WATER THERAPY

• **Baths** The best and most pleasant way of absorbing herbal compounds through the skin is by bathing in a full body bath with 500ml/1pt of infusion or decoction added to the water. Alternatively, you can also take a foot or hand bath, in which case you would use the preparations in undiluted form.

Any herb that can be taken internally can also be used in a bath. There are many herbs and they can be used on their own or in combination to make different kinds of bath with different properties. For a bath that is relaxing and at the same time exquisitely scented, infusions can be made of *Lavender Flowers, Lemon Balm, Elder Flowers* or *Rosemary Leaves.* For a bath that will bring about a restful and healing sleep, add an infusion of either *Valerian, Lime Blossom* or *Hops* to the bath water. For children with sleep problems or when babies are teething, try either *Chamomile* or *Lime Blossom,* as the herbs mentioned above may be too strong. In feverish conditions or to help the circulation, stimulating and diaphoretic herbs can be used, such as *Cayenne, Boneset, Ginger* or *Yarrow.*

These are just some of the possibilities. Try out others for yourself. There are also ideas in books about aromatherapy, a healing system based on the external application of herbs in the form of essential oils. These oils can also be used in baths by putting a few drops of oil into the bathwater.

Instead of preparing an infusion of the herb beforehand, a handful of it can be placed in a muslin bag which is suspended from the hot water tap so that the water flows through it.

• **Douches** Another method of using herbs externally is a douche, the application of herbs to the vagina, which is particularly indicated for local infections. Whenever possible, prepare a new infusion or decoction for each douche. Allow the liquid to cool to a temperature that will be comfortable internally. Pour it into the container of a douche bag and insert the applicator vaginally. Allow the liquid to rinse the inside of the vagina. Note that the liquid will run out of the vagina, so it is easiest to douche sitting on the toilet. It is not necessary to actively hold in the liquid. In most conditions it is advisable to use the liquid undiluted for a number of days, three times daily. If, however, a three to seven day course of douching (along with the appropriate internal herb remedies) has not noticeably improved a vaginal infection, see a qualified practitioner for a diagnosis.

SURFACE THERAPY

• **Ointments** or salves are semi-solid preparations that can be applied to the skin. Depending on the purpose for which they are designed, there are innumerable ways of making ointments; they can vary in texture from very greasy to a thick paste, depending on what base is used and what compounds are mixed together.

Any herb can be used for making ointments, but *Arnica, Chickweed, Comfrey Root, Cucumber, Elder Flower, Golden Seal, Greater Plantain, Lady's Mantle, Marigold Flower, Marshmallow Root, Slippery Elm Bark, Woundwort* and *Yarrow* are particularly good for use in external healing mixtures. Note that *Arnica* is not advisable on open wounds. For the specific use of each herb, please refer to The Herbal section.

The simplest way to prepare an ointment is by using petroleum jelly as a base. Whilst this has the disadvantage of being an inorganic base, it also has a number of advantages. Petroleum jelly is easy to handle so a simple ointment can be made very quickly. Besides this it has the advantage of not being absorbed itself by the skin, making it useful for instance as the base for the anti-catarrhal balm described later. Here the petroleum jelly acts merely as a carrier for the volatile oils, which can thus evaporate and enter the nasal cavities without being absorbed through the skin.

The basic method for a petroleum jelly ointment is to simmer two tablespoonfuls of a herb in 200g/7oz of petroleum jelly for about ten minutes. A single herb, or a mixture of fresh or dried roots, leaves or flowers can be used.

In more traditional ointments, instead of using petroleum jelly a combination of oils is used that acts as a vehicle for the remedies and helps them to be absorbed through the skin, plus hardening agents to

---

MARIGOLD BALM

This is a recipe for a simple *Marigold* ointment, which is excellent for cuts, sores or minor burns. Take 60g/2oz (or about a handful) of freshly picked *Marigold Flowers,* add to 200g/7oz melted petroleum jelly and bring the mixture to the boil. Simmer it very gently for about ten minutes, stirring well. Then sift it through fine gauze and press out all the liquid from the flowers. Pour the liquid into a container and seal it after it has cooled.

---

create the texture desired. The following example is the prescription for 'Unguentum Simplex', a simple ointment from the *British Pharmacopoeia* of 1867:

White wax 2oz (60g)
Lard 3oz (90g)
Almond oil 3 fluid oz (90ml)

'Melt the wax and lard in the oil on a water bath, remove from heat when melted, add almond oil and stir until cool.'

TO MAKE A HERBAL OINTMENT

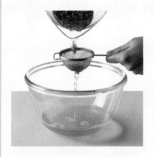

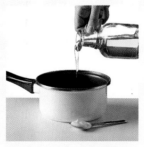

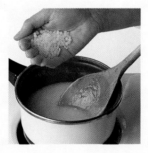

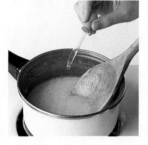

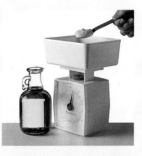

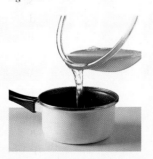

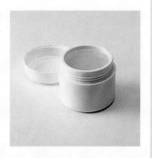

1 Make 500ml/1pt of the appropriate water extract (infusion or decoction), strain off the liquid for use in step 4.

2 Measure out the fat and oil for the base.

3 Pour 90ml/3fl.oz olive or almond oil into the pan. Mix the fat and oil together.

4 Add the strained herbal extract and stir into the base.

5 Simmer until the water has completely evaporated and the extract has become incorporated into the oil. You might find it easier to place the pan in a larger pan of water to prevent burning. Be careful not to overheat the mixture and watch particularly for the point when all the water has evaporated and the bubbling stops. If additional thickeners (such as beeswax) need to be incorporated, they can be added at this point and melted with the base, heating slowly and stirring until blended.

6 If a perishable base is used (such as lard) a drop of tincture of benzoin should be added for each 30g/1oz of base.

7 Pour the mixture into a container.

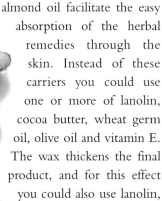

In this basic recipe, the lard and the almond oil facilitate the easy absorption of the herbal remedies through the skin. Instead of these carriers you could use one or more of lanolin, cocoa butter, wheat germ oil, olive oil and vitamin E. The wax thickens the final product, and for this effect you could also use lanolin, cocoa butter or, most ideally, beeswax, depending on the final consistency you want to achieve.

Ranunculus ficaria Pilewort *is a specific for hemorrhoids, as its name indicates.*

• **Suppositories** are designed to enable the insertion of remedies into the orifices of the body. While they can be shaped to be used in the nose or the ears, they are most commonly used for rectal or vaginal problems. They act as carriers for any herbs that it is appropriate to use, and there are three general categories for these. Firstly, there are herbs acting to soothe the mucous membranes, such as the root and the leaf of *Comfrey,* the root of *Marshmallow* and of *Golden Seal,* and the bark of *Slippery Elm.*

Secondly, there are the astringent herbs that can help in the reduction of discharge or in the treatment of hemorrhoids, such as *Periwinkle, Pilewort, Witch Hazel* and *Yellow Dock.*

And thirdly there are remedies to stimulate the peristalsis of the intestines to overcome chronic constipation, or in other words the laxatives. In any of these three categories it will often be appropriate to include one of the anti-microbial herbs with whatever combination of herbs you are using.

As with ointments, you can choose from different bases, keeping in mind that they have to be firm enough to be inserted into the orifice, while at the same time being able to melt at body temperature once inserted, to liberate the herbs they contain. The herbs should be distributed uniformly in the base – particularly important when you are using a powdered herb, the easiest form for this. The kind of suppository you make depends on whether you need the herb material to enter the body or not. A simple recipe and method are given in the box opposite.

• **Compresses** A compress or fomentation is an excellent way to apply a remedy to the skin to

TO MAKE A SUPPOSITORY

Simple suppositories can be made by mixing a finely powdered herb with a good base such as cocoa butter, and moulding it as below. A more complex method has to be used if you want to avoid the introduction of powdered plant material into the body. The simplest way uses gelatine and glycerine and either an infusion, a decoction or a tincture, in the following proportions.

Gelatine	10 parts
Water (or infusion, decoction, tincture)	40 parts
Glycerine	15 parts

Soak the gelatine for a while in the water-based material. Gently heat the mixture until the gelatine dissolves. Add the glycerine and heat the whole mixture in a water bath to evaporate. The final consistency depends on how much water is removed through evaporation. If it is removed completely, a very firm consistency will be achieved.

The easiest way to prepare a mould is to use aluminium foil shaped as you need. The best shape is a torpedo-like, 2.5cm/1in long suppository.

Pour the molten base into the mould and let it cool; store the suppositories in the moulds in a refrigerator for a while, though it is always preferable to make them when they are needed.

accelerate the healing process. To make a compress, use a clean cloth – made either of linen, gauze, cotton wool or cotton – and soak it in a hot infusion or decoction. Place this as hot as possible upon the affected area. As heat enhances the action of the herbs, either change the compress when it cools down or cover the cloth with plastic or waxed paper and place on it a hot-water bottle, which is changed when necessary. All the vulnerary herbs make good compresses, as do stimulants and diaphoretics in many situations.

Bellis perennis Daisy, known as 'the English Arnica', is a vulnerary herb that can be particularly useful in compresses to comfort wounds and bruises.

• **Poultices** The action of a poultice is very similar to that of a compress, but instead of using a liquid extract, the solid plant material is used for a poultice.

Either fresh or dried herbs can be used to make a poultice. With the fresh plant you apply the bruised leaves or root material either directly to the skin or place them between thin gauze. Dried herbs must be made into a paste by adding either hot water or apple cider vinegar until the right consistency is obtained. To keep the poultice warm, you can use the same method as for the compress and place a hot-water bottle on it.

When you are applying the herb directly to the skin, it is often helpful first to cover the skin with a small amount of oil, as this will protect it and make removal of the poultice easier.

Poultices can be made from warming and stimulating herbs, from vulneraries, astringents and also from emollients, which are demulcents that are soothing and softening on the skin, such as *Comfrey Root, Flax Seed, Marshmallow Root, Oatmeal, Quince Seed* and *Slippery Elm Bark.*

Poultices are often used to draw pus out of the skin and there are a multitude of old recipes. Some of them use cabbage, which is excellent, others use bread and milk, some even soap and sugar.

• **Liniments** are specifically formulated to be easily absorbed through the skin, as they are used in massages that aim at the stimulation of muscles and ligaments. They must only be used externally, never internally. To carry the herbal components to the muscles and ligaments, liniments are usually made of a mixture of the herb with alcohol or occasionally with apple cider vinegar, sometimes with an addition

OLD FASHIONED LINIMENT

The following liniment is described by Jethro Kloss in his book *Back to Eden.*

'Combine 2oz powdered *Myrrh,* 1oz powdered *Golden Seal,* 1/2oz *Cayenne Pepper,* one quart rubbing alcohol (70%). Mix together and let stand seven days; shake well every day, decant off, and bottle in corked bottles. If you do not have *Golden Seal,* make it without.' Another excellent liniment that warms and relaxes muscles at the same time is made from equal parts of *Lobelia* and *Cramp Bark* plus a pinch of *Cayenne.* This is made into a tincture or liniment in the same way.

Mentha x *piperita* Peppermint *produces aromatic volatile oil, useful for the treatment of nasal catarrh.*

of herbal oils. The main ingredient of a liniment is usually *Cayenne,* which may be combined with *Lobelia* or other remedies.

• **Oils** As you can see in The Herbal section of the book, many herbs are rich in essential oils. There are herbs like *Peppermint,* where the oils are volatile, which makes the plant aromatic, and there are also those whose oils are not particularly aromatic, such as *St John's Wort.*

Herbal oils can be used in two forms, depending on the mode of extraction. First of all there are the pure essential oils, which are extracted from the herb by a complex and careful process of distillation. Only an expert can make these at home. These oils are best obtained from specialist suppliers (see Useful Addresses page 251), who distil them as the basis for aromatherapy and as such take care that they are as pure as possible.

The second way of extracting oils is much simpler and resembles the method of cold infusion. Instead of infusing the herb in water, it is put into an oil, whereby a solution of the essential oil is obtained in the oilbase.

The best oils to use are pure plant oils such as olive, sunflower or almond oil, but any good pressed vegetable oil can be used and these are preferable to mineral oils.

To make a herbal oil, first cut the herb finely, cover it with oil and put in a clear glass container. Place this in the sun or leave in a warm place for two to three weeks, shaking the container daily. After that time, filter the liquid into a dark glass container and store the extracted oil.

A typical and very soothing example of such an oil is *St John's Wort* oil, which makes a very red oil that can be used externally for massages and to help sunburns and heal wounds. It can also be taken internally in very small doses to ease stomach pains. (Instructions for making the oil are given on page 104.)

THE CHEMISTRY OF HERBS

Plants contain a vast range of chemicals, ranging from water and inorganic salts, sugars and carbohydrates to highly complex proteins and alkaloids. We will focus here on the role these substances have to play, not in the plant itself, but in the body. We will mainly concentrate on the groups that act medicinally, though we shall look at some which are important nutrients and thus influence the body.

We will look at plant pharmacology, briefly examining the various groupings that the numerous constituents have been divided into, looking at their function, and giving some examples of where they occur. These groupings are referred to throughout the book and, as far as they are known, the relevant constituents are given in The Herbal section. The groupings followed here are based on the structure of the constituents rather than on their function, which is dealt with in the section on The Actions of Herbs *(pages 36–9)*.

A knowledge of plant pharmacology is not essential to a herbalist, but is a great help in understanding the plant.

PLANT ACIDS

Weak organic acids are found throughout the plant kingdom. A typical example is the citric acid found in citrus fruits such a lemons.

The organic acids can be divided into those based on a carbon chain, and those containing a carbon ring in their structure, but they all have a -COOH group in common.

The chain acids (or aliphatic acids) range from the simple formic acid we can feel in the sting of *Nettles* to the more complex ones such as citric acid and valeric acid, the latter being the basis for a sedative that is used in allopathic medicine.

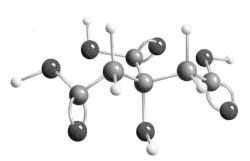

The molecular structure of citric acid, a weak organic chain acid found in lemons and many other plants.

The ring acids (aromatic acids) are an important pharmacological group. The simplest aromatic acid, benzoic acid, can be found in many resins and balsams such as Gum Benzoin, *Balsum of Tolu,* Peru Balsam and also in Cranberries. It can be used as a lotion or an ointment, can be a beneficial inhalant for chronic bronchial problems, and has antiseptic, anti-pyretic and diuretic actions. Friar's Balsam is a well-known form of benzoic acid.

ALCOHOLS

Alcohols are found in various forms in plants, often as constituents of volatile oils or as sterols, like the alcohol oil geraniol in attar of Rose and menthol in *Peppermint* oil. Other common forms of alcohol are waxes, combinations of alcohols and fatty acids, which are found in plants in the coating of leaves and in other parts. The commonly used Carnauba Wax for instance is obtained from the palm *Copernicia cerifera*.

VOLATILE OILS

Most of the volatile oils are based on simple molecules like isoprene or isopentane, which can combine in many different ways to form terpenes, containing multiples of the basic 5-carbon molecules, sometimes with slight variation, making up the volatile oils.

We can find the volatile oils in the aromatic plants such as *Peppermint* or *Thyme,* where different oils – sometimes up to 50 or more – combine to give the plant its particular smell. Depending on the combination the smell will vary and may even be slightly different within the same species, depending on the concentration of oils.

By extracting these oils, the so-called essential or aromatic oils are produced, which can be used therapeutically, but which also are used to a large extent for the production of perfumes.

The range of aromatic oils is very large and they each have unique properties, but they also share some common actions worth mentioning.

All aromatic oils are antiseptics, good examples being Eucalyptus oil, *Garlic* oil and *Thyme* oil. As the

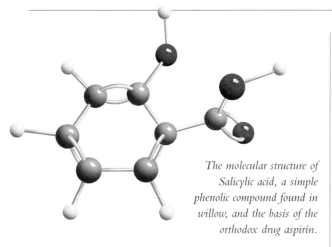

The molecular structure of Salicylic acid, a simple phenolic compound found in willow, and the basis of the orthodox drug aspirin.

oils are very easily transported and distributed throughout the body, they act both locally and on the whole system. When they are taken internally or applied externally, they will soon show up in the urinary system, the lungs and the bronchials, and in secretions like sweat, saliva, tears or the vaginal fluids.

They can even occur in mothers' milk or travel through the placenta into the fetus. Besides their direct antiseptic actions they also stimulate the production of white blood-cells, thereby augmenting the body's own natural defence system.

The volatile oils stimulate the tissue they come in contact with, either leading to slight 'irritations' (as in the case of *Mustard* oil) or to a numbing (as with menthol and camphor). They aid digestion by stimulating the lining of the colon, which sets off a reflex that increases the flow of gastric juices and induces a feeling of hunger. Also they can help to ease griping pains by relaxing the peristalsis in the lower part of the intestines.

The volatile oils also act on the central nervous system. Some will relax and sedate, like *Chamomile,* others will stimulate, like *Peppermint,* and all tend to induce a state of inner ease and wellbeing, thus reducing tension and depression. When aromatic oils are applied externally, part of their effect is due to their actions on the nose, as the olfactory nerves pick up scent molecules from them and transmit the smell to the brain, where a reaction is triggered off.

The molecular structure of menthol, the alcoholic constituent of the volatile oil found in Peppermint.

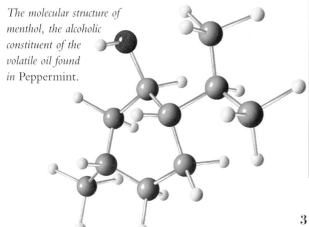

As volatile oils evaporate very easily, herbs containing these oils have to be stored carefully in well-sealed containers.

CARBOHYDRATES

A great variety of carbohydrates can be found in plants, either in the form of sugars such as glucose and fructose, or as starches, where they serve as the main energy store. They also occur in the more complex form of cellulose, the structural support of plants.

The large polysaccharides, such as cellulose, can further bond with other chemicals and produce molecules like pectin, found for instance in apples, or seaweed gums like algin, agar or carragum, found in *Irish Moss.* They are all very viscous and demulcent and are used to produce gels that are utilized in medicine and in food preparations.

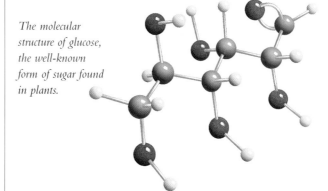

The molecular structure of glucose, the well-known form of sugar found in plants.

Gums and mucilages, which are very complex carbohydrates, are contained in some excellent soothing and healing herbs, like the demulcents *Coltsfoot, Plantain* and *Marshmallow.* Their action relaxes the lining of the gut, triggering a reflex that runs through the spinal nerves to those areas that are related embryologically, such as the lungs and the urinary system.

In this way the mucilages work in a twofold manner: they reduce irritation and inflammation in the whole of the alimentary canal, reduce the sensitivity to gastric acid, prevent diarrhea and reduce peristalsis; they also work via a reflex on the respiratory system, reducing tension and coughing and increasing the secretion of watery mucus.

PHENOLIC COMPOUNDS

Phenol is a basic building block of many important plant constituents. Phenolic compounds may be simple in structure, or a complex combination of a range of basic molecules. One of the simple phenolics is salicylic acid, which is found often in combination with sugar, forming a glycoside, as in *Willow, Cramp Bark, Wintergreen* and *Meadowsweet*. This chemical has antiseptic, pain-killing and anti-inflammatory properties, and is used by allopathic medicine in the form of acetylsalicylic acid, better known as aspirin.

Eugenol, the pain-killing oil found in *Cloves,* and thymol from oil of *Thyme* both have similar effects to salicylic acid. Part of the antiseptic action of *Bearberry* on the urinary system can be explained by the presence of the phenol hydroquinone.

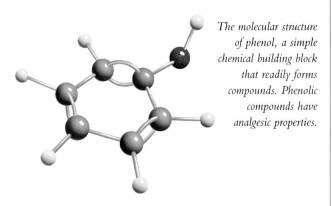

The molecular structure of phenol, a simple chemical building block that readily forms compounds. Phenolic compounds have analgesic properties.

TANNINS

Tannins in herbs cause an astringent action. They act on proteins and some other chemicals and form a protective layer on the skin and the mucous membranes. Thus they can for instance bind the tissue of the gut and reduce diarrhea or internal bleeding. Externally they are useful in the treatment of burns, for sealing wounds and to reduce inflammation. Tannins can be used in infections of the eye (conjunctivitis), mouth, vagina, cervix and rectum.

COUMARINS

The highly evocative smell of new-mown hay has its basis in the coumarin group of chemicals. It is, of course, not just grass that contains these beautifully aromatic constituents; *Sweet Woodruff* is another example. Coumarin itself has limited effects on the body, but one of its metabolites, di-coumarol, is a powerful anti-clotting agent. Allopathic medicine has used the coumarins as a basis for warfarin, an anti-clotting drug used in large doses as a rat poison and in small doses as a guard against thrombosis.

ANTHRAQUINONES

Plants containing anthraquinones are known to be effective purgatives and they also happen to be good natural dyes. They appear usually in the form of glycosides (in a chemical combination with a sugar) and are found for instance in *Rhubarb, Yellow Dock,*

Senna, Buckthorn and *Aloe.* They work by gently stimulating the colon after about eight to twelve hours of ingestion by stimulating the peristalsis of the intestines, but they can do this only when natural bile is present. As there may be a tendency to colic pains through an over-stimulation of the colon wall, they are often given in combination with carminative herbs.

FLAVONES AND FLAVONOID GLYCOSIDES

One of the most common groups of plant constituents in herbs are the flavones and the flavonoid glycosides, and we will refer to them throughout The Herbal section. They are known to have a wide range of activities, from anti-spasmodic and diuretic to circulatory and cardiac stimulants. Some, for instance, like rutin, hesperidin and the bio-flavonoid vitamin P, reduce permeability and fragility of the capillaries and so help the body to strengthen the circulatory system and to lower the blood pressure. *Buckwheat* is a good example of a useful herb for such problems. The bio-flavonoids are also essential for the complete absorption of vitamin C and occur in nature wherever vitamin C is present. Another flavonoid, present in *Milk Thistle,* is responsible for its action in aiding the liver.

SAPONINS

The saponins have attracted the attention of pharmaceutical chemists as they can be used in the synthesis of cortisone – a strong anti-inflammatory drug – and in the synthesis of sex hormones. While the saponins contained in herbs do not directly act in the same way, the body can use them as raw material to build up appropriate chemicals. To show the similarity between a natural saponin and the more potent synthesized drugs, we can compare cortisone with diosgenin from *Wild Yam* and see that they are very similar.

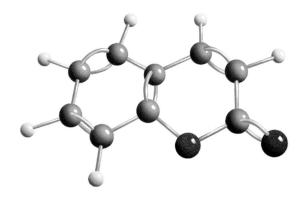

The molecular structure of coumarin, a powerful aromatic chemical compound and anti-clotting agent.

Typical anti-inflammatory herbs that contain saponins include *Golden Rod, Chickweed, Figwort* and *Wild Yam.*

Another important action of saponins is their expectorant action through the stimulation of a reflex of the upper digestive tract, which occurs in remedies such as *Primrose, Mullein, Violet* and *Daisy.*

CARDIAC GLYCOSIDES

Very similar to the saponins are the cardiac glycosides. These have been the object of intensive investigation ever since they were discovered in Foxglove, in 1785, when it was recognized by medicine that these glycosides can support the failing heart.

The cardiac glycosides are formed by a combination of a sugar and a steroidal agylcone. The main activity is defined by the shape and structure of the agylcone, but it is the sugar that determines the bioavailability of the active agylcone.

Many flowering plants contain cardiac glycosides. The best known sources are Foxglove, *Lily of the Valley,* Squill and the *Strophanthus* family. In herbal medicine, *Lily of the Valley* is preferred over Foxglove, as Foxglove is potentially poisonous, whereas *Lily of the Valley,* quite as effective, does not lead to a build-up of toxic components in the body.

Therapeutically, the cardiac glycosides have the incredible ability to increase the force and power of the heart beat without increasing the amount of oxygen needed by the heart muscle. They can thus increase the efficiency of the heart and at the same time steady excess heart beats without strain to the organ.

BITTER PRINCIPLES

The bitter principles represent a grouping of chemicals that have an exceedingly bitter taste. Chemically they show a wide diversity of structure, with most bitters belonging to the iridoids, some to the terpenes (see the section on volatile oils) and some to other groups.

The bitter principles have been shown to have valuable therapeutic effects. Through a reflex action via the tastebuds, they stimulate the secretion of all the digestive juices and also stimulate the activity of the liver, aiding hepatic elimination. The value of these actions is explored elsewhere in the book, particularly in the section on the digestive system. Much pharmaceutical research is going on at the moment regarding these bitter principles, as they often show antibiotic, anti-fungal and even also anti-tumour actions. Research from China suggests that the bitter principle

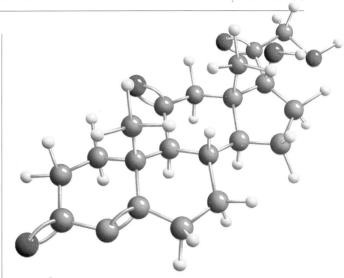

The molecular structure of cortisone, an orthodox anti-inflammatory drug that is based on naturally occurring plant compounds called saponins.

of *Gossypium* may have a role as a male contraceptive by reducing the level of sperm production.

The property of bitterness imparted to plants by these principles is usually part of the overall activity of the herb, and we find sedatives such as *Hops* and *Valerian,* cough remedies like *White Horehound,* anti-inflammatories such as *Bogbean* and *Devil's Claw,* and the vulnerary *Marigold* all sharing this valuable action.

ALKALOIDS

The alkaloids are perhaps the most potent group of plant constituents that act upon the human body and mind. They include the hallucinogen mescaline at one extreme and the deadly poison brucine at the other. There are alkaloids that act on the liver, the nerves, the lungs and the digestive system. Many of the most valued plants in the herbalists' repertoire contain these potent chemicals.

However, within the plants themselves there appears to be no important function for them, apart from possibly being a store for excess nitrogen. Rather, they seem to be provided as a source of healing agents by Planet Earth for humanity and the animal realms through their interaction with the plant realm.

The alkaloids as a group are very diverse in structure. They have nitrogen in their structure and all have a marked physiological activity. Chemically they are divided into thirteen groups based upon their structure, and the activities they show are as diverse as these structures, which makes it almost impossible to say anything in general about them. In the course of the book, individual alkaloids are discussed whenever relevant.

THE ACTION OF HERBS

A great deal of pharmaceutical research has gone into analysing the active constituents of herbs to find out how and why they work. A much older approach is to categorize herbs by looking at what kinds of problems they can treat. The understanding of the actions of herbs and the way they may be used in combination is fundamental to a holistic approach.

In some cases, for instance, the action is due to a specific chemical or combination of chemicals present in the herb – the sedative *Valerian* is an example – or it may be due to a complex synergistic interaction between various constituents of the plant. However, it is best to view the actions as an attribute of the herb as a whole, and any understanding of its chemical basis as an aid in prescription.

To understand this approach let us look at a couple of examples. *Peppermint* for instance, is an anti-catarrhal, an aromatic, an anti-microbial, a carminative, a diaphoretic, an emmenagogue, a febrifuge, a nervine and a stimulant. *Boneset* is also an anti-catarrhal, a diaphoretic and a febrifuge as well as being a bitter, a diuretic, an emetic and a tonic which *Peppermint* is not. If you needed an anti-catarrhal that was at the same time a diuretic, you could use *Boneset*, and if a stimulating anti-catarrhal was needed you could use *Peppermint*. And the two could be combined for a wider effect.

Both herbs play a part in the treatment of a whole range of problems; they not only work on specifics but have a spectrum of actions, which really makes them into the holistic tools they are. Each herb has its own spectrum of actions, so it is important to take care in combining the herbs to cover a range of related problems and to treat the cause as well as symptoms.

In this section a list of actions has been put together and the most useful representatives in each category indicated. The more important of the herbs are underlined. They are in alphabetical order, not necessarily in order of importance. More information can be found in The Herbal section, where the actions of each herb are given. Actions not described on these pages are defined in the glossary.

ALTERATIVE

Alteratives are herbs that will gradually restore the proper function of the body and increase health and vitality. They were at one time known as 'blood cleansers'.
Bladderwrack, *Blue Flag*, Bogbean, *Burdock*, *Cleavers*, *Echinacea*, *Figwort*, Fringetree, *Fumitory*, Garlic, Guaiacum, Golden Seal, *Mountain Grape*, *Nettles*, Pasque Flower, Poke Root, *Queen's Delight*, *Red Clover*, *Sarsaparilla*, Sassafras, Wild Indigo, *Yellow Dock*. ❧

Menyanthes trifoliata
Bogbean, *an alterative and anti-inflammatory*

ANALGESIC, ANODYNE

Analgesics are herbs that reduce pain and are either applied externally or taken internally.
Hops, *Jamaican Dogwood*, *Lady's Slipper*, *Passion Flower*, Red *Poppy*, *Skullcap*, *St John's Wort*, Valerian. ❧

ANTHELMINTIC

Anthelmintics will destroy or expel worms from the digestive system. Unfortunately many of the most effective anthelmintics are no longer available since the Medicines Act of 1968, as they can be toxic in high dosage. Therefore those are not listed here.
Aloe, Garlic, Pomegranate, Tansy, Thuja, Wormwood, Rue. ❧

ANTI-BILIOUS

The anti-bilious herbs help the body to remove excess bile and can thus be beneficial in cases of biliary and jaundice conditions. Compare also cholagogues and hepatics.
Balmony, *Barberry*, *Dandelion*, *Fringetree*, *Golden Seal*, Mugwort, *Vervain*, Wild Yam, Wormwood. ❧

ANTI-CATARRHAL

The anti-catarrhal herbs help the body to remove excess catarrhal build-ups, whether these occur in the sinus area or in other parts of the body.
American Cranesbill, *Bearberry*, *Boneset*, Cayenne, Coltsfoot, *Echinacea*, Elder, Elecampane, *Eyebright*, *Garlic*, *Golden Seal*, *Golden Rod*, *Hyssop*, Iceland Moss, Irish Moss, Marshmallow, *Mullein*, Peppermint, *Sage*, Thyme, *Wild Indigo*, *Yarrow*. ❧

ANTI-EMETIC

The anti-emetics can reduce a feeling of nausea and can help to relieve or prevent vomiting.
Balm, *Black Horehound*, Cayenne, Cloves, Dill, Fennel, Lavender, *Meadowsweet*, Peach Leaves. ❧

ANTI-INFLAMMATORY

The anti-inflammatory herbs help the body to combat inflammations.

Herbs mentioned under demulcents, emollients and vulneraries will often act in this way, especially when they are applied externally.

Black Willow, Bogbean, Chamomile, Devil's Claw, Marigold, Meadowsweet, St John's Wort, White Poplar, Witch Hazel. ❦

Artemisia absinthum Wormwood, *bitter and anthelmintic*

ANTI-LITHIC

The anti-lithic herbs prevent the formation of stones or gravel in the urinary system and can help the body in their removal.

Bearberry, Buchu, Corn Silk, Couchgrass, Gravel Root, Hydrangea, Parsley Piert, Pellitory of the Wall, Sea Holly, Stone Root, Wild Carrot. ❦

ANTI-MICROBIAL

The anti-microbial herbs can help the body to destroy or resist pathogenic micro-organisms.

Aniseed, Bearberry, Caraway Oil, Cayenne, Clove, Coriander, Echinacea, Elecampane, Garlic, Gentian, Juniper, Marigold, Marjoram, Myrrh, Peppermint, Rosemary, Rue, Sage, Southernwood, Thyme, Wild Indigo, Wormwood. ❦

ANTI-SPASMODIC

The anti-spasmodic herbs can prevent or ease spasms or cramps.

Black Cohosh, Black Haw, Chamomile, Cramp Bark, Lady's Slipper, Lime Blossom, Lobelia, Mistletoe, Motherwort, Pasque Flower, Skullcap, Skunk Cabbage, Thyme, Valerian, Vervain, Wild Lettuce, Wild Yam. ❦

APERIENT

Aperient herbs are very mild laxatives. *See* 'Laxatives'.

AROMATIC

The aromatic herbs have a strong and often pleasant odour and can stimulate the digestive system. They are often used to add aroma and taste to other medicines.

Angelica, Aniseed, Balm, Caraway, Cardamon, Celery, Chamomile, Cinnamon, Cloves, Coriander, Dill, Fennel, Hyssop, Ginger, Meadowsweet, Pennyroyal, Peppermint, Rosemary, Valerian, Wood Betony. ❦

ASTRINGENT

Astringents contract tissue by precipitating proteins and can thus reduce secretions and discharges. They contain tannins.

Agrimony, American Cranesbill, Avens, Bayberry, Bearberry, Beth Root, Bistort, Black Catechu, Bugleweed, Eyebright, Golden Rod, Ground Ivy, Kola, Lungwort, Meadowsweet, Mouse Ear, Oak, Periwinkle, Pilewort, Plantain, Raspberry, Red Sage, Rhubarb Root, Rosemary, Slippery Elm, St John's Wort, Tormentil, Wild Cherry, Witch Hazel, Yarrow. ❦

BITTER

Herbs that taste bitter act as stimulating tonics for the digestive system through a reflex via the taste-buds.

Barberry, Boneset, Centaury, Chamomile, Gentian, Golden Seal, Hops, Rue, Southernwood, Tansy, White Horehound, Wormwood, Yarrow. ❦

CARDIAC TONIC

Cardiac tonics affect the heart. Their specific function should be looked up in The Herbal section.

Hawthorn, Motherwort, Night Blooming Cereus. ❦

CARMINATIVE

The carminatives are rich in volatile oils and by their action stimulate the peristalsis of the digestive system and relax the stomach, thereby supporting the digestion and helping against gas in the digestive tract.

Angelica, Aniseed, Balm, Black Mustard, Caraway, Cardamon, Cayenne, Cinnamon, Chamomile, Coriander, Dill, Fennel, Galangal, Garlic, Ginger, Hyssop, Juniper, Peppermint, Sage, Thyme, Valerian. ❦

CHOLAGOGUE

The cholagogues stimulate the release and secretion of bile from the gall-bladder, which can be a marked benefit in gall-bladder problems. They also have a laxative effect on the digestive system since they increase the amount of bile in the duodenum and bile is our internally produced, all-natural laxative.

Balmony, Barberry, Black Root, Blue Flag, Boldo, Dandelion, Fringetree, Fumitory, Gentian, Golden Seal, Mountain Grape, Wahoo, Wild Yam. ❦

DEMULCENT

Demulcents are usually rich in mucilage and can soothe and protect irritated or inflamed internal tissue.

Inula helenium Elecampane, *astringent and anti-catarrhal*

Coltsfoot, Comfrey, Corn Silk, Couchgrass, Flax Seed, Irish Moss, Lungwort, Licorice, Mallow, Marshmallow, Mullein, Oats, Parsley Piert, Slippery Elm. ❦

DIAPHORETIC

Diaphoretics aid the skin in the elimination of toxins and promote perspiration.

Angelica, Bayberry, Boneset, Buchu, Cayenne, Chamomile, Elder, Fennel, Garlic, Ginger, Golden Rod, Guaiacum, Lime Blossom, Peppermint, Pleurisy Root, Prickly Ash, Thuja, Thyme, White Horehound, Yarrow. 🌿

DIURETIC

Diuretics increase the secretion and elimination of urine.

Agrimony, Bearberry, Blue Flag, Boldo, Boneset, Borage, Broom, Buchu, Bugleweed, Burdock, Celery Seed, Cleavers, Corn Silk, Couchgrass, Dandelion, Elder, Gravel Root, Hawthorn Berries, Juniper, Kola, Lily of the Valley, Lime Blossom, Night Blooming Cereus, Parsley, Parsley Piert, Pellitory of the Wall, Saw Palmetto, Sea Holly, Stone Root, Wild Carrot, Yarrow. 🌿

EMETIC

Emetics cause vomiting. Most of the herbs listed cause vomiting only when taken in high dosage. Safe dosages are given for each herb in The Herbal section.

Blood Root, Boneset, Elder Flowers, Ipecacuanha, Lobelia, Senega, Squill. 🌿

EMMENAGOGUE

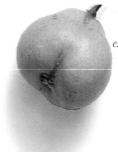

Tropaeolum majus Nasturtium, *a powerful anti-microbial*

Emmenagogues both stimulate and normalize menstrual flow. The term is often employed in the wider context of remedies that act as tonics to the female reproductive system.

Beth Root, Black Cohosh, Black Haw, Blessed Thistle, Blue Cohosh, Chamomile, Chaste Tree, Cramp Bark,

Cydonia oblonga Quince, *an excellent emollient*

False Unicorn Root, Fenugreek, Gentian, Ginger, Golden Seal, Juniper Berry, Marigold, Motherwort, Mugwort, Parsley, Pasque Flower, Pennyroyal, Peppermint, Raspberry, Red Sage, Rosemary, Rue, Southernwood, Squaw Vine, Tansy, True Unicorn Root, Vervain, Wormwood, Yarrow. 🌿

EMOLLIENT

Emollients are applied to the skin to soften, soothe or protect it. They act externally in a manner similar to the way demulcents act internally.

Borage, Chickweed, Coltsfoot, Comfrey, Elecampane, Fenugreek, Flax Seed, Licorice, Mallow, Marshmallow, Mullein, Plantain, Quince Seed, Slippery Elm. 🌿

EXPECTORANT

The expectorants support the body in the removal of excess amounts of mucus from the respiratory system.

Aniseed, Balm of Gilead, Balsam of Tolu, Blood Root, Coltsfoot, Comfrey, Elder Flower, Elecampane, Garlic, Golden Seal, Grindelia, Hyssop, Iceland Moss, Irish Moss, Licorice, Lobelia, Lungwort, Marshmallow, Mouse Ear, Mullein, Pleurisy Root, Senega, Skunk Cabbage, Squill, Thuja, Thyme, Vervain, White Horehound, Wild Cherry. 🌿

FEBRIFUGE, ANTI-PYRETIC

The febrifuges help the body to bring down fevers.

Angelica, Balm, Blessed Thistle, Boneset, Borage, Cayenne, Elder Flower, Hyssop, Pennyroyal, Peppermint, Peruvian Bark,

Pleurisy Root, Prickly Ash, Raspberry, Red Sage, Thyme, Vervain. 🌿

GALACTOGOGUE

The galactogogues can help the breast-feeding mother to increase the flow of milk.

Aniseed, Blessed Thistle, Centaury, Fennel, Goat's Rue, Vervain. 🌿

HEPATIC

The hepatics aid the liver. Their use tones and strengthens it and increases the flow of bile.

Agrimony, Aloe, Balm, Balmony, Barberry, Black Root, Blue Flag, Boldo, Bogbean, Cascara Sagrada, Celery, Centaury, Cleavers, Dandelion, Elecampane, Fennel, Fringetree, Fumitory, Gentian, Golden Seal, Horseradish, Hyssop, Motherwort, Mountain Grape, Prickly Ash, Wahoo, Wild Indigo, Wild Yam, Wormwood, Yarrow, Yellow Dock. 🌿

HYPNOTIC

Hypnotics will induce sleep (not a hypnotic trance).

Chamomile, Californian Poppy, Hops, Jamaican Dogwood, Mistletoe, Passion Flower, Skullcap, Valerian, Wild Lettuce. 🌿

LAXATIVE

The laxatives promote the evacuation of the bowels.

Balmony, Barberry, Buckthorn, Burdock, Cascara Sagrada, Cleavers, Dandelion, Flax Seed, Fringetree, Mountain Grape, Pellitory of the Wall, Rhubarb Root, Senna, Wahoo, Yellow Dock. 🌿

NERVINE

The nervines have a beneficial effect on the nervous system and tone and strengthen it. Some act as stimulants, some as relaxants. Please refer to The Herbal section for more detailed information.

Balm, Black Cohosh, Black Haw, Blue Cohosh, Bugleweed, Chamomile,

Cramp Bark, Damiana, Ginseng, Hops, Kola, Lady's Slipper, Lavender, Lemon Balm, Lime Blossom, Lobelia, Mistletoe, Motherwort, Oats, Pasque Flower, Passion Flower, Peppermint, Red Clover, Rosemary, Skullcap, Valerian, Vervain, Wild Lettuce. ❦

OXYTOCIC

The oxytocics stimulate the contraction of the uterus and can thereby help in childbirth.

Beth Root, Blue Cohosh, Golden Seal, Squaw Vine. ❦

PECTORAL

Pectorals have a general strengthening and healing effect on the respiratory system.

Angelica, Aniseed, Balm of Gilead, Balsam of Tolu, Blood Root, Coltsfoot, Comfrey, Elder, Elecampane, Garlic, Golden Seal, Hyssop, Iceland Moss, Irish Moss, Licorice, Lungwort, Marshmallow, Mouse Ear, Mullein, Pleurisy Root, Senega, Skunk Cabbage, Vervain, White Horehound. ❦

RUBEFACIENT

When rubefacients are applied to the skin they cause a gentle local irritation and stimulate the dilation of the capillaries, thus increasing circulation in the skin. The blood is drawn from deeper parts of the body into the skin and thus often internal pains are relieved.

Black Mustard, Cayenne, Garlic, Ginger, Horseradish, Nettles, Peppermint Oil, Rosemary Oil, Rue. ❦

SEDATIVE

The sedatives calm the nervous system and reduce stress and nervousness throughout the body. They can thus affect tissue of the body that has been irritated by nervous problems.

Black Cohosh, Black Haw, Blue Cohosh, Boldo, Bugleweed, Chamomile, Cowslip, Cramp Bark, Hops, Jamaican Dogwood, Lady's Slipper, Lobelia, Motherwort, Pasque Flower, Passion Flower, Red Clover, Red Poppy, Skullcap, St John's Wort, Valerian, Wild Cherry, Wild Lettuce. ❦

Passiflora incarnata
Passion Flower, analgesic, hypnotic and nervine

SIALAGOGUE

The sialagogues stimulate the secretion of saliva from the salivary glands.

Blue Flag, Cayenne, Centaury, Gentian, Ginger, Prickly Ash, Senega. ❦

SOPORIFIC

The soporifics induce sleep; compare with 'Hypnotics'.

STIMULANT

Stimulants quicken and enliven the physiological functions of the body.

Angelica, Balm of Gilead, Balmony, Bayberry, Black Mustard, Caraway, Cardamon, Cayenne, Cinnamon, Galangal, Garlic, Gentian, Ginseng, Ground Ivy, Horseradish, Juniper, Pennyroyal, Peppermint, Prickly Ash, Rosemary, Rue, Sage, Southernwood, Tansy, White Horehound, Wormwood, Yarrow. ❦

Fumaria officinalis
Fumitory, laxative and alterative

STYPTIC

Styptics reduce or stop external bleeding by their astringency. See 'Astringents'.

TONIC

The tonic herbs strengthen and enliven either specific organs or the whole body. This long list makes more sense when read in conjunction with the section on tonics given for each body system.

Agrimony, Angelica, Aniseed, Balm, Balmony, Bayberry, Bearberry, Beth Root, Black Cohosh, Black Haw, Black Mustard, Black Root, Bogbean, Boldo, Boneset, Buchu, Bugleweed, Burdock, Calumba, Carline Thistle, Cayenne, Centaury, Chamomile, Cleavers, Coltsfoot, Comfrey, Condurango, Couchgrass, Damiana, Dandelion, Echinacea, Elecampane, Eyebright, False Unicorn Root, Fringetree, Fumitory, Garlic, Gentian, Ginseng, Golden Seal, Gravel Root, Grindelia, Hawthorn, Horsechestnut, Hydrangea, Hyssop, Iceland Moss, Lady's Slipper, Licorice, Lime Blossom, Marigold, Motherwort, Mountain Grape, Mugwort, Myrrh, Nettles, Oats, Parsley, Poke Root, Raspberry, Red Clover, Sarsaparilla, Skullcap, Squaw Vine, Tamarind, Thyme, Vervain, Virginia Snake Root, Wood Betony, Wormwood, Yarrow, Yellow Dock. ❦

VULNERARY

Vulneraries are applied externally and aid the body in the healing of wounds and cuts.

Aloe, American Cranesbill, Arnica, Bistort, Black Willow, Burdock, Chickweed, Cleavers, Comfrey, Daisy, Elder, Elecampane, Fenugreek, Flax Seed, Garlic, Golden Seal, Greater Plantain, Horsetail, Hyssop, Irish Moss, Marigold, Marshmallow, Mullein, Myrrh, Shepherd's Purse, Slippery Elm, St John's Wort, Thyme, Witch Hazel, Wood Betony, Yarrow. ❦

FIGHTING OFF INVADERS

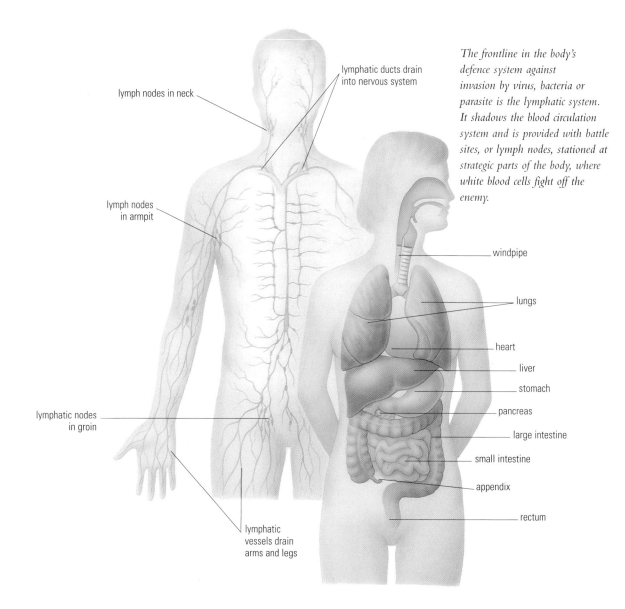

lymphatic ducts drain
into nervous system

lymph nodes in neck

lymph nodes
in armpit

lymphatic nodes
in groin

lymphatic
vessels drain
arms and legs

windpipe

lungs

heart

liver

stomach

pancreas

large intestine

small intestine

appendix

rectum

The frontline in the body's defence system against invasion by virus, bacteria or parasite is the lymphatic system. It shadows the blood circulation system and is provided with battle sites, or lymph nodes, stationed at strategic parts of the body, where white blood cells fight off the enemy.

Infections – whether of bacteria, viruses or fungi – will only occur when the body's defences are weakened. Their natural strength can be diminished by many factors. Physical influences such as an unhealthy diet, a drug therapy or a pre-existing disease can weaken the system. Emotional and mental factors are also crucial. Stress and tension can obviously reduce our energy to a level that allows infections to manifest, but 'catching a cold' or getting other infections can also often be a message from our body asking us to stop and look at what we are doing. To approach infectious diseases herbally we have to recognize that we do not 'catch' them out of thin air but that we create the opportunity and the environment for the infection to thrive. It is not the bacteria's fault! To treat an infection in any real way we aim at restoring the normal resistance of the body, so a whole

treatment ensuring health and vitality of all bodily systems is called for. In many cases it is best to forget about the specific infection and to concentrate on supporting the body doing what it is designed to do – protecting itself. This may take a few days and may even interfere with our all-important worldly commitments, but the need and the message are clear – it is time to give our body and our way of life some attention and care.

Infections often arise as part of an 'epidemic'. When there is a widespread disease attacking many people simultaneously in a community, it may be valid to consider the whole community as a multifaceted group-being that acts in the same way as an individual.

Infestation by parasites is also more likely to happen when the body is weakened. Building up the body's resistance helps it to rid itself of such invaders.

ANTIBIOTICS

There are, no doubt, situations where it is strongly advisable to use drugs like antibiotics. They are an invaluable gift to humanity, saving lives and improving the quality of existence when they are used with discretion and where their use is appropriate. In cases such as meningitis and other potentially lethal infections, they have saved countless lives. Unfortunately, they are often used just because they are convenient and work fast, without paying too much attention to their overall effect and the consequences of their indiscriminate use.

When it is appropriate to resort to antibiotics, some steps can be taken to lessen their impact upon the system. Take at least 2g of vitamin C a day (until about a week after finishing with the antibiotics) and plenty of vitamin B-complex. Both these vitamins help the body to deal with stress – from the infection and from the antibiotics – and increase our natural resistance.

As some antibiotics destroy the natural bacterial flora of the intestines, live yoghurt should be eaten in abundance to support this system against chemical onslaught, as it helps to restore friendly bacteria and balance the ecology of the gut.

While you take antibiotics, rest and be at ease, for you are under attack from powerful chemicals which should be treated with respect. However, be thankful that they are there to help you and express that gratitude to yourself in some meaningful way. To develop a sense of guilt about taking drugs – even though their use is appropriate – would only weaken you and block a deeper healing. When they must be taken, work with them, not against them.

Herbs can be used to help the antibiotic treatment. They can be used during the treatment to augment the action of the drugs and to aid the body and protect it against possible damage. The particular herbs will vary depending on the site of the infection and the person involved and should be chosen accordingly (see pages 42–5 for more information). Herbs can also be used after a drug therapy to tone the system with the aid of bitters and possibly nervine tonics. Cleansing the system with alteratives, diuretics and lymphatic herbs is also important. Whilst specific ones should be chosen according to individual needs, herbs such as *Cleavers, Echinacea, Gentian, Golden Seal, Nettles, Oats* and *Wormwood* are often indicated.

Hydrastis canadensis Golden Seal *can be used in combination with orthodox antibodies to clear bacterial debris from the body.*

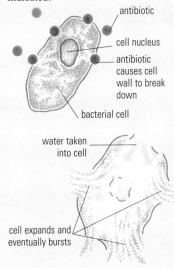

antibiotic
cell nucleus
antibiotic causes cell wall to break down
bacterial cell
water taken into cell
cell expands and eventually bursts

Antibiotics work by locating a disease cell, weakening its walls and then penetrating them. The breached walls allow fluid in and the damaged cell eventually bursts and disintegrates. Herbal remedies can support antibiotic treatment by helping to eliminate the broken down disease cells from the body.

More people died in the influenza epidemic that followed the First World War than were killed in the war itself. This can be put down to problems of hygiene, sanitation and nutrition following that tragic time, but it can also be seen as an outcome of deep communal wounds affecting the collective consciousness of humanity. It is not enough to be individually whole and healthy. The society we are part of must also radiate these qualities or we are part of an unhealthy system and so open to epidemics. These epidemics may be of influenza or Aids, or of fear, alienation and meaninglessness. Our health depends upon wholeness at all these levels.

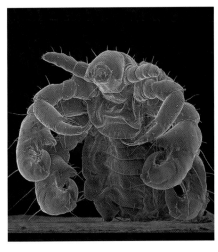

Looking like an alien, the crab louse Pthirus pubis is an extremely irritating blood-sucking parasite, with biting mouth parts and massive crab-like claws.

HERBS FOR INFECTIONS AND INFESTATIONS

Herbs can be used in two ways for infections and infestations; through their anti-microbial action they work directly against microbes and in addition they augment and vitalize the body's own defences.

Fortunately, in most cases they will be performing both functions at the same time.

Myrrh is an example of a herb which combines direct toxic action on bacteria with the ability to stimulate our body's production of white corpuscles – the leucocytes – which are responsible for doing the majority of the defensive work in the body system.

Other actions that are indicated are those that help to eliminate toxins, such as diaphoretics, laxatives and diuretics. Any accumulation of waste material and toxins is a prime environment for microbes to breed in. Most herbs can play a role in treating infections or infestations, but here we will concentrate on the anti-microbials, diaphoretics and anthelmintics.

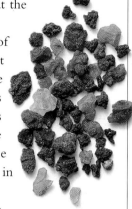

Commiphora molmol
Myrrh, *a powerful anti-microbial*

Anti-Microbials

Many plants have a direct toxic effect upon microbes. The first effective antibiotic drug, penicillin, was discovered in a plant, a fungus. Interestingly enough, an old Welsh remedy for festering sores is based upon mouldy bread. For years this was mocked by the medical profession as an 'old-wives' tale', until it became clear that there is a definite biochemical basis for this seemingly outlandish prescription, as the mould is caused by fungi.

Herbs work in complex ways that cannot always be explained – as not enough research has been done – and the processes whereby they deal with infections are numerous. The best anti-microbials that can be used safely to combat infections include *Echinacea, Garlic, Myrrh, Nasturtium, Thyme, Wild Indigo* and *Wormwood.*

Garlic oil is another powerful anti-microbial worth mentioning. It was used on the wounded during the First World War as an antiseptic applied with a Sphagnum Moss dressing.

HERBAL ANTISEPTIC POWER

In the early part of this century, the antiseptic power of some plant oils was compared with that of phenol, a commonly used chemical antiseptic. It was found that many volatile oils are stronger than phenol, with *Thyme* oil being the strongest. The experiment looked at the antiseptic action on beef tea which had been infected with water from a sewage system, and determined at what dilution there was no more antiseptic action. The chart below shows at what dilution (in parts per 1000 parts) antiseptic action ceased. It can be seen that *Thyme* oil proved to be eight times stronger than phenol. Many other plants were also stronger than phenol.

Thyme	0.7	
Sweet Orange	1.2	
Verbena	1.6	
Rose	1.8	
Clove	2.0	
Eucalyptus	2.2	
Peppermint	2.5	
Orris	3.8	
Anise	4.3	
Rosemary	4.3	
Lavender	5.0	
Phenol	**5.6**	
Fennel	6.4	
Lemon	7.0	
Sassafras	7.5	
Lime	8.4	
Angelica	10.0	

Diaphoretics (Febrifuges)

A diaphoretic is a remedy that induces the body to increase its amount of perspiration. This in turn increases elimination of toxins through the skin and helps to cleanse the body. Diaphoretics are indicated in a wide range of conditions, but nowhere more than in the treatment of fevers and of infections affecting the whole system. (Their use in influenza is discussed in the section on ears, nose, throat and eyes.) With their strengthening and healing properties they can often enable the body to rid itself of infections or fevers in an astoundingly short time.

Diaphoretics speed up and augment the vital healing process without suppressing any part of it. They may be used individually or as part of a wider therapy. The most useful ones are *Angelica, Boneset, Catnip, Cayenne, Elder Flowers* (or *Berries*), *Ginger, Hyssop, Pennyroyal, Peppermint, Pleurisy Root, Thyme* and *Yarrow*.

Anthelmintics (Vermifuges)

Anthelmintics rid the body of parasites and are used internally or externally. Some anthelmintics kill the parasites, others expel them from the body, and most of them are very powerful herbs, some even potentially toxic if taken in large doses. Great care should be taken not to overdose with them.

Legislation in some countries restricts the sale or use by herbalists of some of the more powerful plants. Unfortunately, among them are the more effective anthelmintics like *Kousso, Male Fern* and *Santonica*. Limitations placed on the use of *Male Fern* are most regrettable, since it is very effective against tapeworm and not as potentially dangerous as *Kousso* or *Santonica*. These plants are still widely used by orthodox doctors and veterinarians. Other useful anthelmintics include *Garlic, Pomegranate, Pumpkin Seeds, Quassia, Southernwood, Tansy* and *Wormwood*. In all cases consult The Herbal section to see which herb or combination of herbs is suitable for the circumstances.

Sambucus nigra Elder Flowers *and* Elder Berries, *both very useful stimulants to elimination through perspiration*

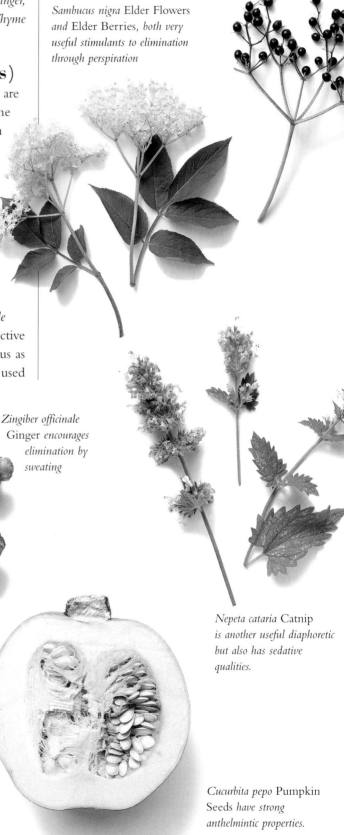

Punica granatum Pomegranate, *a specific remedy for worm infestation*

Zingiber officinale Ginger *encourages elimination by sweating*

Nepeta cataria Catnip *is another useful diaphoretic but also has sedative qualities.*

Cucurbita pepo Pumpkin Seeds *have strong anthelmintic properties.*

Treating Infections

With infections it is particularly important to treat the underlying cause and not to suppress the symptoms. Fever should not be viewed simply as a manifestation of disease that needs to be 'cured' no matter what. The fever may be a symptom of the healing process itself, which should be supported, not suppressed. A basic mixture that helps the body to work through the fever is as follows.

Boneset	2 parts	
Yarrow	2 parts	
Echinacea	1 part	

Drink half a cup as hot as possible every two hours.

Echinacea is included to help the body deal with any microbes, but the simple use of diaphoretics like Boneset or Yarrow will often suffice. If the diaphoretic strength needs to be increased, add a pinch of Cayenne. If the glands are swollen, indicating lymphatic involvement, then Marigold or Cleavers can be included. And if the mucous membranes are involved, Golden Seal can be added as a useful general tonic and a specific help to the membranes. If there is much restlessness, nervine relaxants like Chamomile or Skullcap can be included. These mixtures can be used not only in fevers where the cause is not clear, but also in diseases such as chicken-pox,

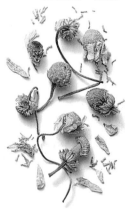

Chamaemelum nobile
Chamomile *helps to relax restless patients suffering from any infection.*

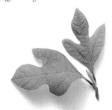

Sassafras albidum
Sassafras *is recommended for skin problems and so can help clear up the after-effects of lice.*

measles, scarlet fever or the like. This is because herbs do not merely halt the named disease, they also bring balanced healing to a pattern of imbalance. Thus the same herbs and actions may suit a range of people with a range of infectious diseases. Where there is catarrhal involvement, as in measles, refer to the advice given in the section on ear, nose, throat and eyes. If the skin is itching, the irritation may be eased by sponging the body with diluted distilled Witch Hazel. In more intransigent viral infections such as glandular fever, a most beneficial mixture that can help even if the problem has turned into a low level, debilitating weakness that might go on for months, is as follows.

Echinacea	2 parts	
Poke Root	2 parts	
Wild Indigo	2 parts	
Wormwood	2 parts	
Myrrh	1 part	

The mixture should be drunk three times a day. If you do not like its unpleasant taste, you can mask it by the use of Licorice.

In any infection, the intake of vitamin C should be raised to at least 2g daily, vitamin B-complex should be taken and Garlic should be considered as an additional remedy, preferably eaten raw. A cleansing diet based on fruit and fruit juices should be the basis of

nutrition. Sometimes fasting is advisable during an infection. It is best to continue with the medication for a short while after recovery.

For specific infections refer to the sections on the body system in which the infections occur.

Treating Infestations

We live in a very close and ecological relationship with numerous organisms. They not only live around but also inside us, and our interaction with them is for the most part symbiotic and mutually beneficial; we exist in homeostatic harmony. Many

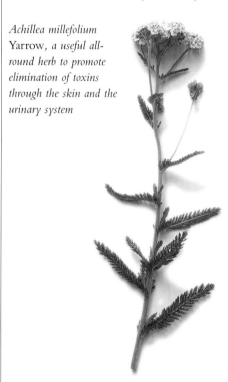

Achillea millefolium
Yarrow*, a useful all-round herb to promote elimination of toxins through the skin and the urinary system*

species of bacteria, for instance, defend our body against the invasion of unfriendly microbes or parasites, such as certain bacteria on the skin or in the intestines. However, this ecological harmony can easily be disrupted, thus opening the gates for the invasion of parasites. The best prevention of such an invasion lies in the maintenance of a natural

Echinacea angustifolia
Echinacea *is a front line remedy for fighting off both bacterial and viral infections.*

and healthy outer and inner environment, in the maintenance of health and well-being and in appropriate hygiene.

INTESTINAL WORMS

A number of animal species can become parasites in the human intestine. Each area on this planet with its own unique ecology has its local variety of parasites, and as we are truly part of our own environment, we sometimes harbour them. The most important intestinal parasites in Western societies are worms: roundworm, tapeworm and threadworm.

Roundworm and tapeworm can be treated in basically the same fashion. The famous American herbalist, Dr Shook, advises that, rather than fasting, we should eat foods that the worms do not like for a couple of days, thus weakening them before taking anthelmintics. Such foods are onions, garlic, pickles and salty things. After eating these (together with your normal food) for some days, drink a strong cup of *Wormwood* tea in the morning and at night for three days. On the fourth day take a cup of *Senna* tea to cleanse the bowels of the dead parasites. *Licorice* can be added to the *Senna* tea to prevent griping pains that might occur and

Senna alexandrina
Senna *helps clear dead internal parasites from the body.*

instead of taking *Wormwood* any other anthelmintic may be used if it seems to be more appropriate. If tapeworm proves to be more tenacious, *Wormwood* might have to be used for a longer period or might have to be exchanged for the stronger *Pomegranate Seeds* or even *Male Fern* (keeping in mind the limitations on its use). As threadworms inhabit the rectum, a different approach is needed and enemas have to be used. The best herb to use is *Quassia*. Pour 500ml/1pt of boiling water onto 30g/1oz of *Quassia* chips and let it infuse until it reaches body temperature, when it will be ready for use. Besides using this infusion for enemas, two teaspoonfuls of it, flavoured with *Licorice* if necessary, should be taken before meals three times a day. Another traditional remedy is to insert a peeled clove of *Garlic* into the rectum at night, but make sure the first skin under the peel is unbroken, otherwise it might be too strong and be irritating.

LICE AND FLEAS

It is possible to rid the body of lice and fleas by using herbal remedies, but only when we maintain a good diet and scrupulous hygiene at the same time. The whole environment of the parasite has to be taken care of, and the treatment has to be an ecological approach. If lifestyle is not attended to, herbs by themselves will not be powerful enough and the only effective way of ridding the body of the parasite will lie in the use of drugs.

Lice can be treated through the use of oils of *Aniseed, Sassafras* or *Quassia,* with *Sassafras* oil being the most effective. For external use, mix one part of *Sassafras* oil with two parts of *Olive* oil, rub it into the scalp and hair and comb with a fine tooth comb to remove the dead lice and eggs. This process has to be repeated daily until the hair is completely cleared of lice and eggs.

SCABIES

This little animal can be very intransigent and must be treated with the greatest respect – and with rigorous hygiene. Bedding linen must be boiled after every use and in extreme cases has to be burned.

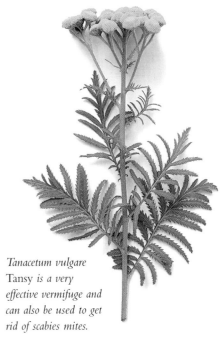

Tanacetum vulgare
Tansy *is a very effective vermifuge and can also be used to get rid of scabies mites.*

As an external remedy, a strong decoction of *Tansy* should be applied liberally, either in the bath or sponged over the body often. Bitters and nervines should be taken internally for a few days and after the last scabies appear to have gone. This helps the body to return to a state of ease with itself.

Gentian and *Skullcap* are ideal nervines, but select the ones that are most appropriate to the individual involved.

A THERAPEUTIC INDEX

The index lists herbs that can be considered as treatment for specific diseases. The diseases or conditions are listed alphabetically. The most useful herbs, or the specifics, for each category are listed first and underlined; others follow. Specifics are those herbs which are considered to be the best and most effective remedies to relieve a particular condition or disease state.

ABSCESS
Echinacea, _Garlic_, _Marshmallow_, _Myrrh_, _Wild Indigo_, Blue Flag, Cleavers, Coltsfoot, Fenugreek, Golden Seal, Mallow, Poke Root. ❦

ACNE
Blue Flag, _Cleavers_, _Echinacea_, _Garlic_, _Poke Root_, _Wild Indigo_. ❦

ADENOIDS
Cleavers, _Echinacea_, _Garlic_, _Golden Seal_, _Marigold_, _Poke Root_, _Wild Indigo_. ❦

ANGINA PECTORIS
Hawthorn, Motherwort. ❦

ANXIETY
Californian Poppy, _Chamomile_, _Mistletoe_, _Motherwort_, _Pasque Flower_, _St John's Wort_, _Skullcap_, _Valerian_, _Wild Lettuce_, Balm, Betony, Cowslip, Damiana, Hops, Hyssop, Oats, Passion Flower, Peppermint, Vervain. ❦

APPENDICITIS
Agrimony, American Cranesbill, Golden Seal, Wild Yam. ❦

APPETITE LOSS
Calamus, _Centaury_, _Condurango_, _Gentian_, _Mugwort_, _Wormwood_, Balmony, Blessed Thistle, Calumba, Caraway, Cardamon, Chamomile, Galangal, Golden Seal, Quassia, Southernwood, Tansy, White Poplar. ❦

ARTERIOSCLEROSIS
Lime, Hawthorn, Mistletoe. ❦

ARTHRITIS
Black Cohosh, _Bogbean_, _Celery Seed_, _Guaiacum_, _Prickly Ash_, _Wild Yam_, Bittersweet, Daisy, Juniper, Meadowsweet, Scots Pine, Silver Birch, White Poplar, Wintergreen, Yarrow. ❦

ASTHMA
Elecampane, _Ephedra_, _Grindelia_, _Lobelia_, _Pill-bearing Spurge_, _Sundew_, _Wild Cherry_, Balsam of Tolu, Black Cohosh, Black Haw, Blood Root, Blue Cohosh, Butterbur, Coltsfoot, Mullein, Pasque Flower, Senega. ❦

BLOOD PRESSURE (HIGH)
Hawthorn, _Lime Blossom_, _Mistletoe_, _Yarrow_, Balm, Black Haw, Cramp Bark, Garlic. ❦

BOILS
Blue Flag, _Echinacea_, _Garlic_, _Myrrh_, _Pasque Flower_, _Poke Root_, _Wild Indigo_, Chickweed, Cleavers, Coltsfoot, Comfrey, Fenugreek, Figwort, Flax Seed, Greater Plantain, Mallow, Marshmallow. ❦

BRONCHITIS
Blood Root, _Coltsfoot_, _Echinacea_, _Elecampane_, _Garlic_, _Grindelia_, _Lobelia_, _Mouse Ear_, _Mullein_, _Pill-bearing Spurge_, _Pleurisy Root_, _Senega_, _Sundew_, _White Horehound_, Angelica, Aniseed, Balm of Gilead, Balsam of Tolu, Caraway, Carline Thistle, Comfrey, Cowslip, Ephedra, Fennel, Fenugreek, Flax Seed, Greater Plantain, Ground Ivy, Horseradish, Hyssop, Iceland Moss, Ipecacuanha, Irish Moss, Licorice, Mallow, Marshmallow, Nasturtium, Pansy, Scots Pine, Soapwort, Squill, Sweet Violet, Thyme, Wild Cherry. ❦

BRUISES
Arnica, _Elder_, Chickweed, Cucumber, Lady's Mantle, Marigold, St John's Wort. ❦

BURNS
Aloe, _Elder_, _Marigold_, _Greater Plantain_, _St John's Wort_, Chamomile, Chickweed, Comfrey, Cucumber, Quince Seed. ❦

CATARRH
Echinacea, _Elder_, _Eyebright_, _Garlic_, _Golden Rod_, _Golden Seal_, _Mouse Ear_, _Mullein_, _Peppermint_, _Pine_, _Poke Root_, Avens, Balsam of Tolu, Bistort, Chamomile, Coltsfoot, Daisy, Fenugreek, Grindelia, Ground Ivy, Hyssop, Iceland Moss, Mallow, Myrrh, Pill-bearing Spurge, Sweet Violet, Wild Indigo. ❦

CHILBLAINS
Cayenne, _Ginger_, Black Mustard, Horsetail, Prickly Ash. ❦

CIRCULATION
Cayenne, _Ginger_, _Prickly Ash_, Black Mustard, Horseradish, Rosemary. ❦

COLDS
Angelica, _Cayenne_, _Elder_, _Garlic_, _Ginger_, _Golden Rod_, _Golden Seal_, _Hyssop_, _Peppermint_, _Yarrow_, Avens, Bayberry, Catnip, Cowslip, Echinacea, Eyebright, Fenugreek, Lime Blossom, Marjoram. ❦

COLIC
Angelica, _Boldo_, _Calamus_, _Condurango_, _Cramp Bark_,

Gentian, _Ginger_, _Peppermint_, _Valerian_, _Wild Yam_, Allspice, Aniseed, Avens, Balmony, Blessed Thistle, Blue Cohosh, Butterbur, Caraway, Cardamon, Catnip, Cayenne, Chamomile, Cinnamon, Coriander, Dill, Fennel, Horseradish, Jambul, Juniper, Licorice, Mugwort, Pennyroyal, Rue, Tormentil, Wild Lettuce, Wormwood. ❦

COLITIS
Agrimony, _American Cranesbill_, _Bayberry_, _Comfrey_, _Marshmallow_, Bistort, Black Catechu, Meadowsweet, Oak, Tormentil. ❦

CONJUNCTIVITIS
Chamomile, _Eyebright_, _Golden Seal_, _Marigold_, Fennel. ❦

CONSTIPATION
Balmony, _Barberry_, _Buckthorn_, _Cascara Sagrada_, _Rhubarb Root_, _Senna_, _Yellow Dock_, Aloe, Black Root, Bogbean, Boldo, Butterbur, Figwort, Flax Seed, Wahoo. ❦

COUGH
Angelica, _Aniseed_, _Balm of Gilead_, _Coltsfoot_, _Comfrey_, _Cowslip_, _Elecampane_, _Garlic_, _Golden Seal_, _Grindelia_, _Ground Ivy_, _Hyssop_, _Mouse Ear_, _Mullein_, _Pine_, _Greater Plantain_, _Pleurisy Root_, _Senega_, _Sundew_, _White Horehound_, Balsam of Tolu, Caraway, Carline Thistle, Daisy, Fennel, Fenugreek, Licorice, Mallow, Marjoram, Marshmallow, Myrrh, Red Poppy, Soapwort, Sweet Violet, Thuja, Thyme, Wild Lettuce. ❦

CRAMP
Black Cohosh, _Cramp Bark_, _Pasque Flower_, _Skullcap_, _Valerian_, _Wild Lettuce_, _Wild Yam_, Cayenne, Ginger, Woundwort. ❦

CYSTITIS
Bearberry, _Buchu_, _Couchgrass_, _Echinacea_, _Juniper_, _Yarrow_, Angelica, Silver Birch, Boldo, Carline Thistle, Celery Seed, Cleavers, Coltsfoot, Corn Silk, Golden Rod, Gravel Root, Ground Ivy, Horsetail, Hydrangea, Pansy, Pellitory of the Wall, Sea Holly. ❦

DEBILITY
Balmony, _Blessed Thistle_, _Cayenne_, _Damiana_, _Dandelion_, _Golden Seal_, _Kola_, _Rosemary_, Agrimony, Barberry, Betony, Calamus, Ginger, Life Root, Mugwort, Oats, True Unicorn Root, White Poplar, Wormwood. ❦

DEPRESSION
Damiana, _Kola_, _Oats_, _Skullcap_, _Wormwood_, Balm, Celery, Chamomile, Mistletoe, Mugwort, Rosemary, Southernwood, Valerian, Vervain. ❦

Tropaeolum majus
Nasturtium

DIARRHEA

Agrimony, _American Cranesbill_, _Bayberry_, _Bistort_, _Black Catechu_, _Comfrey_, _Lady's Mantle_, _Meadowsweet_, _Oak_, _Greater Plantain_, _Rhatany_, _Silverweed_, _Tormentil_, Avens, Blessed Thistle, Burr-Marigold, Caraway, Catnip, Cinnamon, Coriander, Daisy, Eyebright, Ground Ivy, Jambul, Kola, Self-Heal. ❦

DIARRHEA (IN CHILDREN)

Meadowsweet, American Cranesbill, Lady's Mantle. ❦

DIVERTICULITIS

Wild Yam, Comfrey, Chamomile, Marshmallow. ❦

EARACHE

(SEE ALSO 'INFECTION')

Pennywort, _Pasque Flower_, Mullein. ❦

ECZEMA

Blue Flag, _Burdock_, _Chickweed_, _Cleavers_, _Figwort_, _Golden Seal_, _Nettles_, _Red Clover_, _Yellow Dock_, Balm of Gilead, Bittersweet, Comfrey, Mountain Grape, Pansy, Sarsaparilla, Sweet Violet. ❦

EPILEPSY

Hyssop, _Skullcap_, Passion Flower, Valerian. ❦

FEVER

Boneset, _Catnip_, _Cayenne_, _Ginger_, _Peruvian Bark_, _Pleurisy Root_, Angelica, Black Mustard, Borage, Carline Thistle, Chamomile, Horseradish, Peppermint, Vervain. ❦

FIBROSITIS

Cayenne, _Ginger_, _Pine_, _Ragwort_, _Wintergreen_, Horseradish, Rosemary, St John's Wort. ❦

FLATULENCE

Angelica, _Calamus_, _Caraway_, _Cardamon_, _Cayenne_, _Cinnamon_, _Condurango_, _Coriander_, _Fennel_, _Gentian_, _Ginger_, Allspice, Aniseed, Balm, Blessed Thistle, Calumba, Catnip, Centaury, Chamomile, Cloves, Galangal, Horseradish, Juniper, Marjoram, Mugwort, Parsley, Pennyroyal, Peppermint, Southernwood, Thyme, Valerian, Wormwood. ❦

FUNGUS INFECTION

Marigold, Golden Seal, Greater Celandine, Myrrh. ❦

GALL-BLADDER PROBLEMS

Balmony, _Black Root_, _Dandelion_, _Fringetree Bark_, _Milk Thistle_, _Vervain_, _Wahoo_, _Wild Yam_, Barberry, Bogbean, Boldo, Golden Seal, Greater Celandine, Marigold. ❦

GASTRITIS

American Cranesbill, _Calamus_, _Comfrey_, _Golden Seal_, _Marshmallow_, _Meadowsweet_, _Slippery Elm_, Chamomile, Iceland Moss, Irish Moss, Licorice, Mallow, Peach Leaves, Quince. ❦

GINGIVITIS

Bistort, _Echinacea_, _Golden Seal_, _Myrrh_, _Oak Bark_, _Poke Root_, _Rhatany_, _Wild Indigo_, Avens, Bayberry, Black Catechu, Garlic, Lady's Mantle, Red Sage, Self-Heal, Silverweed, Tormentil, Vervain. ❦

GLANDS (SWOLLEN)

Cleavers, _Echinacea_, _Poke Root_, Marigold, Wild Indigo. ❦

GLANDULAR FEVER

Echinacea, _Myrrh_, _Poke Root_, _Wormwood_, Garlic, Wild Indigo. ❦

HALITOSIS

Dill, Fennel,

HAYFEVER

Ephedra, _Golden Seal_, Elder, Eyebright, Garlic, Peppermint. ❦

HEADACHE

Betony, _Feverfew_, _Marjoram_, _Rosemary_, _Skullcap_, Chamomile, Cowslip, Hops, Mistletoe, Peppermint, Rue, St John's Wort, Valerian. ❦

HEARTBURN

Comfrey, _Marshmallow_, _Meadowsweet_, Iceland Moss, Irish Moss, Mallow, Slippery Elm. ❦

HEMORRHOIDS

Bistort, _Horsechestnut_, _Lady's Mantle_, _Pilewort_, _Silverweed_, _Tormentil_, American Cranesbill, Balmony, Comfrey, Greater Plantain, Ground Ivy, Oak, Rhatany. ❦

HYPERSENSITIVITY

Ephedra. ❦

INCONTINENCE (URINARY)

Ephedra, _Horsetail_, Agrimony. ❦

INDIGESTION

Balm, _Calamus_, _Cayenne_, _Centaury_, _Chamomile_, _Condurango_, _Fennel_, _Ginger_, _Peppermint_, _Valerian_, _Wild Yam_, _Wormwood_, Allspice, Agrimony, Balmony, Blessed Thistle, Boldo, Caraway, Cardamon, Catnip, Cinnamon, Cloves, Dill, Galangal, Gentian, Iceland Moss, Marjoram, Mugwort, Quassia, Red Sage, Rosemary, Thyme, True Unicorn Root, Wild Lettuce. ❦

INFECTION

Cleavers, _Echinacea_, _Garlic_, _Golden Seal_, _Myrrh_, _Wild Indigo_, Cayenne, Fenugreek, Ginger, Nasturtium, Thyme, Wormwood. ❦

INFLUENZA

Boneset, _Cayenne_, _Echinacea_, _Garlic_, _Golden Seal_, _Pleurisy Root_, Angelica, Balm, Black Mustard, Carline Thistle, Elder, Ginger, Horseradish, Lime, Marjoram, Myrrh, Nasturtium, Peppermint, White Poplar, Yarrow. ❦

INSOMNIA

Californian Poppy, _Hops_, _Jamaican Dogwood_, _Passion Flower_, _Valerian_, _Wild Lettuce_, Chamomile, Cowslip, Lime Blossom, Pasque Flower, Skullcap. ❦

ITCHING

Chickweed, _Golden Seal_, _Marigold_, Chamomile, Cleavers, Cucumber, Peppermint, St John's Wort. ❦

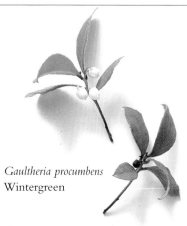

Gaultheria procumbens
Wintergreen

JAUNDICE

Balmony, _Barberry_, _Black Root_, _Dandelion_, _Vervain_, _Wahoo_, _Yellow Dock_, Bittersweet, Centaury, Golden Seal, Mountain Grape, Wild Yam. ❦

KIDNEY STONES

Bearberry, _Corn Silk_, _Couchgrass_, _Gravel Root_, _Hydrangea_, _Pellitory of the Wall_, _Stone Root_, Dandelion, Sea Holly, Wild Carrot, Yarrow. ❦

LABOUR PAINS (FALSE)

Black Cohosh, _Cramp Bark_, _Motherwort_, _Wild Yam_, Blue Cohosh, Valerian, Wild Lettuce. ❦

LARYNGITIS

Balm of Gilead, _Blood Root_, _Echinacea_, _Golden Seal_, _Myrrh_, _Oak_, _Red Sage_, _Thyme_, Agrimony, Bayberry, Bistort, Black Catechu, Caraway, Cayenne, Chamomile, Fenugreek, Golden Rod, Lady's Mantle, Mallow, Poke Root, Tormentil, Wild Indigo. ❦

LEUCORRHEA

American Cranesbill, _Bayberry_, _Beth Root_, _Golden Seal_, _Lady's Mantle_, _Life Root_, _Myrrh_, _Nasturtium_, Wild Indigo, Avens, Bearberry, Bistort, Black Catechu, Ground Ivy, Oak. ❦

LIVER TONIC

Balmony, _Black Root_, _Blue Flag_, _Centaury_, _Dandelion_, _Wahoo_, _Yellow Dock_, Bogbean, Burdock, Garlic, Golden Seal, Mountain Grape, Wild Yam. ❦

LUMBAGO

Black Mustard, _Cayenne_, _Ragwort_, _Wintergreen_. ❦

MENOPAUSE

Black Cohosh, _Chaste Tree_, _False Unicorn Root_, _Golden Seal_, _St John's Wort_, Beth Root, Life Root. ❦

MENSTRUATION (DELAYED)

Blue Cohosh, _Chaste Tree_, _False Unicorn Root_, _Life Root_, _Parsley_, _Pennyroyal_, _Rue_, _Tansy_, _Southernwood_, _Wormwood_, Marigold, Motherwort, Mugwort, Thuja, Yarrow. ❦

MENSTRUATION (EXCESSIVE)

American Cranesbill, _Beth Root_, _Periwinkle_, Golden Seal, Lady's Mantle. ❦

MENSTRUATION (PAINFUL)
Black Cohosh, *Black Haw*, *Cramp Bark*, *Jamaican Dogwood*, *Pasque Flower*, *St John's Wort*, *Skullcap*, *Valerian*, *Wild Lettuce*, Blue Cohosh, Butterbur, Caraway, Chaste Tree, False Unicorn Root, Marigold, Squaw Vine, Wild Yam. ❦

METRORRHAGIA
American Cranesbill, *Beth Root*, *Golden Seal*, *Periwinkle*, Lady's Mantle. ❦

MIGRAINE
Feverfew, Jamaican Dogwood, Kola, Mistletoe, Peppermint, Skullcap, Wormwood. ❦

MILK STIMULATION (BREAST)
Goat's Rue, *Milk Thistle*, Borage, Caraway, Dill, Fennel, Fenugreek. ❦

MISCARRIAGE (THREATENED)
Blue Cohosh, *False Unicorn Root*, Black Haw, Cramp Bark. ❦

MOUTH ULCERS
Myrrh, *Red Sage*, Bistort, Chamomile, Lady's Mantle, Oak. ❦

NAUSEA
Black Horehound, *Chamomile*, *Meadowsweet*, *Peppermint*, Avens, Cayenne, Cinnamon, Cloves, Fennel, Galangal, Marshmallow. ❦

NEURALGIA
Betony, *Black Cohosh*, *Jamaican Dogwood*, *Mistletoe*, *Passion Flower*, *St John's Wort*, *Skullcap*, *Valerian*, Hops, Pasque Flower, Rosemary. ❦

NOSEBLEED
Lady's Mantle, *Witch Hazel*, Marigold, Tormentil. ❦

OVARIAN PAIN
Jamaican Dogwood, *Pasque Flower*, *Valerian*, Passion Flower, St John's Wort, Skullcap, Wild Yam. ❦

PAIN
Black Cohosh, *Black Willow*, *Jamaican Dogwood*, *Valerian*, *Wild Lettuce*, Cramp Bark, Guaiacum, Hops, Rosemary, Skullcap. ❦

PALPITATIONS
Motherwort, Skullcap, Valerian. ❦

PHLEBITIS
Hawthorn, *Horsechestnut*, Lime Blossom, Mistletoe. ❦

PREGNANCY TONIC
Raspberry Leaves, Squaw Vine. ❦

PREGNANCY (VOMITING)
Black Horehound, *False Unicorn Root*, *Meadowsweet*, Blue Cohosh, Peppermint. ❦

PRE-MENSTRUAL TENSION
Chaste Tree, *Skullcap*, *Valerian*, Lime Blossom, Pasque Flower. ❦

PROSTATE
Damiana, *Horsetail*, *Hydrangea*, *Saw Palmetto*, Corn Silk, Couchgrass, Sea Holly. ❦

PSORIASIS
Blue Flag, *Burdock*, *Cleavers*, *Figwort*, *Mountain Grape*, *Red Clover*, *Sarsaparilla*, *Yellow Dock*, Balm of Gilead, Chickweed, Flax Seed, Sassafras, Thuja. ❦

RHEUMATISM
Angelica, *Black Cohosh*, *Bogbean*, *Celery Seed*, *Guaiacum*, *Meadowsweet*, *Prickly Ash*, *White Poplar*, *Wild Lettuce*, *Wild Yam*, *Wintergreen*, *Yarrow*, Arnica, Bittersweet, Black Mustard, Blue Cohosh, Burdock, Cayenne, Couchgrass, Daisy, Dandelion, Elder, Fennel, Gravel Root, Horseradish, Horsetail, Juniper, Poke Root, Ragwort, St John's Wort, Sarsaparilla, Sassafras, Scots Pine, Silver Birch, Thuja, Wild Carrot. ❦

SCIATICA
Black Cohosh, *Jamaican Dogwood*, *St John's Wort*, Yarrow. ❦

SHINGLES
Jamaican Dogwood, *Mistletoe*, *Passion Flower*, *St John's Wort*, Flax Seed, Hops, Skullcap, Valerian, Wild Lettuce, Wild Yam. ❦

SINUSITIS
Elder, *Eyebright*, *Garlic*, *Golden Rod*, *Golden Seal*, *Poke Root*, *Scots Pine*, *Wild Indigo*, Chamomile, Myrrh, Peppermint, Thyme, Yarrow. ❦

SORE THROAT
Balm of Gilead, *Echinacea*, *Garlic*, *Golden Seal*, *Oak*, Agrimony, Bayberry, Cayenne, Chamomile, Ginger, Golden Rod, Myrrh, Poke Root, Silverweed, Thyme. ❦

SPOTS
Blue Flag, *Cleavers*, *Echinacea*, *Figwort*, *Garlic*, *Poke Root*. ❦

STRESS
Damiana, *Lime Blossom*, *Mistletoe*, *St John's Wort*, *Skullcap*, Balm, Betony, Borage, Chamomile, Cowslip, Hops, Oats, Pasque Flower, Passion Flower, Valerian, Wild Lettuce, Wormwood. ❦

SUNBURN
Aloe, *Marigold*, Eyebright, St John's Wort. ❦

TENSION
Betony, *Cowslip*, *Jamaican Dogwood*, *Lime Blossom*, *Mistletoe*, *Motherwort*, *Pasque Flower*, *Passion Flower*, *St John's Wort*, *Skullcap*, *Valerian*, *Vervain*, *Wild Lettuce*, Balm, Californian Poppy, Damiana, Hops, Peppermint. ❦

Stellaria media
Chickweed

TINNITUS
Black Cohosh, *Golden Seal*, Golden Rod, Ground Ivy. ❦

TONSILLITIS
Cleavers, *Echinacea*, *Garlic*, *Golden Seal*, *Myrrh*, *Poke Root*, *Red Sage*, Thyme, Wild Indigo. ❦

TOOTHACHE
Cloves. ❦

TRAVEL SICKNESS
Black Horehound, Galangal, Peppermint. ❦

TUMOURS
Cleavers, Comfrey, Elder, Fenugreek, Greater Celandine, Red Clover, Sweet Violet, Thuja. ❦

ULCERS (PEPTIC)
American Cranesbill, *Comfrey*, *Marshmallow*, *Meadowsweet*, *Slippery Elm*, Calamus, Golden Seal, Irish Moss, Licorice, Mallow. ❦

ULCERS (SKIN)
Chickweed, *Comfrey*, *Golden Seal*, *Marigold*, Echinacea, Marshmallow. ❦

VARICOSE ULCERS
Golden Seal, *Horsechestnut*, *Marigold*, Comfrey, Marshmallow. ❦

VARICOSE VEINS
Horsechestnut, Hawthorn, Lime Blossom, St John's Wort, Witch Hazel. ❦

VOMITING
Black Horehound, *Meadowsweet*, Cinnamon, Cloves, Comfrey, False Unicorn Root, Iceland Moss, Peppermint, Rosemary. ❦

WARTS
Greater Celandine, Thuja. ❦

WATER RETENTION
Bearberry, *Broom*, *Buchu*, *Dandelion*, *Gravel Root*, *Juniper Berries*, *Pellitory of the Wall*, *Wild Carrot*, Burr-Marigold, Carline Thistle, Celery Seed, Corn Silk, Horsetail, Parsley, Sea Holly, Silver Birch, Stone Root, Yarrow. ❦

WHOOPING COUGH
Coltsfoot, *Grindelia*, *Lobelia*, *Mouse Ear*, Black Cohosh, Ephedra, Garlic, Mullein, Pansy, Red Clover, Sundew, Wild Cherry. ❦

WORMS
Cucumber, Garlic, Kousso, Male Fern, Pomegranate, Pumpkin, Quassia, Santonica, Tansy, Wormwood. ❦

WOUNDS
Chickweed, *Comfrey*, *Elder*, *Golden Seal*, *Marigold*, *Greater Plantain*, *St John's Wort*, *Self-Heal*, *Woundwort*, Carline Thistle, Chamomile, Fenugreek, Garlic, Horsetail, Lady's Mantle, Marshmallow, Mouse Ear, Red Sage, Tormentil. ❦

HERBAL REMEDIES IN THE HOME

There are well over two thousand plants which can be used in herbal medicine in the Western world. The planet-wide list is far greater. So what can you realistically provide in the home? A daunting prospect faces the fledgling herbalist, yet by using the actions approach presented in this book, it is possible to stock a small herbal medicine chest which will fulfil most day-to-day needs.

The list of herbs shown below includes representatives of all the main actions, but also specific ones as well. The herbs are listed in alphabetical order of their Latin names.

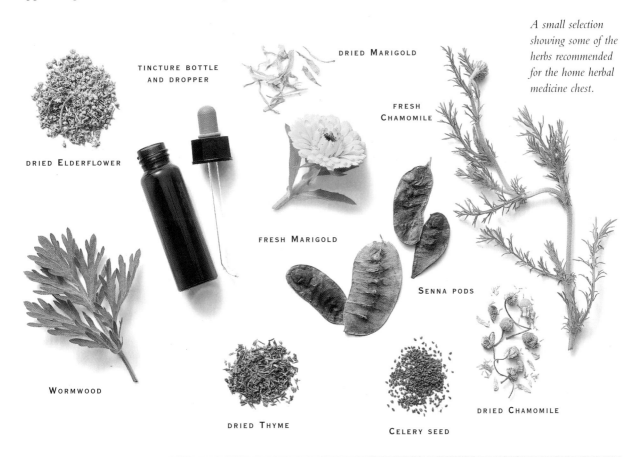

A small selection showing some of the herbs recommended for the home herbal medicine chest.

TINCTURE BOTTLE AND DROPPER

DRIED MARIGOLD

FRESH CHAMOMILE

DRIED ELDERFLOWER

FRESH MARIGOLD

SENNA PODS

WORMWOOD

DRIED CHAMOMILE

DRIED THYME

CELERY SEED

A BASIC HERBAL MEDICINE CHEST

Achillea millefolium Yarrow
Althaea officinalis Marshmallow
Apium graveolens Celery Seed
Arctium lappa Burdock Root
Artemisia absinthum Wormwood
Capsicum annuum Cayenne
Chamaelirium luteum
   False Unicorn Root
Chamaemelum nobile Chamomile
Echinacea angustifolia Echinacea
Eupatorium perfoliatum Boneset
Filipendula ulmaria Meadowsweet
Galium aparine Cleavers

Mentha x *piperita* Peppermint
Pimpinella anisum Aniseed
Rumex crispus Yellow Dock
Salix nigra Black Willow
Sambucus nigra Elder
Scutellaria laterifolia Skullcap
Senna alexandrina Senna Pods
Symphytum officinale Comfrey
Taraxacum officinale Dandelion
Thymus vulgaris Thyme
Tussilago farfara Coltsfoot
Urtica dioica Nettle
Valeriana officinalis Valerian

In addition to these specific herbs, it will be helpful to have the following in the medicine chest, in the form of ointments:
Arnica montana Arnica
Calendula officinalis Marigold
Stellaria media Chickweed
Symphytum officinale Comfrey
You should also include distilled
Hamamelis virginiana
Witch Hazel, obtainable from pharmacies.

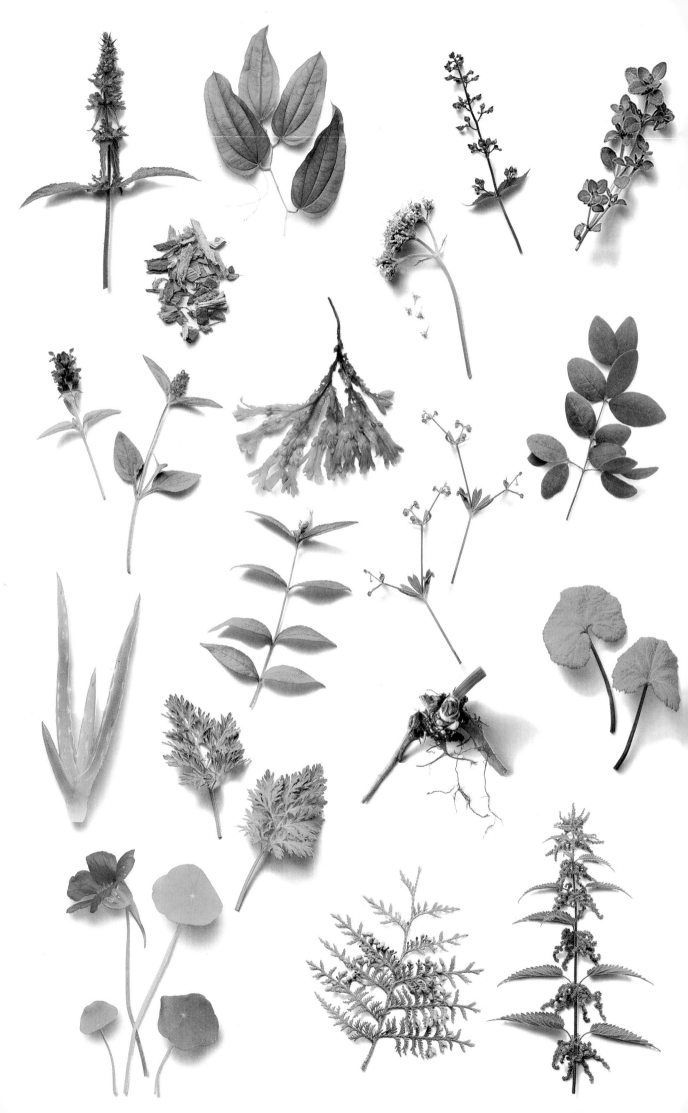

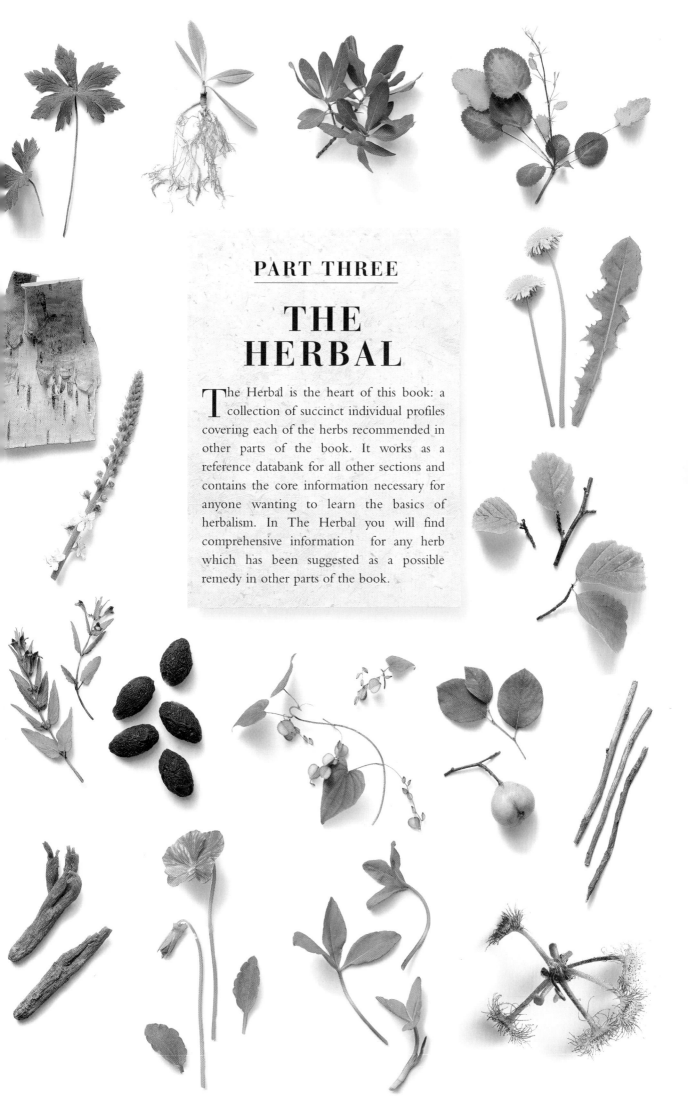

PART THREE

THE HERBAL

The Herbal is the heart of this book: a collection of succinct individual profiles covering each of the herbs recommended in other parts of the book. It works as a reference databank for all other sections and contains the core information necessary for anyone wanting to learn the basics of herbalism. In The Herbal you will find comprehensive information for any herb which has been suggested as a possible remedy in other parts of the book.

INTRODUCING THE HERBAL

Herbs can be used freely and safely as part of one's lifestyle without thinking of them as 'medicines'. For specific health needs, their best use would be preventative – to prevent problems appearing. There are specific herbs which strengthen and tone specific organs and systems. These may be used where a tendency towards illness is recognized but no overt disease is present. By using herbs it may well be possible to overcome any weakness.

To find out which herb or herbs are recommended for a particular disease, refer first to the Therapeutic Index *(pages 46–8)* and then consult The Herbal for more information. Self-diagnosis is not advisable.

Consult a herbalist, if there is one available, or a doctor to ascertain the nature of your problems.

The normal dosage for an adult is given for each herb. For children under twelve this should be reduced by a quarter, and for children under seven by a half. For adults over 65 there should be a quarter reduction and a reduction to half the full dose for people over 70. These are very broad guidelines, and will be less important for a very large, strong person of 75 than for a small, frail person of 65.

There is usually little to fear in combining herbs with chemical drugs, but there are some important exceptions, so consult your doctor and an herbalist.

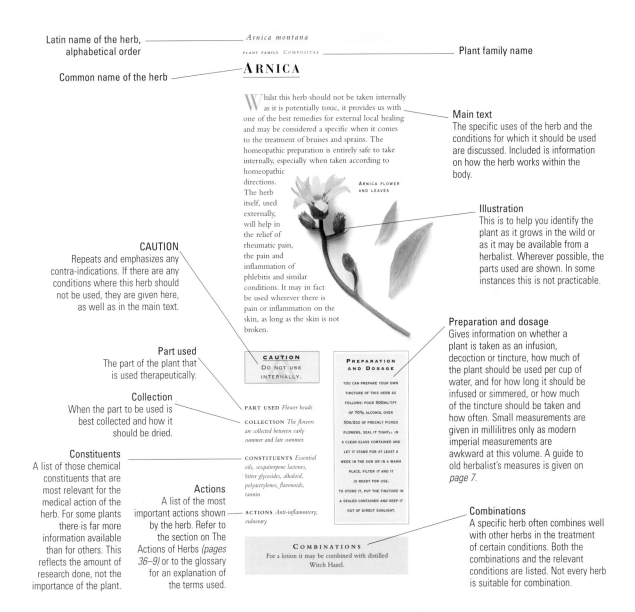

Latin name of the herb, alphabetical order — *Arnica montana*

PLANT FAMILY COMPOSITAE — Plant family name

Common name of the herb — **ARNICA**

Whilst this herb should not be taken internally as it is potentially toxic, it provides us with one of the best remedies for external local healing and may be considered a specific when it comes to the treatment of bruises and sprains. The homeopathic preparation is entirely safe to take internally, especially when taken according to homeopathic directions. The herb itself, used externally, will help in the relief of rheumatic pain, the pain and inflammation of phlebitis and similar conditions. It may in fact be used wherever there is pain or inflammation on the skin, as long as the skin is not broken.

ARNICA FLOWER AND LEAVES

Main text
The specific uses of the herb and the conditions for which it should be used are discussed. Included is information on how the herb works within the body.

Illustration
This is to help you identify the plant as it grows in the wild or as it may be available from a herbalist. Wherever possible, the parts used are shown. In some instances this is not practicable.

CAUTION
Repeats and emphasizes any contra-indications. If there are any conditions where this herb should not be used, they are given here, as well as in the main text.

CAUTION
DO NOT USE INTERNALLY.

Part used
The part of the plant that is used therapeutically.

PART USED *Flower heads*

Collection
When the part to be used is best collected and how it should be dried.

COLLECTION *The flowers are collected between early summer and late summer.*

Constituents
A list of those chemical constituents that are most relevant for the medical action of the herb. For some plants there is far more information available than for others. This reflects the amount of research done, not the importance of the plant.

CONSTITUENTS *Essential oils, sesquiterpene lactones, bitter glycosides, alkaloid, polyacetylenes, flavonoids, tannin*

Actions
A list of the most important actions shown by the herb. Refer to the section on The Actions of Herbs *(pages 36–9)* or to the glossary for an explanation of the terms used.

ACTIONS *Anti-inflammtory, vulnerary*

PREPARATION AND DOSAGE
YOU CAN PREPARE YOUR OWN TINCTURE OF THIS HERB AS FOLLOWS: POUR 500ML/1PT OF 70% ALCOHOL OVER 50G/2OZ OF FRESHLY PICKED FLOWERS. SEAL IT TIGHTLY IN A CLEAR GLASS CONTAINER AND LET IT STAND FOR AT LEAST A WEEK IN THE SUN OR IN A WARM PLACE. FILTER IT AND IT IS READY FOR USE. TO STORE IT, PUT THE TINCTURE IN A SEALED CONTAINER AND KEEP IT OUT OF DIRECT SUNLIGHT.

Preparation and dosage
Gives information on whether a plant is taken as an infusion, decoction or tincture, how much of the plant should be used per cup of water, and for how long it should be infused or simmered, or how much of the tincture should be taken and how often. Small measurements are given in millilitres only as modern imperial measurements are awkward at this volume. A guide to old herbalist's measures is given on *page 7.*

COMBINATIONS
For a lotion it may be combined with distilled Witch Hazel.

Combinations
A specific herb often combines well with other herbs in the treatment of certain conditions. Both the combinations and the relevant conditions are listed. Not every herb is suitable for combination.

Acacia catechu

PLANT FAMILY LEGUMINOSAE

BLACK CATECHU

Black Catechu is a powerful astringent used in chronic diarrhea, dysentery and mucous colitis. As a douche it is used in leucorrhea. As a mouthwash or gargle it is used in gingivitis, stomatitis, pharyngitis and laryngitis.

PART USED *Dried extract prepared from the heart-wood of the tree*

COLLECTION *The heart of the tree is collected after felling.*

CONSTITUENTS *20–35% Catechutannic acid, acacatechin, quercitin*

ACTIONS *Astringent, antiseptic*

PREPARATION AND DOSAGE

INFUSION

POUR A CUP OF BOILING WATER ONTO 1 TEASPOONFUL OF THE DRIED HERB AND LEAVE TO INFUSE FOR 10–15 MINUTES. THIS SHOULD BE DRUNK THREE TIMES A DAY.

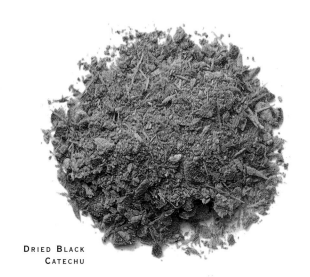

DRIED BLACK CATECHU

COMBINATIONS

In conditions of the colon it combines well with Calamus, Meadowsweet, Agrimony and Peppermint. As a mouthwash it combines well with Myrrh.

Achillea millefolium

PLANT FAMILY COMPOSITAE

YARROW

Yarrow is one of the best diaphoretic herbs and is a standard remedy for aiding the body to deal with fevers. It lowers blood pressure due to a dilation of the peripheral vessels. It stimulates the digestion and tones the blood vessels. As a urinary antiseptic it is indicated in infections such as cystitis. Used externally it will aid in the healing of wounds. It is considered to be a specific in thrombotic conditions associated with high blood pressure.

YARROW SHOOT, FLOWERS AND LEAVES

PART USED *Aerial parts*

COLLECTION *The whole of the plant above ground should be gathered when in flower between early summer and early Fall.*

CONSTITUENTS *Up to 0.5% volatile oil, flavonoids, tannins, a bitter alkaloid*

ACTIONS *Diaphoretic, hypotensive, astringent, diuretic, antiseptic, anti-catarrhal, emmenagogue, hepatic, stimulant, tonic*

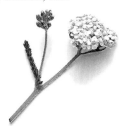

PREPARATION AND DOSAGE

INFUSION

POUR A CUP OF BOILING WATER ONTO 1–2 TEASPOONFULS OF THE DRIED HERB AND LEAVE TO INFUSE FOR 10–15 MINUTES. THIS SHOULD BE DRUNK HOT THREE TIMES A DAY. WHEN FEVERISH IT SHOULD BE DRUNK HOURLY.

TINCTURE

TAKE 2–4ML OF THE TINCTURE THREE TIMES A DAY.

COMBINATIONS

For fevers it will combine well with Elder Flower, Peppermint, Boneset, Cayenne and Ginger. For raised blood pressure it may be used with Hawthorn, Lime Blossom and Mistletoe.

Acorus calamus

PLANT FAMILY ARACEAE

CALAMUS

Calamus, or Sweet Flag, combines demulcent effects of the mucilage with the carminative effect of the volatile oil and the stimulating effect of the bitters. It is thus an excellent tonic for the whole gastro-intestinal tract. It may be used in dyspepsia of all kinds, in gastritis and gastric ulcers. It will stimulate a flagging appetite and help to ease exhaustion and weakness when there is a digestive involvement. It may be considered a specific in colic resulting from flatulence.

CALAMUS LEAVES
AND YOUNG RHIZOME

PART USED
Dried rhizome

COLLECTION *The rhizome should be harvested between early Fall and mid-Fall. A hook may be needed to extract it from muddy soil. Free the rhizome from leaves and root and clean it thoroughly. Halve it along its length and dry it in the shade.*

CONSTITUENTS *Mucilage, up to 3% volatile oil, bitter principles, glycoside, tannin*

ACTIONS *Carminative, demulcent, anti-spasmodic*

PREPARATION AND DOSAGE

INFUSION

POUR A CUP OF BOILING WATER ONTO 2 TEASPOONFULS OF THE DRIED HERB AND LEAVE TO INFUSE FOR 10–15 MINUTES. DRINK A CUP HALF AN HOUR BEFORE MEALS.

TINCTURE

TAKE 2–4ML OF THE TINCTURE THREE TIMES A DAY.

COMBINATIONS
In flatulent colic it combines well with Ginger and Wild Yam. In gastric conditions it is best combined with Meadowsweet and Marshmallow.

Aesculus hippocastanum

PLANT FAMILY HIPPOCASTANACEAE

HORSECHESTNUT

The unique actions of Horsechestnut are on the vessels of the circulatory system. It seems to increase the strength and tone of the veins in particular. It may be used internally to aid the body in the treatment of problems such as phlebitis, inflammation in the veins, varicosity and hemorrhoids. Externally it may be used as a lotion for the same conditions; it is also very effective for leg ulcers.

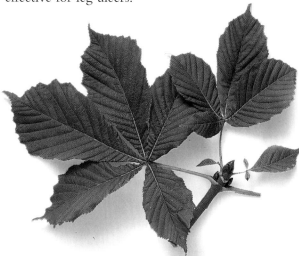

PART USED *Fruit, that is, the Horsechestnut itself*

HORSECHESTNUT
LEAVES

COLLECTION *The ripe chestnuts should be gathered as they fall from the trees in early Fall and mid-Fall.*

CONSTITUENTS *Saponins, tannin, flavones, starch, fatty oil, the glycosides, aesculin and fraxin*

ACTIONS *Astringent, circulatory tonic*

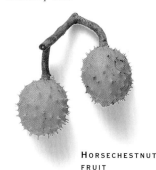

HORSECHESTNUT
FRUIT

PREPARATION AND DOSAGE

INFUSION

POUR A CUP OF BOILING WATER ONTO 1–2 TEASPOONFULS OF THE DRIED FRUIT AND LEAVE TO INFUSE FOR 10–15 MINUTES. THIS SHOULD BE DRUNK THREE TIMES A DAY OR USED AS A LOTION.

TINCTURE

TAKE 1–4ML OF THE TINCTURE THREE TIMES A DAY.

Agathosma betulina

PLANT FAMILY RUTACEAE

BUCHU

Buchu may be used in any infection of the genito-urinary system, such as cystitis, urethritis and prostatitis. Its healing and soothing properties indicate its use together with other relevant remedies in any condition of this system. It can be especially useful in painful and burning urination.

> ### PREPARATION AND DOSAGE
>
> #### INFUSION
>
> POUR A CUP OF BOILING WATER ONTO 1–2 TEASPOONFULS OF THE LEAVES AND LET INFUSE FOR 10 MINUTES. THIS SHOULD BE DRUNK THREE TIMES A DAY.
>
> #### TINCTURE
>
> TAKE 2–4ML OF THE TINCTURE THREE TIMES A DAY.

PART USED *Leaves*

COLLECTION *The leaves should be collected during the flowering and fruiting stage.*

CONSTITUENTS *Up to 2.5% volatile oils which contain diosphenol, limonene and methone*

ACTIONS *Diuretic, urinary antiseptic, anti-lithic, diaphoretic, tonic*

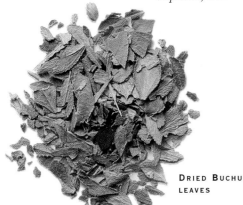

DRIED BUCHU LEAVES

COMBINATIONS

In cystitis it may be used with Yarrow or Couchgrass, in burning urination with Marshmallow or Corn Silk.

Agrimonia eupatoria

PLANT FAMILY ROSACEAE

AGRIMONY

The combination of astringency and bitter tonic properties makes Agrimony a valuable remedy, particularly when an astringent action on the digestive system is needed, as its tonic action is due to the bitter stimulation of digestive and liver secretions. It is a specific in childhood diarrhea. Its properties give it a role in the treatment of mucous colitis. Agrimony is the herb of choice in appendicitis. It may be used in indigestion. There is a long tradition of its use as a spring tonic. It may be used in urinary incontinence and cystitis. As a gargle it is beneficial in the relief of sore throats and laryngitis. As an ointment it will aid the healing of wounds and bruises.

AGRIMONY SHOOT, FLOWERS AND LEAVES

PART USED *Dried aerial parts*

COLLECTION *The whole of the plant above ground should be collected when the flowers are just blooming. It should be dried in the shade and not above 40°C/104°F.*

CONSTITUENTS *Tannins, glycosidal bitters, nicotinic acid, silicic acid, iron, vitamins B and K, essential oil*

ACTIONS *Astringent, tonic, diuretic, vulnerary, cholagogue, hepatic*

> ### PREPARATION AND DOSAGE
>
> #### INFUSION
>
> POUR A CUP OF BOILING WATER ONTO 1–2 TEASPOONFULS OF THE DRIED HERB AND LEAVE TO INFUSE FOR 10–15 MINUTES. THIS SHOULD BE DRUNK THREE TIMES A DAY.
>
> #### TINCTURE
>
> TAKE 1–3ML OF THE TINCTURE THREE TIMES A DAY.

COMBINATIONS

It is often used with carminatives for digestive problems.

Agropyron repens

PLANT FAMILY GRAMINACEAE

COUCHGRASS

Couchgrass may be used in urinary infections such as cystitis, urethritis and prostatitis. Its demulcent properties soothe irritation and inflammation. It is of value in the treatment of enlarged prostate glands. It may also be used in kidney stones and gravel. As a tonic diuretic, Couchgrass has been used with other herbs in the treatment of rheumatism.

PREPARATION AND DOSAGE

DECOCTION

PUT 2 TEASPOONFULS OF THE CUT RHIZOME IN A CUP OF WATER, BRING TO THE BOIL AND LET SIMMER FOR 10 MINUTES. THIS SHOULD BE DRUNK THREE TIMES A DAY.

TINCTURE

TAKE 3–6ML OF THE TINCTURE THREE TIMES A DAY.

PART USED *Rhizome*

COLLECTION *Unearth the rhizome in spring or early Fall. Wash carefully and dry in sun or shade.*

CONSTITUENTS *Triticin, mucilage, silicic acid, potassium, inositol, mannitol, glycoside, an anti-microbial substance*

ACTIONS *Diuretic, demulcent, anti-microbial, anti-lithic, tonic*

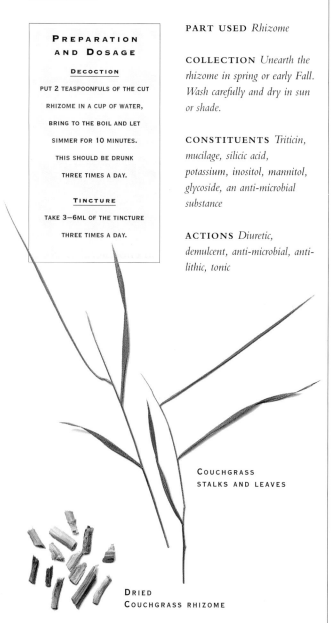

COUCHGRASS STALKS AND LEAVES

DRIED COUCHGRASS RHIZOME

COMBINATIONS

For cystitis, urethritis and prostatitis it may be used with Buchu, Bearberry or Yarrow. It can be combined with Hydrangea for prostate problems.

Alchemilla mollis

PLANT FAMILY ROSACEAE

LADY'S MANTLE

Lady's Mantle and other species of Alchemilla have been widely used in folk medicine throughout Europe. This plant will help reduce pains associated with periods as well as ameliorating excessive bleeding. It also has a role to play in easing the changes of the menopause. As an emmenagogue it stimulates the proper menstrual flow if there is any resistance. Its astringency provides it with a role in the treatment of diarrhea, as a mouthwash for sores and ulcers and as a gargle for laryngitis.

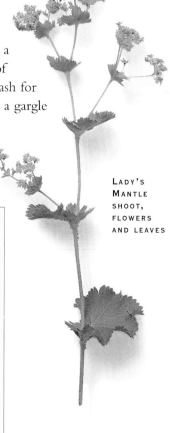

LADY'S MANTLE SHOOT, FLOWERS AND LEAVES

PREPARATION AND DOSAGE

INFUSION

POUR A CUP OF BOILING WATER ONTO 2 TEASPOONFULS OF THE DRIED HERB AND LEAVE TO INFUSE FOR 10–15 MINUTES. THIS SHOULD BE DRUNK THREE TIMES A DAY. TO HELP DIARRHEA AND AS A MOUTHWASH OR LOTION, A STRONGER DOSAGE IS MADE BY BOILING THE HERB FOR A FEW MINUTES TO EXTRACT ALL THE TANNIN.

TINCTURE

TAKE 2–4ML OF THE TINCTURE THREE TIMES A DAY.

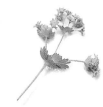

PART USED *Leaves and flowering shoots*

COLLECTION *The leaves and stems are collected between mid-summer and late summer.*

CONSTITUENTS *Tannin, bitter principle, traces of essential oil, salicylic acid*

ACTIONS *Astringent, diuretic, anti-inflammatory, emmenagogue, vulnerary*

Aletris farinosa

PLANT FAMILY LILIACEAE

TRUE UNICORN ROOT

This herb should not be confused with False Unicorn Root *(Chamaelirium luteum)*. It is an excellent remedy for sluggish digestion, which may give rise to dyspepsia, flatulence and debility. Its bitter nature will stimulate the digestive process and so it often relieves anorexia (appetite loss). Another name for True Unicorn Root is Colic Root, which shows its value in the treatment of digestive colic. As all these conditions often have a nervous involvement, this herb has been called a nervine. However, its benefit in anxiety is based on an easing of the physical aspects rather than on a direct relaxation of the nerves. It is reported to be of value in threatened miscarriage, but most herbalists prefer to use False Unicorn Root.

PART USED
Rhizome and root

COLLECTION *The underground parts are unearthed at the end of flowering in late summer, washed and cut into pieces and then dried.*

CONSTITUENTS
Bitter principle

ACTIONS *Bitter, anti-spasmodic, sedative, emmenagogue*

PREPARATION AND DOSAGE

DECOCTION

PUT ½–1 TEASPOONFUL OF THE ROOT IN A CUP OF WATER, BRING TO THE BOIL AND SIMMER FOR 10 MINUTES. THIS SHOULD BE DRUNK THREE TIMES A DAY.

INFUSION

POUR A CUP OF BOILING WATER ONTO 1–2 TEASPOONFULS OF THE DRIED HERB AND LEAVE TO INFUSE FOR 10–15 MINUTES. THIS SHOULD BE DRUNK THREE TIMES A DAY.

TINCTURE

1–2ML OF THE TINCTURE THREE TIMES A DAY.

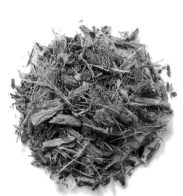

DRIED TRUE UNICORN ROOT

Allium sativum

PLANT FAMILY LILIACEAE

GARLIC

GARLIC BULB

Garlic is among the few herbs that have a universal usage and recognition. Its daily usage aids and supports the body in ways that no other herb does. It is one of the most effective anti-microbial plants available, acting on bacteria, viruses and alimentary parasites. The volatile oil is an effective agent and as it is largely excreted via the lungs, it is used in respiratory infections such as chronic bronchitis, catarrh, recurrent colds and influenza. It may be helpful in the treatment of whooping cough and as part of a broader approach to bronchitic asthma. It may be used as a preventative for most infectious conditions, digestive as well as respiratory. For the digestive tract Garlic will support the development of the natural bacterial flora whilst killing pathogenic organisms. In addition it will reduce blood pressure when taken over a period of time as well as reducing blood cholesterol levels. It has been used externally for the treatment of ringworm and threadworm.

PART USED *Bulb*

COLLECTION *The bulb with its numerous cloves should be unearthed when the leaves begin to wither in early Fall.*

CONSTITUENTS *Volatile oil, mucilage, glucokinins, germanium*

ACTIONS *Antiseptic, anti-microbial, diaphoretic, cholagogue, hypotensive, anti-spasmodic, alterative, anthelmintic, anti-catarrhal, carminative, expectorant, pectoral, rubefacient, stimulant, tonic, vulnerary*

PREPARATION AND DOSAGE

A CLOVE SHOULD BE EATEN THREE TIMES A DAY. IF THE SMELL BECOMES A PROBLEM, USE GARLIC OIL CAPSULES.
TAKE THREE ONCE A DAY AS A PROPHYLACTIC OR THREE TIMES A DAY WHEN AN INFECTION OCCURS.

GARLIC CLOVE

COMBINATIONS
For microbial infections it will combine well with Echinacea.

Aloe vera

PLANT FAMILY LILIACEAE

ALOE

Aloe may be used internally where a powerful cathartic is needed. In a small dosage it increases the menstrual flow. Externally the juice is used fresh for minor burns, sunburn, insect bites, etc.

CAUTION

AS ALOE STIMULATES UTERINE CONTRACTIONS, IT SHOULD BE AVOIDED DURING PREGNANCY. AS IT IS EXCRETED IN THE MOTHER'S MILK, IT SHOULD BE AVOIDED DURING BREASTFEEDING, OR IT MAY BE PURGATIVE TO THE CHILD.

PART USED *Solidified gel from the leaves*

COLLECTION *The liquid that drains from freshly cut leaves dries to a thick consistency.*

CONSTITUENTS *Aloins, anthraquinones, resin*

ACTIONS *Cathartic, vulnerary, emmenagogue, vermifuge, hepatic. External demulcent, vulnerary*

PREPARATION AND DOSAGE

FOR INTERNAL USE TAKE 0.1– 0.3G OF THE JUICE.

FOR EXTERNAL USE, PUT SOME OF THE FRESH JUICE ONTO THE AFFLICTED AREA.

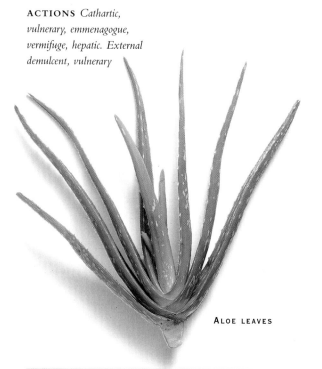

ALOE LEAVES

COMBINATIONS

If it is used internally to increase menstrual flow, it should be combined with carminatives to reduce griping.

Alpinia officinarum

PLANT FAMILY ZINGIBERACEAE

GALANGAL

Like many other valuable plants, Galangal is little used today. It provides us with a useful stimulating carminative that aids flatulence, dyspepsia and nausea, especially where due to a sluggish metabolism. It is reported to help in allaying sea-sickness. The reputed herbalist Mrs Grieve tells us that the Arabs 'use it to make their horses fiery'.

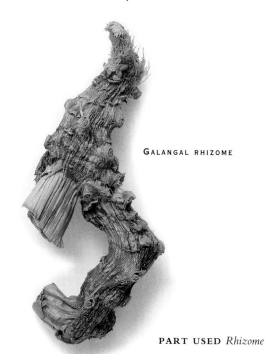

GALANGAL RHIZOME

PART USED *Rhizome*

COLLECTION *The herb is cultivated in China where the rhizomes are unearthed in late summer and early Fall, washed, cut into segments and dried.*

CONSTITUENTS *Volatile oil, acrid resin, galangol, kaempferol, galangin, alpinin*

ACTIONS *Stimulant, carminative*

PREPARATION AND DOSAGE

INFUSION

POUR A CUP OF BOILING WATER ONTO ½ TEASPOONFUL OF THE POWDERED RHIZOME AND LEAVE TO INFUSE FOR 10–15 MINUTES. THIS SHOULD BE DRUNK THREE TIMES A DAY.

TINCTURE

TAKE 1–2ML OF THE TINCTURE THREE TIMES A DAY.

Althaea officinalis

PLANT FAMILY MALVACEAE

MARSHMALLOW

The high mucilage content of Marshmallow makes it an excellent demulcent. The root is used primarily for digestive problems, inflammations of the digestive tract and on the skin, whilst the leaf is used for the lungs and the urinary system. For bronchitis, respiratory catarrh and irritating coughs consider Marshmallow Leaf. It is very soothing in urethritis and urinary gravel. Externally, the root is indicated in varicose veins and ulcers as well as abscesses and boils.

MARSHMALLOW LEAVES

PART USED
Root and leaf

COLLECTION *The leaves should be collected in summer after flowering and the root is unearthed in late Fall. It is cleaned of root fibres and cork and should be dried immediately.*

CONSTITUENTS *Root: 25–35% mucilage, tannins, pectin, asparagine Leaf: Mucilage, trace of an essential oil*

ACTIONS
Root: demulcent, diuretic, emollient, vulnerary Leaf: demulcent, expectorant, diuretic, emollient, anti-catarrhal, pectoral

---

PREPARATION AND DOSAGE

DECOCTION

PUT 1 TEASPOONFUL OF THE CHOPPED ROOT INTO A CUP OF WATER AND BOIL IT GENTLY FOR 10–15 MINUTES. THIS SHOULD BE DRUNK THREE TIMES A DAY.

INFUSION

POUR BOILING WATER ONTO 1–2 TEASPOONFULS OF THE DRIED LEAF AND LET INFUSE FOR 10 MINUTES. THIS SHOULD BE DRUNK THREE TIMES A DAY ALSO.

COMPRESS

A VALUABLE COMPRESS OR POULTICE CAN BE MADE FROM THIS HERB.

TINCTURE

TAKE 1–4ML OF THE TINCTURE THREE TIMES A DAY.

COMBINATIONS
In ulcerative conditions, internal or external, it may be used with Comfrey. For bronchitis use with Licorice and White Horehound. It is often mixed with Slippery Elm to make ointments.

Anethum graveolens

PLANT FAMILY UMBELLIFERAE

DILL

Dill is an excellent remedy for flatulence and the colic that is sometimes associated with it. This is the herb of choice in the colic of children. It will stimulate the flow of milk in nursing mothers. Chewing the seeds will clear up bad breath (halitosis).

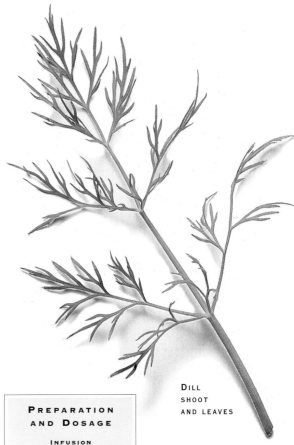

DILL SHOOT AND LEAVES

PREPARATION AND DOSAGE

INFUSION

POUR A CUP OF BOILING WATER ONTO 1–2 TEASPOONFULS OF THE GENTLY CRUSHED SEEDS AND LET INFUSE FOR 10–15 MINUTES. FOR THE TREATMENT OF FLATULENCE TAKE A CUP BEFORE MEALS.

TINCTURE

TAKE 1–2ML OF THE TINCTURE THREE TIMES A DAY.

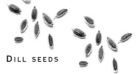

DILL SEEDS

PART USED *Seeds*

COLLECTION *The seeds should be collected when fully ripe, that is, when they have turned brown. Spread out to dry, but not in artificial heat.*

CONSTITUENTS
4% volatile oil which includes carvone and limonene

ACTIONS
Carminative, aromatic, anti-spasmodic, galactogogue, anti-emetic

Angelica archangelica

PLANT FAMILY UMBELLIFERAE

ANGELICA

This herb is a useful expectorant for coughs, bronchitis and pleurisy, especially when they are accompanied by fever, colds or influenza. The leaf can be used as a compress in inflammations of the chest. Its content of carminative essential oil explains its use in easing intestinal colic and flatulence. As a digestive agent it stimulates appetite and may be used in anorexia nervosa. It has been shown to help ease rheumatic inflammations. In cystitis it acts as a urinary antiseptic.

PART USED *Roots and leaves are used medicinally, the stem and seeds are used in confectionery*

COLLECTION *The root is collected in the Fall of its first year. If it is very thick it can be cut longitudinally to speed its drying. The leaves should be collected in early summer.*

CONSTITUENTS *Essential oils including phellandrene and pinene, angelica acid, coumarin compounds, bitter principle, tannin*

ACTIONS *Carminative, anti-spasmodic, expectorant, diuretic, diaphoretic, aromatic, pectoral, stimulant, tonic*

> ### PREPARATION AND DOSAGE
>
> #### DECOCTION
> PUT 1 TEASPOONFUL OF THE CUT ROOT IN A CUP OF WATER, BRING TO THE BOIL AND SIMMER FOR 2 MINUTES. TAKE IT OFF THE HEAT AND LET IT STAND FOR 15 MINUTES. TAKE ONE CUP THREE TIMES A DAY.
>
> #### TINCTURE
> TAKE 2–5ML OF THE TINCTURE THREE TIMES A DAY.

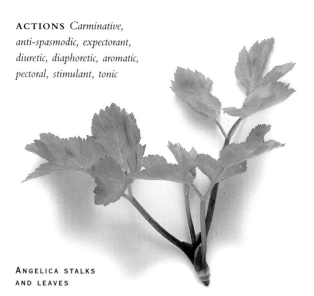

ANGELICA STALKS AND LEAVES

> ### COMBINATIONS
> For bronchial problems it combines well with Coltsfoot and White Horehound; for indigestion, flatulence and loss of appetite with Chamomile.

Aphanes arvensis

PLANT FAMILY ROSACEAE

PARSLEY PIERT

This delicate little plant is commonly used for the removal of kidney and urinary stones and gravel. Through its potent diuretic action associated with soothing demulcence of the urinary tract it will help in all cases of painful urination. It may be used where there is water retention, especially where this is due to kidney or liver problems.

DRIED PARSLEY PIERT

PART USED *Aerial parts*

COLLECTION *It should be collected in summer when in flower.*

CONSTITUENTS *Tannins*

ACTIONS *Diuretic, demulcent, anti-lithic*

> ### PREPARATION AND DOSAGE
>
> #### INFUSION
> POUR A CUP OF BOILING WATER ONTO 1–2 TEASPOONFULS OF THE DRIED HERB AND LEAVE TO INFUSE FOR 10–15 MINUTES. THIS SHOULD BE DRUNK THREE TIMES A DAY.
>
> #### TINCTURE
> TAKE 2–4ML OF THE TINCTURE THREE TIMES A DAY.

> ### COMBINATIONS
> It will combine well with Pellitory of the Wall or Buchu in cases of kidney stones or gravel.

Apium graveolens

PLANT FAMILY UMBELLIFERAE

CELERY

Celery Seeds find their main use in the treatment of rheumatism, arthritis and gout. They are especially useful in rheumatoid arthritis where there is an associated mental depression. Their diuretic action is obviously involved in rheumatic conditions, but they are also used as a urinary antiseptic, largely because of the volatile oil apiol.

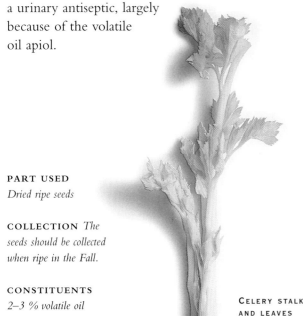

PART USED
Dried ripe seeds

COLLECTION *The seeds should be collected when ripe in the Fall.*

CONSTITUENTS
2–3 % volatile oil

CELERY STALK
AND LEAVES

ACTIONS *Anti-rheumatic, diuretic, carminative, sedative, aromatic*

PREPARATION AND DOSAGE

INFUSION

POUR A CUP OF BOILING WATER ONTO 1–2 TEASPOONFULS OF FRESHLY CRUSHED SEEDS. LEAVE TO INFUSE FOR 10–15 MINUTES. THIS SHOULD BE DRUNK THREE TIMES A DAY.

TINCTURE

TAKE 2–4ML OF THE TINCTURE THREE TIMES A DAY.

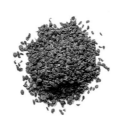

CELERY SEEDS

COMBINATIONS

In rheumatic conditions the seeds combine well with Bogbean. They appear to work better in combination with Dandelion.

Arctium lappa

PLANT FAMILY COMPOSITAE

BURDOCK

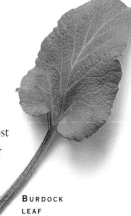

BURDOCK
LEAF

Burdock is a most valuable remedy for the treatment of skin conditions which result in dry and scaly skin. It may be most effective for psoriasis if used over a long period of time. Similarly, all types of eczema (though primarily the dry kinds) may be treated effectively if Burdock is used over a period of time. It will be useful as part of a wider treatment for rheumatic complaints, especially where they are associated with psoriasis. Part of the action of this herb is through the bitter stimulation of the digestive juices and especially of bile secretion. Thus it will aid digestion and appetite. It has been used in anorexia nervosa to aid kidney function and to heal cystitis. In general, Burdock will move the body to a state of health, removing such indicators of systemic imbalance as skin problems and dandruff. Externally it may be used as a compress or poultice to speed up the healing of wounds and ulcers. Eczema and psoriasis may also be treated this way externally, but such skin problems can only be healed by internal remedies.

PREPARATION AND DOSAGE

DECOCTION

PUT 1 TEASPOONFUL OF THE ROOT INTO A CUP OF WATER, BRING TO THE BOIL AND SIMMER FOR 10–15 MINUTES. THIS SHOULD BE DRUNK THREE TIMES A DAY. FOR EXTERNAL USE SEE FURTHER INFORMATION IN THE CHAPTER ON THE SKIN.

TINCTURE

TAKE 2–4ML OF THE TINCTURE THREE TIMES A DAY.

PART USED
Roots and rhizome

COLLECTION *The roots and rhizome should be unearthed in early Fall or mid-Fall.*

CONSTITUENTS *Flavonoid glycosides, bitter glycosides, alkaloid, anti-microbial substance, inulin*

ACTIONS *Alterative, diuretic, bitter, laxative, tonic, vulnerary*

COMBINATIONS

For skin problems, combine with Yellow Dock, Red Clover or Cleavers.

Arctostaphylos uva-ursi

PLANT FAMILY ERICACEAE

BEARBERRY

Bearberry has a specific antiseptic and astringent effect upon the membranes of the urinary system. It will generally soothe, tone and strengthen them. It is specifically used where there is gravel or ulceration in the kidney or bladder. It may be used in the treatment of infections such as pyelitis and cystitis or as part of a holistic approach to more chronic kidney problems. It has a useful role to play in the treatment of gravel or a calculus in the kidney. With its high astringency it is used in some forms of bed-wetting. As a douche it may be helpful in vaginal ulceration and infection.

BEARBERRY
SHOOTS AND LEAVES

PREPARATION AND DOSAGE

INFUSION

POUR A CUP OF BOILING WATER
ONTO 1–2 TEASPOONFULS OF
THE DRIED LEAVES AND LET
INFUSE FOR 10–15 MINUTES.
THIS SHOULD BE DRUNK
THREE TIMES A DAY.

TINCTURE

TAKE 2–4ML OF THE TINCTURE
THREE TIMES A DAY.

PART USED *Leaves*

COLLECTION *Leaves may be collected throughout the year, but preferably in spring and summer.*

CONSTITUENTS *Glycosides, including arbutin and ericolin. 6% tannin, flavonoids and resin*

ACTIONS *Diuretic, astringent, demulcent, anti-catarrhal, anti-lithic, anti-microbial, tonic*

COMBINATIONS
Bearberry may be combined with Couchgrass and Yarrow for urinary infections.

Aristolochia serpentaria

PLANT FAMILY ARISTOLOCHIACEAE

VIRGINIA SNAKEROOT

At one time Virginia Snakeroot was considered one of the most important herbs to come to Europe from America, though today it is not widely used. Its name comes from its use in aiding the body to combat nettle rash, poison ivy and some snake bites. This apparent anti-inflammatory action goes some way to explain its use in the treatment of rheumatism and gout. Its main use has been in the treatment of dyspepsia, nausea, colic pains and similar digestive problems. It will stimulate the digestive system and aid its functions.

PREPARATION AND DOSAGE

INFUSION

POUR A CUP OF BOILING WATER
ONTO 1 TEASPOONFUL OF THE
POWDERED ROOT AND LEAVE TO
INFUSE FOR 10–15 MINUTES.
THIS SHOULD BE DRUNK
THREE TIMES A DAY.

TINCTURE

TAKE 1–2ML OF THE TINCTURE
THREE TIMES A DAY.

PART USED
Rhizome and root

COLLECTION *The underground parts are unearthed in the Fall from woodlands throughout the eastern areas of North America.*

CONSTITUENTS *Aristolochid acid, essential oil, tannin, bitter principle*

ACTIONS *Stimulant, digestive, tonic, diaphoretic*

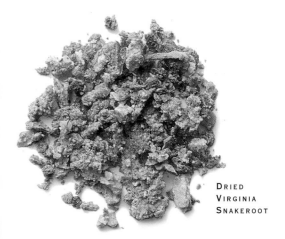

DRIED
VIRGINIA
SNAKEROOT

Armoracia rusticana

PLANT FAMILY CRUCIFERAE

HORSERADISH

Horseradish is an old household remedy useful wherever a stimulating herb is called for. It can be used in influenza and fevers as a rough equivalent to Cayenne Pepper. It stimulates the digestive process whilst easing wind and griping pains. It has been used in cases of urinary infection. Externally it has a stimulating action similar to Mustard Seed. It can be used for rheumatism and as a poultice in bronchitis.

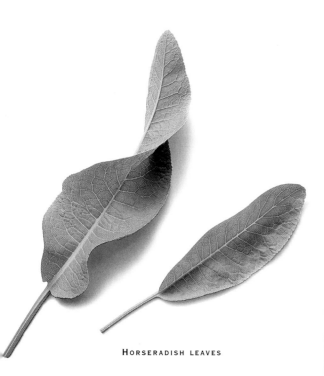

HORSERADISH LEAVES

PART USED *Tap root*

COLLECTION *The roots are collected in the winter and stored in sand.*

CONSTITUENTS *Essential oil that contains mustard oil glycosides; sinigrin*

ACTIONS *Stimulant, carminative, rubefacient, mild laxative, diuretic, hepatic*

PREPARATION AND DOSAGE

THE FRESH ROOT IS OFTEN USED AS A VEGETABLE.

INFUSION

POUR A CUP OF BOILING WATER ONTO 1 TEASPOONFUL OF THE POWDERED OR CHOPPED ROOT. LEAVE TO INFUSE FOR 5 MINUTES. THIS SHOULD BE DRUNK THREE TIMES A DAY OR MORE OFTEN WHEN BEING USED TO TREAT INFLUENZA OR FEVERS.

Arnica montana

PLANT FAMILY COMPOSITAE

ARNICA

Whilst this herb should not be taken internally as it is potentially toxic, it provides us with one of the best remedies for external local healing and may be considered a specific when it comes to the treatment of bruises and sprains. The homeopathic preparation is entirely safe to take internally, especially when taken according to homeopathic directions. The herb itself, used externally, will help in the relief of rheumatic pain, the pain and inflammation of phlebitis and similar conditions. It may in fact be used wherever there is pain or inflammation on the skin, as long as the skin is not broken.

ARNICA FLOWER AND LEAVES

CAUTION
DO NOT USE INTERNALLY.

PART USED *Flower heads*

COLLECTION *The flowers are collected between early summer and late summer.*

CONSTITUENTS *Essential oils, sesquiterpene lactones, bitter glycosides, alkaloid, polyacetylenes, flavonoids, tannin*

ACTIONS *Anti-inflammtory, vulnerary*

PREPARATION AND DOSAGE

YOU CAN PREPARE YOUR OWN TINCTURE OF THIS HERB AS FOLLOWS: POUR 500ML/1PT OF 70% ALCOHOL OVER 50G/2OZ OF FRESHLY PICKED FLOWERS. SEAL IT TIGHTLY IN A CLEAR GLASS CONTAINER AND LET IT STAND FOR AT LEAST A WEEK IN THE SUN OR IN A WARM PLACE. FILTER IT AND IT IS READY FOR USE. TO STORE IT, PUT THE TINCTURE IN A SEALED CONTAINER AND KEEP IT OUT OF DIRECT SUNLIGHT.

COMBINATIONS
For a lotion it may be combined with distilled Witch Hazel.

Artemisia abrotanum

PLANT FAMILY COMPOSITAE

SOUTHERNWOOD

Whilst having the general tonic action of bitters, Southernwood finds most use in aiding menstrual flow. It will act to initiate delayed menstruation (which has given rise to some sexist names for the plant, such as Lad's Love). Its bitter stimulation will also help in removing threadworm in children.

PART USED *Aerial parts*

COLLECTION *It is best collected in late summer and early Fall, ideally with flowering tops, though it rarely flowers in Britain. Dry it with care and ensure that not too much of the volatile oil is lost.*

CONSTITUENTS
Volatile oil

ACTIONS *Bitter, emmenagogue, anthelmintic, antimicrobial, stimulant*

PREPARATION AND DOSAGE

INFUSION

POUR A CUP OF BOILING WATER ONTO 1–2 TEASPOONFULS OF THE DRIED HERB AND LEAVE TO INFUSE FOR 10–15 MINUTES IN A CLOSED CONTAINER. THIS SHOULD BE DRUNK THREE TIMES A DAY. MRS GRIEVE RECOMMENDS A TEASPOONFUL OF THE POWDERED HERB IN TREACLE (YOU COULD USE HONEY) MORNING AND EVENING FOR WORMS IN CHILDREN.

TINCTURE

TAKE 1–4ML OF THE TINCTURE THREE TIMES A DAY.

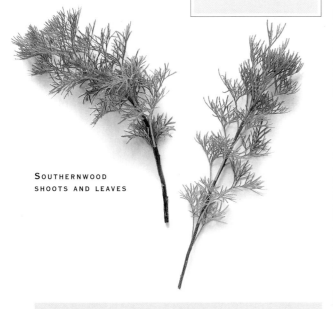

SOUTHERNWOOD
SHOOTS AND LEAVES

COMBINATIONS
Southernwood combines well with False Unicorn Root for delayed menstruation.

Artemisia absinthum

PLANT FAMILY COMPOSITAE

WORMWOOD

WORMWOOD
STALK AND
LEAVES

Traditionally, Wormwood has been used in a wide range of conditions, most of which have been vindicated by analysis of the herb. It is primarily used as a bitter and therefore has the effect of stimulating and invigorating the whole of the digestive process. It may be used where there is indigestion, especially when due to a deficient quantity or quality of gastric juice. It is a powerful remedy in the treatment of worm infestations, especially roundworm and pinworm. It may also be used to help the body deal with fever and infections. Due to the general tonic action it will be of benefit in many diverse conditions because it benefits the body in general.

PREPARATION AND DOSAGE

INFUSION

POUR A CUP OF BOILING WATER ONTO 1–2 TEASPOONFULS OF THE DRIED HERB AND LEAVE TO INFUSE FOR 10–15 MINUTES. THIS SHOULD BE DRUNK THREE TIMES A DAY.

PILL

THE POWDERED HERB MAY BE USED IN PILL FORM TO GET RID OF WORMS, THUS AVOIDING THE EXTREME, BITTER TASTE.

TINCTURE

TAKE 1–4ML OF THE TINCTURE THREE TIMES A DAY.

PART USED *Leaves or flowering tops*

COLLECTION *The leaves and flowering tops are gathered at the end of the flowering period between mid-summer and early Fall.*

CONSTITUENTS *Rich in essential oils including absinthol, thujyl, isovaleric acid; bitter sesquiterpenes, flavonoid glycosides*

ACTIONS *Bitter tonic, carminative, anthelmintic, anti-inflammatory, anti-bilious, anti-microbial, emmenagogue, hepatic, stimulant*

Artemisia cina

PLANT FAMILY COMPOSITAE

SANTONICA

Santonica, or Wormseed, is one of the oldest worm remedies recorded. It proves most effective against roundworm and to a lesser extent threadworm. However, it will do nothing against tapeworm. Due to the potency and to a low-level toxicity of santonin, this herb should only be used under medical supervision.

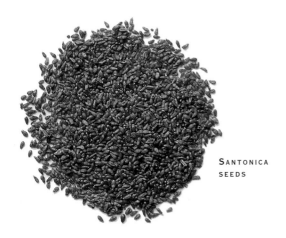

SANTONICA
SEEDS

PART USED *Seeds*

COLLECTION *The seeds are collected in the Fall in areas where they grow, including most of Asia.*

CONSTITUENTS *Santonin, volatile oil, artemisin*

ACTIONS *Anthelmintic*

CAUTION
ONLY USE
SANTONICA
UNDER MEDICAL
SUPERVISION.

PREPARATION
AND DOSAGE
SELF-PRESCRIPTION IS NOT
RECOMMENDED FOR THIS HERB.
CONSULT A QUALIFIED
PRACTITIONER TO PRESCRIBE
AND MAKE UP THE REMEDY.

Artemisia vulgaris

PLANT FAMILY COMPOSITAE

MUGWORT

Mugwort can be used wherever a digestive stimulant is called for. It will aid the digestion through the bitter stimulation of the juices whilst also providing a carminative oil. It has a mildly nervine action in aiding depression and easing tension, which appears to be due to the volatile oil, so it is essential that this is not lost in preparation. Mugwort may also be used as an emmenagogue in the aiding of normal menstrual flow.

PREPARATION
AND DOSAGE

INFUSION
POUR A CUP OF BOILING WATER
ONTO 1–2 TEASPOONFULS OF THE
DRIED HERB AND LEAVE TO INFUSE
FOR 10–15 MINUTES IN A
COVERED CONTAINER. THIS
SHOULD BE DRUNK THREE TIMES A
DAY. MUGWORT IS USED AS A
FLAVOURING IN A NUMBER OF
APERITIF DRINKS, A PLEASANT WAY
TO TAKE IT!

TINCTURE
TAKE 1–4ML OF THE TINCTURE
THREE TIMES A DAY.

PART USED
Leaves or root

COLLECTION *The leaves and flowering stalks should be gathered just at blossoming time, which is between mid-summer and early Fall.*

CONSTITUENTS *Volatile oil containing cineole and thujone; a bitter principle, tannin, resin, inulin*

ACTIONS *Bitter tonic, stimulant, nervine tonic, emmenagogue, anti-bilious*

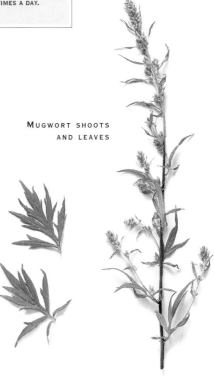

MUGWORT SHOOTS
AND LEAVES

Asclepias tuberosa

PLANT FAMILY ASCLEPIADACEAE

PLEURISY ROOT

Pleurisy Root is effective against respiratory infections, where it reduces inflammations and assists expectoration. It can be used in the treatment of bronchitis and other chest conditions. The addition of diaphoretic and anti-spasmodic powers will show why it is so highly valued in the treatment of pleurisy and pneumonia. It can be used in influenza.

PLEURISY ROOT
LEAVES AND FLOWERS

PART USED *Rhizome*

COLLECTION *The rhizome should be unearthed in early spring or mid-spring. Clean well and split up. Dry in shade or sun.*

CONSTITUENTS *Glycosides including asclepiadin and possibly cardio-active glycosides; essential oil*

ACTIONS *Diaphoretic, expectorant, anti-spasmodic, carminative, pectoral*

PREPARATION AND DOSAGE

INFUSION

POUR A CUP OF BOILING WATER ONTO ½–1 TEASPOONFUL OF THE HERB AND LET INFUSE FOR 10–15 MINUTES. THIS SHOULD BE DRUNK THREE TIMES A DAY.

TINCTURE

TAKE 1–2ML OF THE TINCTURE THREE TIMES A DAY.

COMBINATIONS
It will combine well with Cayenne, Lobelia and Grindelia in the treatment of respiratory congestion.

Avena sativa

PLANT FAMILY GRAMINEAE

OATS

Oats provide one of the best remedies for 'feeding' the nervous system, especially when under stress. The oat remedy is considered a specific in cases of nervous debility and exhaustion when associated with depression. It may be used with most of the other nervines, both relaxant and stimulatory, to strengthen the whole of the nervous system. It is also used in general debility. The high levels of silicic acid in the straw will explain its use as a remedy for skin conditions, especially in external applications.

PREPARATION AND DOSAGE

OATS MAY MOST CONVENIENTLY BE TAKEN IN THE FORM OF PORRIDGE OR OATMEAL.

FLUID EXTRACT

IN LIQUID FORM IT IS MOST OFTEN GIVEN AS A FLUID EXTRACT. TAKE 3–5ML THREE TIMES A DAY.

BATH

A SOOTHING BATH FOR USE IN NEURALGIA AND IRRITATED SKIN CONDITIONS CAN BE MADE: 450G/1LB OF SHREDDED STRAW IS BOILED IN 2L/4PT OF WATER FOR HALF AN HOUR. THE LIQUID IS STRAINED AND ADDED TO THE BATH.

PART USED *Seeds and whole plant*

COLLECTION *The seeds and straw are gathered in late summer at harvest time. The stalks are cut and bound together. Leave them upright to dry and then thresh out the fruit. The straw is just the crushed dry stalks.*

CONSTITUENTS *Seeds: 50% starch, alkaloids including trigonelline and avenine; saponins, flavones, sterols, vitamin B Plant straw: Rich in silicic acid; mucin, calcium*

ACTIONS *Nervine tonic, anti-depressant, nutritive, demulcent, vulnerary*

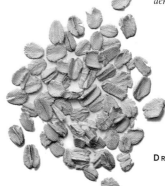

DRIED OATS

COMBINATIONS
For depression it may be used with Skullcap and Lady's Slipper.

Ballota nigra

PLANT FAMILY LABIATAE

BLACK HOREHOUND

Black Horehound – which should not be confused with White Horehound – is an excellent remedy for the settling of nausea and vomiting where the cause lies within the nervous system rather than in the stomach. It may be used with safety in motion sickness, for example, where the nausea is triggered through the inner ear and the central nervous system. This herb will also be of value in helping the vomiting of pregnancy, or nausea and vomiting due to nervousness. This remedy has a reputation as a normalizer of menstrual function and also as a mild expectorant.

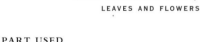

BLACK HOREHOUND SHOOT,
LEAVES AND FLOWERS

PART USED
Dried aerial parts

COLLECTION *The herb should be gathered just as it begins to bloom in mid-summer.*

CONSTITUENTS
Flavonoids

ACTIONS *Anti-emetic, sedative, mild astringent, emmenagogue, expectorant*

PREPARATION AND DOSAGE

INFUSION

POUR A CUP OF BOILING WATER ONTO 1–2 TEASPOONFULS OF THE DRIED HERBS AND LEAVE TO INFUSE FOR 10–15 MINUTES. THIS SHOULD BE DRUNK THREE TIMES A DAY OR AS NEEDED.

TINCTURE

TAKE 1–2ML OF THE TINCTURE THREE TIMES A DAY.

COMBINATIONS

For the relief of nausea and vomiting it may be combined with Meadowsweet and Chamomile.

Baptisia tinctoria

PLANT FAMILY LEGUMINOSAE

WILD INDIGO

Wild Indigo is a herb to be considered wherever there is a focused infection. It is especially useful in the treatment of infections of the nose and sinus. Taken both internally and as a mouthwash it will heal mouth ulcers, gingivitis and help in the control of pyorrhea. Systemically it may be helpful in the treatment of enlarged and inflamed lymph glands (lymphadenitis) and also to reduce fevers. Externally an ointment will help infected ulcers and ease sore nipples. A douche of the decoction will help leucorrhea.

PREPARATION AND DOSAGE

DECOCTION

PUT ½–1 TEASPOONFUL OF THE ROOT IN A CUP OF WATER, BRING TO THE BOIL AND SIMMER FOR 10–15 MINUTES. THIS SHOULD BE DRUNK THREE TIMES A DAY.

TINCTURE

TAKE 1–2ML OF THE TINCTURE THREE TIMES A DAY.

PART USED *Root*

COLLECTION *The root is unearthed in the Fall after flowering has stopped. Clean the root and cut; dry well.*

CONSTITUENTS
Alkaloids, glycosides, oleo-resin

ACTIONS *Anti-microbial, anti-catarrhal, febrifuge, alterative, hepatic*

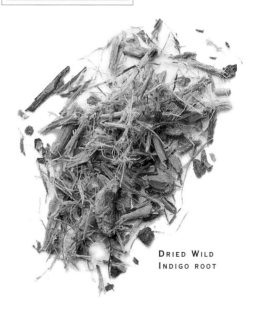

DRIED WILD
INDIGO ROOT

COMBINATIONS

For the treatment of infections it may be used with Echinacea and Myrrh. For lymphatic problems it can be combined with Cleavers and Poke Root.

Bellis perennis

PLANT FAMILY COMPOSITAE

DAISY

Daisy, one of our most common plants, is useful for coughs and catarrh. For all conditions that manifest in these forms, Daisy may be used freely and safely. It has a reputation of value in arthritis and rheumatism as well as in liver and kidney problems. Due to its astringency it is also useful for diarrhea.

PART USED *Fresh or dried flower heads*

COLLECTION *The flowers may be picked between early spring and mid-Fall.*

CONSTITUENTS *Saponins, tannin, essential oil, flavones, bitter principle, mucilage*

ACTIONS *Expectorant, astringent, vulnerary*

PREPARATION AND DOSAGE

INFUSION

POUR A CUP OF BOILING WATER ONTO 1 TEASPOONFUL OF THE DRIED HERB AND LEAVE TO INFUSE FOR 10 MINUTES. THIS SHOULD BE DRUNK THREE OR FOUR TIMES A DAY.

TINCTURE

TAKE 2–4ML OF THE TINCTURE THREE TIMES A DAY.

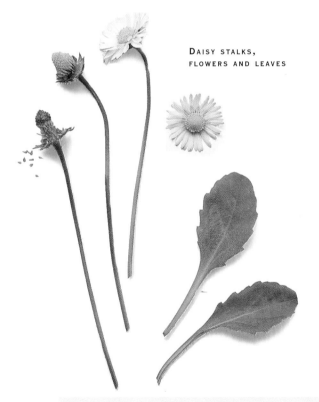

DAISY STALKS, FLOWERS AND LEAVES

COMBINATIONS
For respiratory catarrh it may be used with Golden Rod or Coltsfoot.

Berberis vulgaris

PLANT FAMILY BERBERIDACEAE

BARBERRY

Barberry is one of the best remedies for correcting liver function and promoting the flow of bile. It is indicated when there is an inflammation of the gall-bladder or in the presence of gallstones. When jaundice occurs due to a congested state of the liver, Barberry is also indicated. As a bitter tonic with mild laxative effects, it is used with weak or debilitated people to strengthen and cleanse the system. An interesting action is its ability to reduce an enlarged spleen. It acts against malaria and is also effective in the treatment of protozoal infection due to *Leishmania* spp.

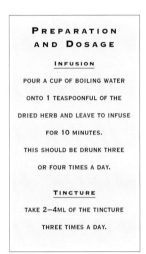

BARBERRY SHOOT AND LEAVES

CAUTION

AVOID DURING PREGNANCY.

PREPARATION AND DOSAGE

DECOCTION

PUT 1 TEASPOONFUL OF THE BARK INTO A CUP OF COLD WATER AND BRING TO THE BOIL. LEAVE FOR 10–15 MINUTES. THIS SHOULD BE DRUNK THREE TIMES A DAY.

TINCTURE

TAKE 2–4ML OF THE TINCTURE THREE TIMES A DAY.

PART USED
Bark of root or stem

COLLECTION *The roots should be unearthed in early spring or late Fall and the stem bark should be collected at the same time. Pare off the bark from root and stem and dry in the shade.*

CONSTITUENTS *Alkaloids, including berberine, oxyancanthine, chelidonic acid and tannins*

ACTIONS *Cholagogue, anti-emetic, bitter tonic, laxative, anti-bilious, hepatic*

COMBINATIONS
In gall-bladder disease it combines well with Fringetree Bark and Black Root.

Betula pendula

PLANT FAMILY BETULACEAE

SILVER BIRCH

Birch leaves act as an effective remedy for cystitis and other infections of the urinary system as well as removing excess water from the body. Perhaps because of this cleansing diuretic activity, the plant has been used for gout, rheumatism and mild arthritic pain. The bark will ease muscle pain if it is applied externally, putting the fresh, wet internal side of the bark against the skin.

PART USED
Young leaves and bark

COLLECTION *The leaves are collected in late spring or summer. When collecting the bark, it is important not to ring-bark the tree – in other words, do not take off the bark all around the circumference; otherwise the tree will die.*

CONSTITUENTS *Tannins, saponins, bitters, glycosides, essential oil, flavonoids*

ACTIONS *Diuretic, antiseptic, tonic*

> ### PREPARATION AND DOSAGE
>
> #### INFUSION
> POUR A CUP OF BOILING WATER ONTO 1–2 TEASPOONFULS OF THE DRIED LEAVES AND LET INFUSE FOR 10 MINUTES. THIS SHOULD BE DRUNK THREE TIMES A DAY.
>
> #### TINCTURE
> TAKE 1–2ML OF THE TINCTURE THREE TIMES A DAY.

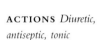

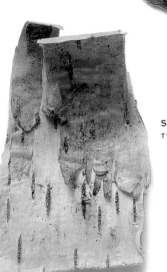

SILVER BIRCH BARK, TWIG AND LEAVES

COMBINATIONS
For urinary infections it may be used with Bearberry, whilst for rheumatic pain it combines well with Black Willow.

Bidens tripartita

PLANT FAMILY COMPOSITAE

BURR-MARIGOLD

Though little used today, Burr-Marigold has a reputation as a valuable astringent used for hemorrhage wherever it occurs. It may be used for fevers and water retention when this is due to a problem in the kidneys. When the dried herb is burnt, the flower heads give off a cedar-like smell that will act as an anti-insect incense.

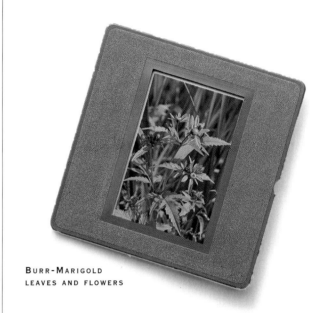

BURR-MARIGOLD LEAVES AND FLOWERS

> ### PREPARATION AND DOSAGE
>
> #### INFUSION
> POUR A CUP OF BOILING WATER ONTO 1–2 TEASPOONFULS OF THE DRIED HERB AND LEAVE TO INFUSE FOR 5–10 MINUTES. THIS SHOULD BE DRUNK THREE TIMES A DAY.
>
> #### TINCTURE
> TAKE 1–2ML OF THE TINCTURE THREE TIMES A DAY.

PART USED *Aerial parts*

COLLECTION *The whole of the plant above ground should be collected when in flower between mid-summer and early Fall.*

CONSTITUENTS *Flavonoids, xanthophyls, sterols, tannins*

ACTIONS *Astringent, diaphoretic, diuretic*

Borago officinalis

PLANT FAMILY BORAGINACEAE

BORAGE

Borage acts as a restorative agent on the adrenal cortex, which means that it will revive and renew the adrenal glands after a medical treatment with cortisone or steroids. There is a growing need for remedies that will aid this gland with the stress it is exposed to, both externally and internally. Borage may be used as a tonic for the adrenals over a period of time. It may be used during fevers and especially during convalescence. It has a reputation as an anti-inflammatory herb used in conditions such as pleurisy. The leaves and seeds stimulate the flow of milk in nursing mothers.

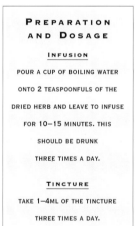

PART USED *Dried leaves*

COLLECTION *The leaves should be gathered when the plant is coming into flower in the early summer. Strip each leaf off singly and reject any that are marked in any way. Do not collect when wet with rain or dew.*

CONSTITUENTS *Saponins, mucilage, tannins, essential oil*

ACTIONS *Diaphoretic, expectorant, tonic, anti-inflammatory, galactogogue, diuretic, emollient*

> ### PREPARATION AND DOSAGE
>
> #### INFUSION
> POUR A CUP OF BOILING WATER ONTO 2 TEASPOONFULS OF THE DRIED HERB AND LEAVE TO INFUSE FOR 10–15 MINUTES. THIS SHOULD BE DRUNK THREE TIMES A DAY.
>
> #### TINCTURE
> TAKE 1–4ML OF THE TINCTURE THREE TIMES A DAY.

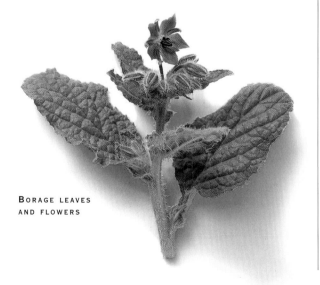

BORAGE LEAVES AND FLOWERS

Brassica nigra

PLANT FAMILY CRUCIFERAE

BLACK MUSTARD

This well-known spice has its main use in medicine as a stimulating external application. The rubefacient action causes a mild irritant to the skin, stimulating the circulation to that area and relieving muscular and skeletal pain. Its stimulating, diaphoretic action can be utilized in the way that Cayenne and Ginger are. For feverishness, colds and influenza, Black Mustard may be taken as a tea, or ground and sprinkled into a bath. The stimulation of circulation will aid chilblains as well as the conditions already mentioned. An infusion or poultice of Black Mustard will aid in cases of bronchitis.

> ### PREPARATION AND DOSAGE
>
> #### POULTICE
> MUSTARD IS MOST COMMONLY USED AS A POULTICE, WHICH CAN BE MADE BY MIXING 120G/4OZ OF FRESHLY GROUND BLACK MUSTARD SEEDS WITH WARM WATER (AT ABOUT 45°C/113°F) TO FORM A THICK PASTE. THIS IS SPREAD ON A PIECE OF CLOTH THE SIZE OF THE BODY AREA THAT IS TO BE COVERED. TO STOP THE PASTE STICKING TO THE SKIN, LAY A DAMPENED GAUZE ON THE SKIN. APPLY THE CLOTH AND REMOVE AFTER 1 MINUTE. THE SKIN MAY BE REDDENED BY THIS TREATMENT, WHICH CAN BE EASED BY APPLYING OLIVE OIL AFTERWARDS.
>
> #### INFUSION
> POUR A CUP OF BOILING WATER ONTO 1 TEASPOONFUL OF MUSTARD FLOUR AND LEAVE TO INFUSE FOR 5 MINUTES. THIS MAY BE DRUNK THREE TIMES A DAY.
>
> #### FOOTBATH
> MAKE AN INFUSION USING 1 TABLESPOON OF BRUISED SEEDS TO 1L/2PT OF BOILING WATER.

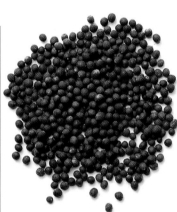

DRIED BLACK MUSTARD SEEDS

PART USED *Seeds*

COLLECTION *The ripe seed pods are collected in the late summer. Tap the seeds out and dry in a thin layer.*

CONSTITUENTS *Mucilage, fixed oil, volatile oil, sinigrin*

ACTIONS *Rubefacient, irritant, stimulant, diuretic, emetic, carminative, tonic*

Calendula officinalis

PLANT FAMILY COMPOSITAE

MARIGOLD

Marigold may be used safely wherever there is an inflammation of the skin, whether due to infection or physical damage. It may be used for any external bleeding or wound,

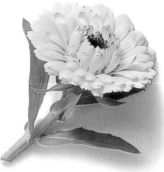

MARIGOLD
FLOWER HEAD

bruising or strains. It is ideal for first-aid treatment of minor burns and scalds, used as a lotion, a poultice or compress. Internally, it may be used in the treatment of gastric and duodenal ulcers. As a cholagogue it helps relieve gall-bladder problems and indigestion. Marigold has anti-fungal activity and may be used internally and externally to combat such infections. It also helps delayed menstruation and painful periods.

**PREPARATION
AND DOSAGE**

INFUSION

POUR A CUP OF BOILING WATER
ONTO 1–2 TEASPOONFULS OF THE
FLORETS AND LEAVE TO INFUSE
FOR 10–15 MINUTES.
THIS SHOULD BE DRUNK
THREE TIMES A DAY.

EXTERNAL USE

SEE THE DIRECTIONS IN THE
CHAPTER ON THE SKIN.

TINCTURE

TAKE 1–4ML OF THE TINCTURE
THREE TIMES A DAY.

PART USED
Yellow petals (florets)

COLLECTION *Either the whole flower tops or just the petals are collected between early summer and early Fall. They should be dried with great care to ensure there is no discolouration.*

CONSTITUENTS *Saponins, carotenoids, bitter principle, essential oil, sterols, flavonoids, mucilage*

ACTIONS
Anti-inflammatory, astringent, vulnerary, anti-microbial, cholagogue, emmenagogue, tonic

---

COMBINATIONS

For digestive problems it may be used with Marshmallow Root and American Cranesbill. As an external soothing application it can be used with Slippery Elm and any other relevant remedy. A useful antiseptic lotion will be produced by combining it with Golden Seal and Myrrh.

Capsella bursa-pastoris

PLANT FAMILY CRUCIFERAE

SHEPHERD'S PURSE

This easily recognized plant may be used wherever a gentle diuretic is called for – in water retention due to kidney problems for instance. As an astringent it will prove effective in the treatment of diarrhea, wounds, nose bleeds and other conditions. It has specific use in the stimulation of the menstrual process whilst also being of use in the reduction of excess flow.

PART USED *Aerial parts*

COLLECTION *The herb can be collected from late winter until mid-Fall.*

CONSTITUENTS *Tyramine, choline acetylcholine, tannin, essential oil, resin, saponins, flavonoids, diosmine, potassium*

ACTIONS *Uterine stimulant, diuretic, astringent, vulnerary*

SHEPHERD'S PURSE
SHOOTS, LEAVES AND
FLOWERS

**PREPARATION
AND DOSAGE**

INFUSION

POUR A CUP OF BOILING WATER
ONTO 1–2 TEASPOONFULS OF THE
DRIED HERB AND LEAVE TO INFUSE
FOR 10 MINUTES.
IF IT IS USED FOR MENSTRUAL
CONDITIONS, IT SHOULD BE DRUNK
EVERY 2–3 HOURS DURING AND
JUST BEFORE THE PERIOD.
OTHERWISE DRINK IT
THREE TIMES A DAY.

TINCTURE

TAKE 1–2ML OF THE TINCTURE
THREE TIMES A DAY.

Capsicum annuum var. *annuum*

PLANT FAMILY SOLANACEAE

CAYENNE

Cayenne is the most useful of the systemic stimulants. It regulates the blood flow, equalizing and strengthening the heart, arteries, capillaries and nerves. It is a general tonic and is specific for the circulatory and digestive system. It may be used in flatulent dyspepsia and colic. If there is insufficient peripheral circulation, leading to cold hands and feet and possibly chilblains, Cayenne may be used. It is used for treating debility and for warding off colds. Externally it is used as a rubefacient in problems like lumbago and rheumatic pains. As an ointment it helps unbroken chilblains, as long as it is used in moderation!

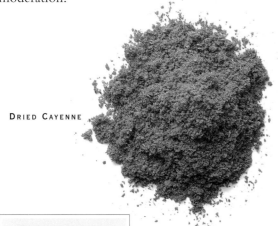

DRIED CAYENNE

PREPARATION AND DOSAGE

INFUSION

POUR A CUP OF BOILING WATER ONTO ½–1 TEASPOONFUL OF CAYENNE AND LEAVE TO INFUSE FOR 10 MINUTES. A TABLESPOONFUL OF THIS INFUSION SHOULD BE MIXED WITH HOT WATER AND DRUNK WHEN NEEDED.

TINCTURE

TAKE ¼–1ML OF THE TINCTURE THREE TIMES A DAY OR WHEN NEEDED.

PART USED *Fruit*

COLLECTION *The fruit should be harvested when fully ripe and dried in the shade.*

CONSTITUENTS *Capsaicin, carotenoids, flavonoids, essential oil, vitamin C*

ACTIONS *Stimulant, carminative, tonic, sialagogue, rubefacient, anti-catarrhal, anti-emetic, anti-microbial, diaphoretic*

COMBINATIONS

As a gargle in laryngitis it combines well with Myrrh. This combination is also a good antiseptic wash.

Carlina vulgaris

PLANT FAMILY COMPOSITAE

CARLINE THISTLE

This beautiful herb has been described as having properties similar to that of Elecampane. It has valuable antiseptic properties when used to aid wound-healing. It may be used in any urinary problem, especially in infections such as cystitis.

PART USED *Root and leaves*

COLLECTION *The root of the perennial plant should be unearthed in the Fall.*

CONSTITUENTS *Essential oil, sesquiterpene, tannin, inulin*

ACTIONS *Diuretic, diaphoretic, vulnerary, tonic*

PREPARATION AND DOSAGE

INFUSION

POUR A CUP OF BOILING WATER ONTO 1 TEASPOONFUL OF THE DRIED LEAVES AND LET INFUSE FOR 10–15 MINUTES. THIS SHOULD BE DRUNK THREE TIMES A DAY.

TINCTURE

TAKE 1–2ML OF THE TINCTURE THREE TIMES A DAY.

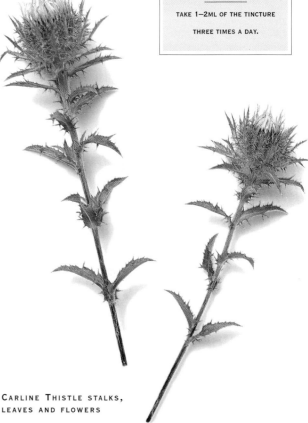

CARLINE THISTLE STALKS, LEAVES AND FLOWERS

Carum carvi

PLANT FAMILY UMBELLIFERAE

CARAWAY

Caraway is used as a calming herb to ease
flatulent dyspepsia and intestinal colic,
especially in children. It will stimulate the appetite.
Its astringency will help in the treatment of
diarrhea as well as in laryngitis as a gargle. It can
be used in bronchitis and bronchial asthma. Its
anti-spasmodic actions help
in the relief of period
pains. It has been used
to increase milk
flow in nursing
mothers.

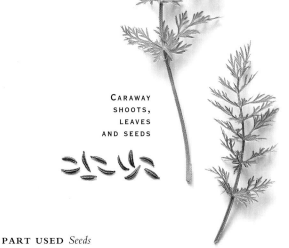

CARAWAY
SHOOTS,
LEAVES
AND SEEDS

PART USED *Seeds*

COLLECTION *Collect the
flowering heads (umbels) in
mid-summer and leave to
ripen. Shake the seeds off
when ready.*

CONSTITUENTS *Up to
6% volatile oil including
carvone and limonene; fatty oil
and tannin*

ACTIONS *Carminative, anti-
spasmodic, expectorant,
emmenagogue, galactagogue,
astringent, aromatic, anti-
microbial, stimulant*

> **PREPARATION
> AND DOSAGE**
>
> **INFUSION**
>
> POUR A CUP OF BOILING WATER
> ONTO 1 TEASPOONFUL OF FRESHLY
> CRUSHED SEEDS AND LEAVE TO
> INFUSE FOR 10–15 MINUTES.
> THIS SHOULD BE DRUNK
> THREE TIMES A DAY.
>
> **TINCTURE**
>
> TAKE 1–4ML OF THE TINCTURE
> THREE TIMES A DAY.

COMBINATIONS
For flatulence and colic Caraway combines well with
Chamomile and Calamus, in diarrhea with Agrimony and
Bayberry and in bronchitis with White Horehound.

Caulophyllum thalictrioides

PLANT FAMILY BERBERIDACEAE

BLUE COHOSH

Blue Cohosh is a plant that comes to us from
the Native North Americans, which shows in
its other names of Squaw Root and Papoose
Root. It is an excellent uterine tonic, which may
be used in any situation where there is a weakness
or loss of tone. It may be used at any time during
pregnancy if there is a threat of miscarriage.
Similarly, because of its anti-spasmodic action, it
will ease false labour pains. However, when labour
does ensue, the use of Blue Cohosh just before
birth will help ensure an easy delivery. In all these
cases it is a safe herb to use. As an emmenagogue
it can be used to bring on a delayed or suppressed
menstruation whilst ensuring that the pain that
sometimes accompanies it is relieved. Blue
Cohosh may be used in cases where an
anti-spasmodic is needed, such as in colic, asthma
or nervous coughs. It has a reputation for easing
rheumatic pain.

PART USED
Rhizome and root

COLLECTION *The roots
and rhizome are collected in the
Fall, as at the end of the
growing season they are richest
in natural chemicals.*

CONSTITUENTS *Steroidal
saponins, alkaloids*

ACTIONS *Uterine tonic,
emmenagogue, anti-spasmodic,
anti-rheumatic, nervine
oxytocic, sedative*

> **PREPARATION
> AND DOSAGE**
>
> **DECOCTION**
>
> PUT 1 TEASPOONFUL OF THE DRIED
> ROOT IN A CUP OF WATER, BRING
> TO THE BOIL AND SIMMER FOR 10
> MINUTES. THIS SHOULD BE DRUNK
> THREE TIMES A DAY.
>
> **TINCTURE**
>
> TAKE 1–2ML OF THE TINCTURE
> THREE TIMES A DAY.

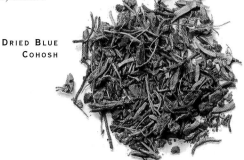

DRIED BLUE
COHOSH

COMBINATIONS
To strengthen the uterus it may be used well with False
Unicorn Root, Motherwort and Yarrow.

73

Centaurium erythraea

PLANT FAMILY GENTIANACEAE

CENTAURY

It may be used whenever a digestive and gastric stimulant is required. It is indicated primarily in appetite loss (anorexia) when it is associated with liver weakness. Centaury is a useful herb in dyspepsia and in any condition where a sluggish digestion is involved.

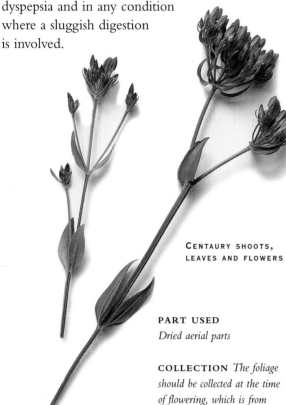

CENTAURY SHOOTS, LEAVES AND FLOWERS

PART USED
Dried aerial parts

COLLECTION *The foliage should be collected at the time of flowering, which is from mid-summer to early Fall. Dry it in the sun.*

CONSTITUENTS
Glycosidal bitter principles gentiopicrin and erythrocentaurine, nicotinic acid compounds, traces of essential oil, oleanolic acid and other acids, resin

ACTIONS *Bitter, aromatic, mild nervine, gastric stimulant, galactagogue, hepatic, sialagogue, tonic*

PREPARATION AND DOSAGE

INFUSION

POUR A CUP OF BOILING WATER ONTO 1 TEASPOONFUL OF THE DRIED HERB AND LEAVE TO INFUSE FOR 5–10 MINUTES. DRINK ONE CUP HALF AN HOUR BEFORE MEALS.

TINCTURE

TAKE 1–2ML OF THE TINCTURE THREE TIMES A DAY.

COMBINATIONS

In dyspepsia it combines well with Meadowsweet, Marshmallow Root and Chamomile. In anorexia nervosa it is indicated with Burdock Root and Chamomile.

Cetraria islandica

PLANT FAMILY PARMELIACEAE

ICELAND MOSS

As a soothing demulcent with a high mucilage content, Iceland Moss finds use in the treatment of gastritis, vomiting and dyspepsia. It is often used in respiratory catarrh and bronchitis. It generally soothes the mucous membranes. In addition its nourishing qualities contribute to the treatment of cachexia, a state of malnourishment and debility.

PREPARATION AND DOSAGE

DECOCTION

PUT 1 TEASPOONFUL OF THE SHREDDED MOSS IN A CUP OF COLD WATER, BOIL FOR 3 MINUTES AND LET STAND FOR 10 MINUTES. A CUP SHOULD BE DRUNK MORNING AND EVENING.

TINCTURE

TAKE 1–2ML OF THE TINCTURE THREE TIMES A DAY.

PART USED *Entire plant. It is a lichen.*

COLLECTION *The lichen may be gathered throughout the year, though between late spring and early Fall is perhaps best. It should be freed from attached impurities and dried in the sun or the shade.*

CONSTITUENTS *Rich in mucilage; bitter fumaric acids, usnic acid, some iodine, traces of vitamin A*

ACTIONS *Demulcent, anti-emetic, expectorant, anti-catarrhal, pectoral, tonic*

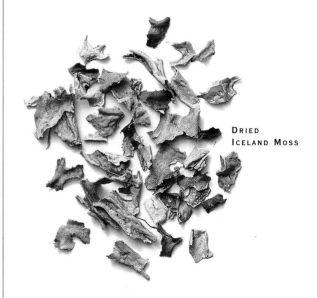

DRIED ICELAND MOSS

COMBINATIONS

For the treatment of nausea and vomiting it can be combined with Black Horehound.

Chamaelirium luteum

PLANT FAMILY LILIACEAE

FALSE UNICORN ROOT

This herb, which comes to us via the Native North Americans, is one of the best tonics and strengtheners of the reproductive system that we have. Though primarily used for the female system, it can be equally beneficial for men. It is known to contain precursors of the estrogens (female hormones). However, it acts in an amphoteric way to normalize function. The body may use this herb to balance and tone and thus it will aid in apparently opposite situations. Whilst being of help in all uterine problems, it is specifically useful in delayed or absent menstruation (amenorrhea). Where ovarian pain occurs, False Unicorn Root may be safely used. It is also indicated in cases of threatened miscarriage and to ease vomiting associated with pregnancy. However, large doses will cause nausea and vomiting.

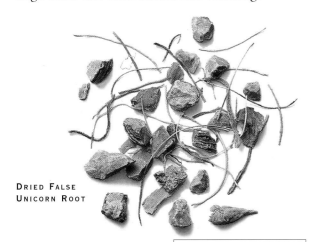

DRIED FALSE UNICORN ROOT

PART USED *Dried rhizome and root*

COLLECTION *The underground parts are unearthed in the Fall.*

CONSTITUENTS *Steroidal saponins which include chamaelirin*

ACTIONS *Uterine tonic, diuretic, anthelmintic, emetic, emmenagogue*

> ### PREPARATION AND DOSAGE
>
> **DECOCTION**
>
> PUT 1–2 TEASPOONFULS OF THE ROOT IN A CUP OF WATER, BRING TO THE BOIL AND SIMMER GENTLY FOR 10–15 MINUTES. THIS SHOULD BE DRUNK THREE TIMES A DAY. FOR THREATENED MISCARRIAGE IT MAY BE DRUNK COPIOUSLY.
>
> **TINCTURE**
>
> TAKE 2–4ML OF THE TINCTURE THREE TIMES A DAY.

Chamaemelum nobile

PLANT FAMILY COMPOSITAE

GARDEN CHAMOMILE

Chamomile is renowned for its medical and household uses. Both Garden Chamomile and German Chamomile *(Matricaria recutita)* can be used. It is an excellent, gentle sedative, safe for use with children. It will contribute its relaxing actions in any combination and is thus used in anxiety and insomnia. Indigestion and inflammations such as gastritis are often eased with Chamomile. It can be used as a mouthwash for mouth inflammations, a gargle for sore throats and an eye-bath for sore eyes. As an inhalation over a steam bath, it will speed recovery from nasal catarrh. Externally it will speed wound healing and reduce swelling. As a carminative with relaxing properties it will ease flatulence and dyspeptic pain.

GARDEN CHAMOMILE STALKS, LEAVES AND FLOWERS

PART USED *Flowers and leaves*

COLLECTION *The flowers should be gathered between late spring and late summer when they are not wet with dew or rain. They should be dried with care at not too high a temperature.*

CONSTITUENTS *Volatile oil which includes chamazulene and isadol; mucilage, coumarin, flavone glycosides*

ACTIONS *Anti-spasmodic, carminative, anti-inflammatory, analgesic, antiseptic, vulnerary, aromatic, bitter, diaphoretic, emmenagogue, nervine, sedative, tonic*

> ### PREPARATION AND DOSAGE
>
> **INFUSION**
>
> POUR A CUP OF BOILING WATER ONTO 2 TEASPOONFULS OF THE DRIED LEAVES AND LET INFUSE FOR 5–10 MINUTES. FOR DIGESTIVE PROBLEMS, THIS TEA SHOULD BE DRUNK AFTER MEALS. A STRONGER INFUSION SHOULD BE USED AS A MOUTHWASH FOR CONDITIONS SUCH AS GINGIVITIS. HALF A CUP OF FLOWERS BOILED IN 2L/4PT OF WATER MAKE A STEAM BATH. COVER YOUR HEAD WITH A TOWEL AND INHALE THE STEAM.
>
> **TINCTURE**
>
> TAKE 2–4ML OF THE TINCTURE THREE TIMES A DAY.

Chelidonium majus

PLANT FAMILY PAPAVERACEAE

GREATER CELANDINE

At therapeutic doses, Greater Celandine is an excellent remedy for the treatment of infections of the gall-bladder and gallstones. At higher doses, this plant is poisonous, causing powerful purging of the digestive tract. It may be used as an anti-spasmodic remedy in stomach pain. Externally the orange latex from the stem may be used in the treatment of verrucae, skin tumours and tinea (a fungal infection of the skin). It has been found that the alkaloid chelidonine inhibits mitosis.

GREATER CELANDINE SHOOT, LEAVES AND FLOWERS

PREPARATION AND DOSAGE

DECOCTION

PUT 2 TEASPOONFULS OF THE HERB OR 1 TEASPOONFUL OF THE ROOT IN A CUP OF COLD WATER, BRING TO THE BOIL AND THEN REMOVE FROM THE HEAT. LET STAND FOR 10 MINUTES. TAKE ONE CUP TWICE A DAY. NOTE: IT IS DANGEROUS TO EXCEED THIS DOSE.

TINCTURE

TAKE 1–2ML OF THE TINCTURE THREE TIMES A DAY.

CAUTION
DO NOT EXCEED THE DOSE GIVEN ABOVE.

PART USED
Roots or aerial parts

COLLECTION *The root should be unearthed in late summer or Fall and dried in the sun or shade. The foliage should be gathered at the time of flowering (late spring to early summer) and dried as quickly as possible in the shade.*

CONSTITUENTS *Root: Alkaloids including chelidonine, chelerythine, coptisine, protopine; chelidonic acid, essential oil, saponin, yellow latex with carotenoid latex*

ACTIONS *Anti-spasmodic, cholagogue, anodyne, purgative, diuretic*

COMBINATIONS
In gall-bladder disease, Greater Celandine combines well with Barberry and Dandelion.

Chelone glabra

PLANT FAMILY SCROPHULARIACEAE

BALMONY

Balmony is an excellent agent for liver problems. It acts as a tonic on the whole digestive and absorptive system. It has a stimulating effect on the secretion of digestive juices, and in this most natural way its laxative properties are produced. Balmony is used in gallstones, inflammation of the gall-bladder and in jaundice. It stimulates the appetite, eases colic, dyspepsia and biliousness and is helpful in debility. Externally it has been used in inflamed breasts, painful ulcers and piles. It is considered a specific in gallstones that lead to congestive jaundice.

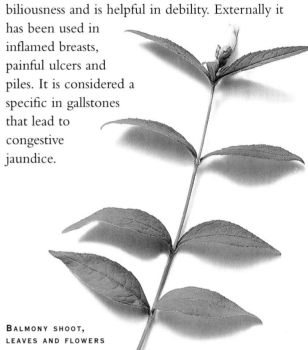

BALMONY SHOOT, LEAVES AND FLOWERS

PART USED
Dried aerial parts

COLLECTION *Collect and dry during the flowering period between mid-summer and early Fall.*

CONSTITUENTS *Resins and bitter iridoids have been reported.*

ACTIONS *Cholagogue, anti-emetic, stimulant, laxative, anti-bilious, hepatic, tonic*

PREPARATION AND DOSAGE

INFUSION
POUR A CUP OF BOILING WATER ONTO 2 TEASPOONFULS OF THE DRIED HERB AND LET INFUSE FOR 10–15 MINUTES. THIS SHOULD BE DRUNK THREE TIMES A DAY.

TINCTURE
TAKE 1–2ML OF THE TINCTURE THREE TIMES A DAY.

COMBINATIONS
For the relief of constipation, Balmony may be combined with Butternut. For jaundice it will best be used with Golden Seal.

Chionanthus virginicus

PLANT FAMILY OLEACEAE

FRINGETREE

This valuable herb may be safely used in all liver problems, especially when they have developed into jaundice. It is a specific for the treatment of gall-bladder inflammation and a valuable part of treating gallstones. It is a remedy that will aid the liver in general and as such it is often used as part of a wider treatment for the whole body. Through its action of releasing bile it acts as a gentle and effective laxative.

PREPARATION AND DOSAGE

INFUSION

POUR A CUP OF BOILING WATER ONTO 1–2 TEASPOONFULS OF THE BARK AND LEAVE TO INFUSE FOR 10–15 MINUTES. THIS SHOULD BE DRUNK THREE TIMES A DAY.

TINCTURE

TAKE 1–2ML OF THE TINCTURE THREE TIMES A DAY.

PART USED *Root bark*

COLLECTION *The roots are unearthed in spring or Fall. Wash carefully and peel the bark. They should be dried with care.*

CONSTITUENTS *Phyllyrin, a lignin glycoside, saponins*

ACTIONS *Hepatic, cholagogue, alterative, diuretic, tonic, laxative, anti-bilious*

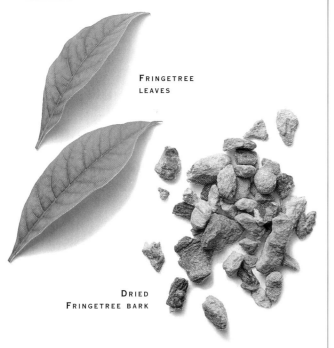

FRINGETREE
LEAVES

DRIED
FRINGETREE BARK

COMBINATIONS

For the treatment of liver and gall-bladder conditions it may be used with Barberry, Wahoo or Wild Yam.

Chondrus crispus

PLANT FAMILY RHODOPHYTA

IRISH MOSS

The mucilage present in Irish Moss, or Carragheen, is used in large quantities by the food industry to make jellies or aspic and to be used as a smooth binder. This very property is the basis of its use in digestive conditions where a demulcent is called for, such as gastritis and ulcers. However, its main use is in respiratory problems such as bronchitis. It finds a use in cosmetics as a skin softener.

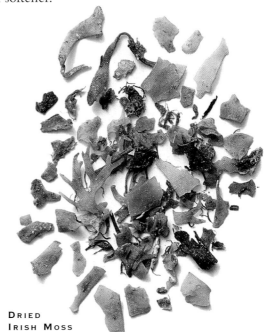

DRIED
IRISH MOSS

PREPARATION AND DOSAGE

INFUSION

POUR A CUP OF BOILING WATER ONTO 1–1½ TEASPOONFULS OF THE DRIED HERB AND LEAVE TO INFUSE FOR 10 MINUTES. THIS SHOULD BE DRUNK THREE TIMES A DAY.

TINCTURE

TAKE 1–2ML OF THE TINCTURE THREE TIMES A DAY.

PART USED *Dried thallus (young shoots). It is a seaweed.*

COLLECTION *It is collected from the rocky coastlines of northwestern Europe, especially Ireland, all year round at low tide.*

CONSTITUENTS *Up to 80% mucilage; carrageenans, iodine, bromide, iron, other mineral salts, vitamin A and B₁.*

ACTIONS *Expectorant, demulcent, anti-catarrhal, pectoral, vulnerary*

Cimicifuga racemosa

PLANT FAMILY RANUNCULACEAE

BLACK COHOSH

Black Cohosh has a most powerful action as a relaxant and a normalizer of the female reproductive system. It may be used beneficially in cases of painful or delayed menstruation, ovarian cramps or cramping pain in the womb. It has a normalizing action on the balance of female sex hormones and may safely be used to regain normal hormonal activity. It is very active in the treatment of rheumatic pains, rheumatoid arthritis, osteo-arthritis, and in muscular and neurological pain. It finds use in sciatica and neuralgia. As a relaxing nervine it may be used in many situations where such an agent is needed. It will be useful in labour to aid uterine activity whilst allaying nervousness. Black Cohosh will reduce spasms and so aid in the treatment of pulmonary complaints such as whooping cough. It has been found beneficial in cases of tinnitus.

BLACK COHOSH
SHOOT AND LEAVES

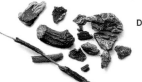

DRIED BLACK COHOSH

PART USED *Root and rhizome; dried, not fresh*

COLLECTION *The roots are unearthed with the rhizome in Fall after the fruits have ripened. They should be cut lengthways and dried carefully.*

CONSTITUENTS *Resin, bitter glycosides, ranunculin (which changes to anemonin upon drying), salicylic acid, tannin, estrogenic principle*

ACTIONS *Emmenagogue, anti-spasmodic, alterative, sedative, nervine, tonic*

PREPARATION AND DOSAGE

DECOCTION

POUR A CUP OF WATER ONTO ½–1 TEASPOONFUL OF THE DRIED ROOT AND BRING TO THE BOIL. LET IT SIMMER FOR 10–15 MINUTES. THIS SHOULD BE DRUNK THREE TIMES A DAY.

TINCTURE

TAKE 2–4ML OF THE TINCTURE THREE TIMES A DAY.

COMBINATIONS
For uterine conditions combine with Blue Cohosh.
For rheumatic problems use with Bogbean.

Cinchona officinalis

PLANT FAMILY RUBIACEAE

PERUVIAN BARK

Peruvian Bark is renowned as a treatment of feverish conditions and especially those that are periodic, such as malaria. It may be used in all fevers, but usually as part of a wider treatment. The bitter action gives this herb a role in the stimulation of the digestive system, aiding the whole process. It will stimulate the secretion of digestive juices and in this way act as a tonic. There is also a distinct action of quieting the heart, reducing palpitations and normalizing the function.

PART USED *Bark*

COLLECTION *The bark is collected by felling the six- to eight-year-old trees and then stripping the bark.*

CONSTITUENTS *Alkaloids including quinine and quinidine; tannins, bitter principle*

ACTIONS *Febrifuge, digestive bitter, anthelmintic, heart relaxant*

PREPARATION AND DOSAGE

INFUSION

POUR A CUP OF BOILING WATER ONTO 1 TEASPOONFUL OF THE BARK AND LEAVE IT TO INFUSE FOR 30 MINUTES. THIS SHOULD BE DRUNK THREE TIMES A DAY.

TINCTURE

TAKE 1–2ML OF THE TINCTURE THREE TIMES A DAY.

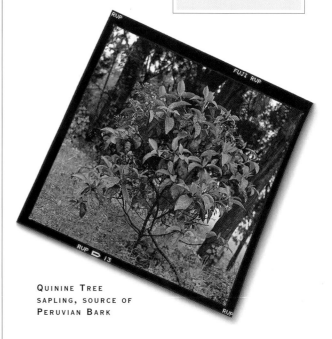

QUININE TREE
SAPLING, SOURCE OF
PERUVIAN BARK

Cinnamomum zeylanicum

PLANT FAMILY LAURACEAE

CINNAMON

Cinnamon is usually used as a carminative addition to other herbs. It relieves nausea and vomiting. Because of its mild astringency it is used against diarrhea.

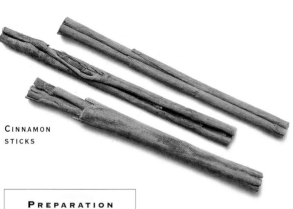

CINNAMON
STICKS

PREPARATION AND DOSAGE

THE BARK, USUALLY POWDERED, MAY BE FREELY USED IN MIXTURES OR BY ITSELF TO FLAVOUR TEAS.

PART USED *Dried inner bark of the shoots*

COLLECTION *The bark is collected commercially throughout the tropics.*

CONSTITUENTS *Volatile oils*

ACTIONS *Carminative, astringent, aromatic, stimulant*

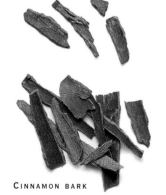

CINNAMON BARK

Cnicus benedictus

PLANT FAMILY COMPOSITAE

BLESSED THISTLE

Through its bitter properties, Blessed Thistle increases the flow of gastric and bile secretions. It may be used with benefit in appetite loss (anorexia), dyspepsia and indigestion and it has a role in any disease of the digestive system which is accompanied by wind and colic. Because of its astringency it may be used in diarrhea or hemorrhage. Externally it is a vulnerary and antiseptic.

BLESSED
THISTLE
STALK, LEAVES
AND FLOWER

PART USED *Dried aerial parts and seeds*

COLLECTION *The leaves and flowering twigs should be gathered when blooming (early summer to late summer). Dry them in the shade and cut them up after drying. The seeds are collected in Fall when the plant has set seed.*

CONSTITUENTS *Bitter glycoside called cnicin, flavonoids, essential oil, mucilage*

ACTIONS *Bitter tonic, astringent, diaphoretic, anti-bacterial, expectorant, emmenagogue, galactagogue*

PREPARATION AND DOSAGE

INFUSION

POUR A CUP OF BOILING WATER ONTO 1 TEASPOONFUL OF THE DRIED HERB AND LEAVE TO INFUSE FOR 10–15 MINUTES. THIS SHOULD BE DRUNK THREE TIMES A DAY.

TINCTURE

TAKE 1–2ML OF THE TINCTURE THREE TIMES A DAY.

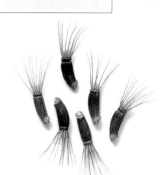

COMBINATIONS

In indigestion, due to a sluggish state of the digestive system, it may be combined with Balmony and Kola; in diarrhea with Meadowsweet and Tormentil.

Cola nitida

PLANT FAMILY STERCULIACEAE

KOLA

Kola has a marked stimulating effect on the human consciousness. It can be used wherever there is a need for direct stimulation, which is less often than is usually thought. Through regaining proper health and therefore right functioning, the nervous system does not need such help. In the short term it may be used in nervous debility in states of atony and weakness. It can act as a specific in nervous diarrhea. It will aid in states of depression and may in some people give rise to euphoric states. In some varieties of migraine it can help greatly. Through the stimulation it will be a valuable part of the treatment for anorexia. It can be viewed as specific in cases of depression associated with weakness and debility.

PREPARATION AND DOSAGE

DECOCTION

PUT 1–2 TEASPOONFULS OF THE POWDERED NUTS IN A CUP OF WATER, BRING TO THE BOIL AND SIMMER GENTLY FOR 10–15 MINUTES. THIS SHOULD BE DRUNK WHEN NEEDED.

TINCTURE

TAKE 1–4ML OF THE TINCTURE THREE TIMES A DAY.

PART USED *Seed kernel*

COLLECTION *The Kola tree grows in tropical Africa and is cultivated in South America. The seeds are collected when ripe and are initially white, turning the characteristic red upon drying.*

CONSTITUENTS *Alkaloids which include more than 1.25% caffeine and theobromine; tannin, volatile oil*

ACTIONS *Stimulant to central nervous system, anti-depressive, astringent, diuretic*

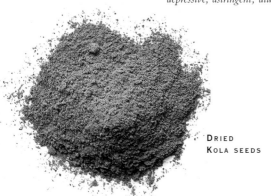

DRIED KOLA SEEDS

COMBINATIONS
Kola will go well with Oats, Damiana and Skullcap.

Collinsonia canadensis

PLANT FAMILY LABIATAE

STONE ROOT

As its name suggests, Stone Root finds its main use in the treatment and prevention of stone and gravel in the urinary system and the gall-bladder. It can be used as a prophylactic but is also excellent when the body is in need of help in passing stones or gravel. It is also a strong diuretic.

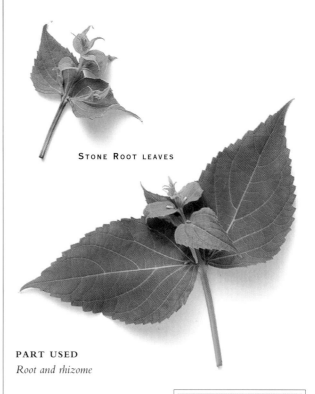

STONE ROOT LEAVES

PART USED
Root and rhizome

COLLECTION Roots and rhizome are unearthed in the Fall.

CONSTITUENTS
Saponins, resin, tannin, organic acid, alkaloid

ACTIONS Anti-lithic, diuretic, diaphoretic

PREPARATION AND DOSAGE

DECOCTION
PUT 1–3 TEASPOONFULS OF THE DRIED ROOT IN A CUP OF WATER, BRING TO THE BOIL AND SIMMER FOR 10–15 MINUTES. THIS SHOULD BE DRUNK THREE TIMES A DAY.

TINCTURE
TAKE 2–4ML OF THE TINCTURE THREE TIMES A DAY.

COMBINATIONS
For urinary stone and gravel it may be combined with Parsley Piert, Gravel Root, Pellitory of the Wall or Hydrangea.

Commiphora molmol

PLANT FAMILY BURSERACEAE

MYRRH

Myrrh is an effective anti-microbial agent that has been shown to work in two complementary ways. Primarily it stimulates the production of white blood corpuscles (with their anti-pathogenic actions) and secondarily it has a direct anti-microbial effect. Myrrh finds specific use in the treatment of infections in the mouth as well as the catarrhal problems of pharyngitis and sinusitis. It may also help with laryngitis and respiratory complaints. Systemically it is of value in the treatment of boils as well as glandular fever and brucellosis. It is often used as part of the treatment of the common cold. Externally it will be healing and antiseptic for wounds and abrasions.

MYRRH RESIN

PREPARATION AND DOSAGE

INFUSION

AS THE RESIN ONLY DISSOLVES IN WATER WITH DIFFICULTY, IT SHOULD BE POWDERED WELL TO MAKE AN INFUSION. POUR A CUP OF BOILING WATER ONTO 1–2 TEASPOONFULS OF THE POWDER AND LEAVE TO INFUSE FOR 10–15 MINUTES. THIS SHOULD BE DRUNK THREE TIMES A DAY.

TINCTURE

AS THE RESIN DISSOLVES MUCH MORE EASILY IN ALCOHOL, THE TINCTURE IS PREFERABLE AND EASILY OBTAINABLE. TAKE 1–4ML OF THE TINCTURE THREE TIMES A DAY.

PART USED
Gum resin

COLLECTION *The gum resin is collected from the bushes that secrete it in the arid regions of East Africa and Arabia.*

CONSTITUENTS *Up to 17% essential oil, up to 40% resin, gums*

ACTIONS *Anti-microbial, astringent, carminative, anti-catarrhal, expectorant, vulnerary, tonic*

COMBINATIONS
It will combine well with Echinacea for infections and as a mouthwash for ulcers and similar problems. For external use it should be combined with distilled Witch Hazel.

Convallaria majalis

PLANT FAMILY LILIACEAE

LILY OF THE VALLEY

Lily of the Valley is perhaps the most valuable heart remedy that the medicinal herbalist uses today. The specifics of its mode of action are discussed in The Circulatory System *(see page 170)*, but it is well to remember that this herb has an action equivalent to Foxglove (*Digitalis*) without its potential toxic effects. Lily of the Valley may be used in the treatment of heart failure and water retention (dropsy) where this is associated with the heart. It will aid the body where there is difficulty with breathing due to congestive conditions of the heart.

PART USED *Dried leaves*

COLLECTION *The leaves are gathered at the time of flowering in late spring and early summer.*

CONSTITUENTS *Cardiac glycosides including convalla-toxin and convallatoxol; saponins including convallarin and convallaric acid; asparagin, flavonoids, essential oil with farnesol*

ACTIONS
Cardio-active, diuretic

CAUTION
USE ONLY UNDER MEDICAL SUPERVISION

PREPARATION AND DOSAGE

INFUSION

AN INFUSION CAN BE MADE BUT SHOULD ONLY BE USED UNDER QUALIFIED SUPERVISION.

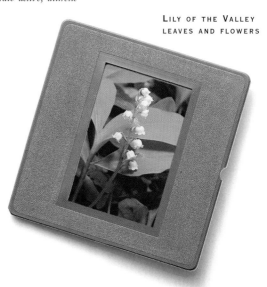

LILY OF THE VALLEY LEAVES AND FLOWERS

COMBINATIONS
It combines well with Motherwort and Hawthorn.

Coriandrum sativum

PLANT FAMILY UMBELLIFERAE

CORIANDER

This exquisite spice is used medicinally as a herb that helps the digestive system get rid of wind and ease the spasm pain (colic) that sometimes accompanies it. It will also ease diarrhea, especially in children. It may be used as an equivalent to 'gripe water', which is usually made from Dill Seeds. The oil acts as a stimulant to the stomach, increasing secretion of digestive juices and thus also stimulating the appetite.

PART USED
Ripe seeds

CORIANDER LEAVES

COLLECTION *The flowering heads (umbels) are collected in late summer and left to ripen. The seeds are then easily collected as they can be shaken off.*

CONSTITUENTS *Essential oil including coriandrol, fatty oil; tannin, sugar*

ACTIONS *Carminative, aromatic, anti-microbial*

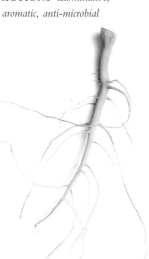

CORIANDER ROOT AND SEEDS

> ### PREPARATION AND DOSAGE
> #### INFUSION
> POUR A CUP OF BOILING WATER ONTO 1 TEASPOONFUL OF THE BRUISED SEEDS AND LET INFUSE FOR 5 MINUTES IN A CLOSED POT. THIS SHOULD BE DRUNK BEFORE MEALS.

Crataegus laevigata

PLANT FAMILY ROSACEAE

HAWTHORN

Hawthorn berries provide us with one of the best tonic remedies for the heart and circulatory system. They act in a normalizing way upon the heart by either stimulating or depressing its activity depending upon the need. In other words, Hawthorn berries will move the heart to normal function in a gentle way. As a long-term treatment they may safely be used in heart failure or weakness. They can similarly be used in cases of palpitations. As a tonic for the circulatory system they find their primary use in the treatment of high blood pressure, arteriosclerosis and angina pectoris. Whilst they can be very effective in the aiding of these conditions, qualified attention is essential.

> ### PREPARATION AND DOSAGE
> #### INFUSION
> POUR A CUP OF BOILING WATER ONTO 2 TEASPOONFULS OF THE BERRIES AND LEAVE TO INFUSE FOR 20 MINUTES. THIS SHOULD BE DRUNK THREE TIMES A DAY OVER A LONG PERIOD.
>
> #### TINCTURE
> TAKE 2–4ML OF THE TINCTURE THREE TIMES A DAY.

HAWTHORN BERRIES

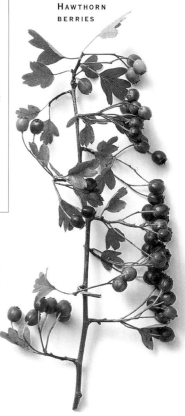

PART USED *Ripe fruits*

COLLECTION *The berries are collected in early Fall and mid-Fall.*

CONSTITUENTS *Saponins, glycosides, flavonoids, acids including ascorbic acid, tannin*

ACTIONS *Cardiac tonic, hypotensive, diuretic*

> ### COMBINATIONS
> For the treatment of high blood pressure and the circulatory system they can be combined with Lime Blossom, Mistletoe and Yarrow.

Cucumis sativus

PLANT FAMILY CUCURBITACEAE

CUCUMBER

The seeds of the Cucumber are similar in effect to those of Pumpkin as they also possess anti-tapeworm properties. The main use of Cucumber is as a cosmetic. The juice of fresh fruit is cooling, healing and soothing to the skin.

CUCUMBER
SEEDS

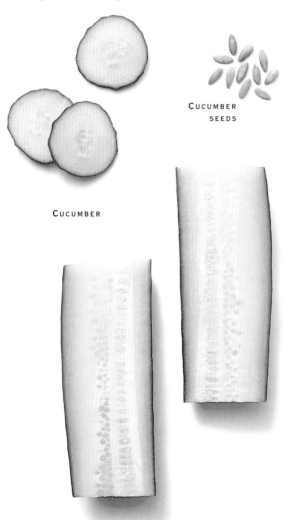

CUCUMBER

PART USED *Whole fruit, the seeds*

COLLECTION *The seeds are collected from fresh cucumbers.*

ACTIONS *Demulcent, vulnerary, mild diuretic Seeds: anthelmintic*

PREPARATION AND DOSAGE

FOR TREATING TAPEWORM INFESTATIONS TAKE 60G/2OZ OF GROUND SEEDS AND MIX THEM WITH SUGAR OR HONEY. THIS SHOULD BE TAKEN WHILST FASTING AND BE FOLLOWED AFTER 2 HOURS BY A CATHARTIC.

Cucurbita pepo

PLANT FAMILY CUCURBITACEAE

PUMPKIN

The seeds of this valuable vegetable have long been used as a remedy for worms and tapeworms. The effect appears to be a mechanical one. The seeds should be used when ripe and fresh.

PART USED *Seeds*

COLLECTION *The seeds are removed from the pulp inside the pumpkin, which should be harvested in late summer.*

CONSTITUENTS *Fatty oil, cucurbitin, albumin, lecithin, resin, phytosterin*

ACTIONS *Anthelmintic*

PREPARATION AND DOSAGE

MRS GRIEVE GIVES THE FOLLOWING RECIPE. 'A MIXTURE IS MADE BY BEATING 2OZ OF THE SEEDS WITH AS MUCH SUGAR AND MILK, OR WATER, ADDED TO MAKE A PINT, AND THIS MIXTURE IS TAKEN FASTING, IN THREE DOSES, ONE EVERY TWO HOURS, CASTOR OIL BEING TAKEN A FEW HOURS AFTER THE LAST DOSE.'

PUMPKIN
AND SEEDS

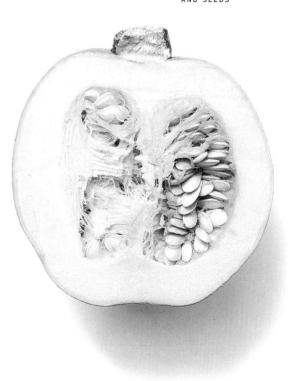

Cydonia oblonga

PLANT FAMILY ROSACEAE

QUINCE

Quince seeds can act as an effective and gentle laxative in cases of constipation as well as a soothing astringent in conditions such as gastritis and enteritis. As a mouthwash they will ease soreness and inflammation in the mouth. They can also be used with good effect in dry, irritating coughs where an expectorant is called for. Externally they may be applied to minor burns.

PART USED *Seeds*

COLLECTION *The seeds are taken out of the Quince fruit, which is collected in the Fall.*

CONSTITUENTS *Mucilage, tannin, fatty oil, pectin, amygdalin, vitamin C*

ACTIONS *Astringent, anti-inflammatory, demulcent, laxative, emollient*

PREPARATION AND DOSAGE

INFUSION

THE SEEDS SHOULD BE SOAKED IN WATER FOR 3–5 HOURS TO GET A SOLUTION OF SLIME FROM THE OUTER COATS OF THE SEEDS. THIS SHOULD BE DRUNK AS NEEDED OR THREE TIMES A DAY.

TINCTURE

TAKE 1–2ML OF THE TINCTURE THREE TIMES A DAY OR AS NEEDED.

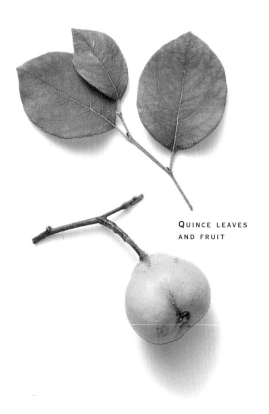

QUINCE LEAVES
AND FRUIT

Cypripedium calceolus var. *pubescens*

PLANT FAMILY ORCHIDACEAE

LADY'S SLIPPER

Lady's Slipper is one of the most widely applicable nervines that we possess in the materia medica. It may be used in all stress reactions, emotional tension and anxiety states. It will help elevate the mood, especially where depression is present. It can help in easing nervous pain, though it is best used in combination with other herbs for this purpose. It is perhaps at its best when treating anxiety that is associated with insomnia.

LADY'S SLIPPER
LEAVES AND FLOWER

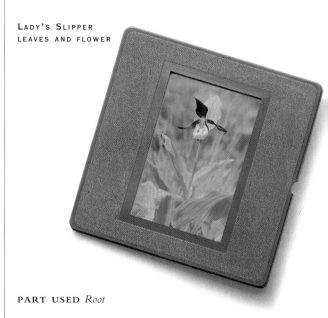

PART USED *Root*

COLLECTION *Lady's Slipper is a protected plant in the United Kingdom and so should never be collected if found wild.*

CONSTITUENTS
Volatile oil, resin, glucosides, tannin

ACTIONS *Sedative, hypnotic, anti-spasmodic, nervine tonic, analgesic*

PREPARATION AND DOSAGE

INFUSION

POUR A CUP OF BOILING WATER ONTO 1–2 TEASPOONFULS OF THE ROOT AND LET INFUSE FOR 10–15 MINUTES. THIS SHOULD BE DRUNK AS REQUIRED.

TINCTURE

TAKE 1–4ML OF THE TINCTURE THREE TIMES A DAY.

COMBINATIONS

It combines well with Oats and Skullcap.
For nerve pain it may be used with Jamaican Dogwood,
Passion Flower and Valerian.

Cytisus scoparius

PLANT FAMILY PAPILIONACEAE

BROOM

Broom is a valuable remedy where there is a weak heart and low blood pressure. Since it is also a diuretic and produces peripheral constriction of the blood vessels while increasing the efficiency of each stroke of the heart, it can be used where water retention occurs due to heart weakness. Broom is used in cases of over-profuse menstruation.

BROOM
LEAVES
AND SEEDPODS

CAUTION

DO NOT USE BROOM IN PREGNANCY OR HYPERTENSION.

PART USED *Flowering tops*

COLLECTION *May be gathered throughout spring, summer and Fall. The tops may be dried in the sun or by heat.*

CONSTITUENTS *Alkaloids including sparteine and cystisine; flavonoid glycosides, tannin, bitter principle, volatile oil*

ACTIONS *Cardioactive, diuretic, hypertensive, peripheral vasoconstrictor, astringent*

PREPARATION AND DOSAGE

INFUSION

POUR A CUP OF BOILING WATER ONTO 1 TEASPOONFUL OF THE DRIED HERB AND LET INFUSE FOR 10–15 MINUTES. THIS SHOULD BE DRUNK THREE TIMES A DAY.

TINCTURE

TAKE 1–2ML OF THE TINCTURE THREE TIMES A DAY.

COMBINATIONS
Broom can be combined with Lily of the Valley and Hawthorn Berries when treating the heart.

Daucus carota

PLANT FAMILY UMBELLIFERAE

WILD CARROT

The volatile oil that is present in Wild Carrot is an active urinary antiseptic, which helps explain its use in the treatment of such conditions as cystitis and prostatitis. It has been considered a specific in the treatment of kidney stones for a long time. In the treatment of gout and rheumatism it is used in combination with other remedies to provide its cleansing diuretic action. The seeds can be used as a settling carminative agent for the relief of flatulence and colic.

PREPARATION AND DOSAGE

INFUSION

POUR A CUP OF BOILING WATER ONTO 1 TEASPOONFUL OF THE DRIED HERB AND LET INFUSE FOR 10–15 MINUTES. THIS SHOULD BE DRUNK THREE TIMES A DAY. TO PREPARE AN INFUSION OF THE SEEDS, USE 1/3–1 TEASPOONFUL TO A CUP OF WATER.

TINCTURE

TAKE 1–2ML OF THE TINCTURE THREE TIMES A DAY.

PART USED *Dried aerial parts and seeds*

COLLECTION *The aerial parts of the herb should be collected between early summer and late summer when in flower or when seeding in late summer and early Fall.*

CONSTITUENTS *Volatile oil, an alkaloid*

ACTIONS *Diuretic, anti-lithic, carminative*

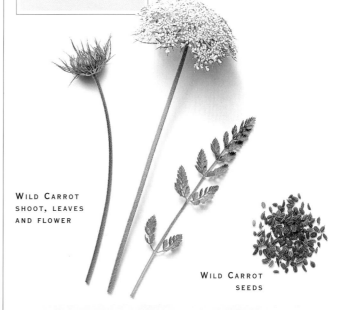

WILD CARROT
SHOOT, LEAVES
AND FLOWER

WILD CARROT
SEEDS

COMBINATIONS
For urinary infections it may be used with Yarrow and Bearberry. For kidney stones use it with Hydrangea, Gravel Root or Pellitory of the Wall.

Dioscorea villosa

PLANT FAMILY DIOSCOREACEAE

WILD YAM

This valuable herb was at one time the sole source of the chemicals that were used as the raw materials for contraceptive hormone manufacture. In herbal medicine Wild Yam is a valuable herb that can be used to relieve intestinal colic, to sooth diverticulitis, ease dysmenorrhea and ovarian and uterine pains. It is of great use in the treatment of rheumatoid arthritis, especially the acute phase where there is intense inflammation.

PART USED *Dried underground parts*

COLLECTION *This tropical plant is uprooted in the Fall, most stocks coming from west Africa.*

CONSTITUENTS *Steroidal saponins including dioscine; phytosterols, alkaloids, tannins, much starch*

ACTIONS *Anti-spasmodic, anti-inflammatory, anti-rheumatic, cholagogue, anti-bilious, hepatic*

PREPARATION AND DOSAGE

DECOCTION

PUT 1–2 TEASPOONFULS OF THE HERB IN A CUP OF WATER, BRING TO THE BOIL AND SIMMER GENTLY FOR 10–15 MINUTES. THIS SHOULD BE DRUNK THREE TIMES A DAY.

TINCTURE

TAKE 2–4ML OF THE TINCTURE THREE TIMES A DAY.

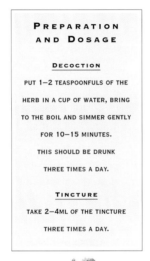

DRIED
WILD YAM
ROOT

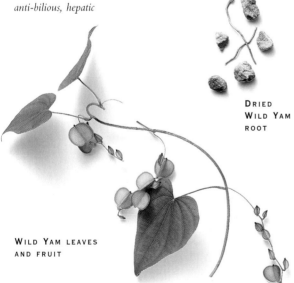

WILD YAM LEAVES
AND FRUIT

COMBINATIONS

To relieve intestinal colic it may be combined with Calamus, Chamomile and Ginger. For rheumatoid arthritis it may be used with Black Cohosh.

Drosera rotundifolia

PLANT FAMILY DROSERACEAE

SUNDEW

Sundew may be used with great benefit in bronchitis and whooping cough. The presence of plumbagin helps to explain this, as it has been shown to be active against streptococcus, staphylococcus and pneumococcus bacteria. Sundew will also help with infections in other parts of the respiratory tract. Its relaxing effect upon involuntary muscles helps in the relief of asthma. In addition to the pulmonary conditions it has a long history in the treatment of stomach ulcers.

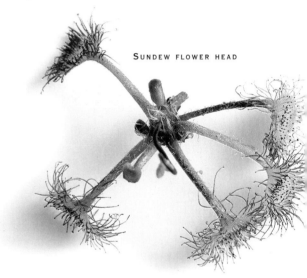

SUNDEW FLOWER HEAD

PART USED *Entire plant*

COLLECTION *The whole of the plant is gathered during the flowering period in mid-summer or late summer.*

CONSTITUENTS *Naphthaquinones including plumbagin; flavonoids, tannins, citric and malic acid*

ACTIONS *Anti-spasmodic, demulcent, expectorant*

PREPARATION AND DOSAGE

INFUSION

POUR A CUP OF BOILING WATER ONTO 1 TEASPOONFUL OF THE DRIED HERB AND LEAVE TO INFUSE FOR 10–15 MINUTES. THIS SHOULD BE DRUNK THREE TIMES A DAY.

TINCTURE

TAKE 1–2ML OF THE TINCTURE THREE TIMES A DAY.

COMBINATIONS

In the treatment of asthma Sundew may be used with Grindelia and Pill-bearing Spurge.

Dryopteris filix-mas

PLANT FAMILY POLYPODIACEAE

MALE FERN

Male Fern is one of the most effective treatments for killing tapeworm. It is, however, potentially poisonous in overdose and should only be used under medical supervision.

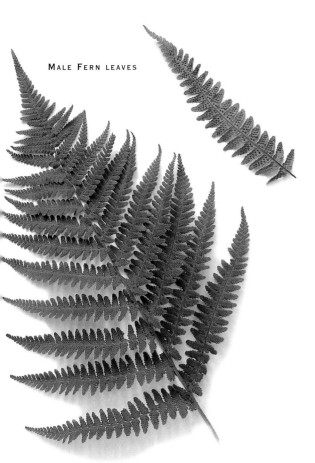

MALE FERN LEAVES

PART USED *Rhizome freed of root*

COLLECTION *The rhizome is unearthed in the Fall.*

CONSTITUENTS *Filicin, filixid acid, tannin, phloroglucin derivatives, traces of essential oil*

ACTIONS *Vermifuge*

CAUTION

USE ONLY UNDER MEDICAL SUPERVISION.

PREPARATION AND DOSAGE

DO NOT MAKE HOME REMEDIES WITH THIS HERB.

Echinacea angustifolia

PLANT FAMILY COMPOSITAE

ECHINACEA

Echinacea is the prime remedy to help the body rid itself of microbial infections. It is effective against both bacterial and viral attacks. It may be used in conditions such as boils, septicemia and other infections of that sort. In conjunction with other herbs it may be used for any infection anywhere in the body. For example, in combination with Yarrow or Bearberry it will effectively stop cystitis. It is especially useful for infections of the upper respiratory tract such as laryngitis, tonsillitis, and for catarrhal conditions of the nose and sinus. In general it may be used widely and safely. The tincture or decoction may be used as a mouthwash in the treatment of pyorrhea and gingivitis. As a lotion it helps septic sores and cuts.

ECHINACEA
SHOOT AND FLOWER

PREPARATION AND DOSAGE

DECOCTION

PUT 1–2 TEASPOONFULS OF THE ROOT IN ONE CUP OF WATER AND BRING IT SLOWLY TO THE BOIL. LET IT SIMMER FOR 10–15 MINUTES. THIS SHOULD BE DRUNK THREE TIMES A DAY.

TINCTURE

TAKE 1–4ML OF THE TINCTURE THREE TIMES A DAY.

PART USED
Cone flower, roots

COLLECTION *The roots should be unearthed in the Fall. It is suggested that the fresh extract is more effective than the dried root.*

CONSTITUENTS *Volatile oil, glycoside, echinaceine, phenolics*

ACTIONS
Anti-microbial, alterative, anti-catarrhal, tonic

COMBINATIONS
This useful herb may be combined with many different plants.

Elettaria cardamomum

PLANT FAMILY ZINGIBERACEAE

CARDAMON

This valuable culinary herb may be used to treat flatulent dyspepsia and to relieve griping pains. It will stimulate the appetite and the flow of saliva. It is often used as a carminative flavouring agent when purgatives are given.

PREPARATION AND DOSAGE

INFUSION

POUR A CUP OF BOILING WATER ONTO 1 TEASPOONFUL OF THE FRESHLY CRUSHED SEEDS AND LEAVE TO INFUSE FOR 10–15 MINUTES. THIS SHOULD BE DRUNK THREE TIMES A DAY.

IF TREATING FLATULENCE OR LOSS OF APPETITE, DRINK HALF AN HOUR BEFORE MEALS.

PART USED *Seeds*

COLLECTION *The seeds are mainly obtained from commercial plants in Sri Lanka or southern India where the crop is gathered between mid-Fall and early winter.*

CONSTITUENTS *Up to 4% volatile oil including terpineol, cineole, limonene, sabinene and pinene*

ACTIONS *Carminative, sialagogue, orexigenic, aromatic, stimulant*

CARDAMON SEEDS

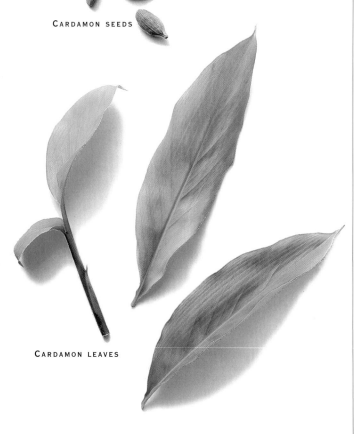

CARDAMON LEAVES

Eleutherococcus senticosus

PLANT FAMILY CRUCIFERAE

SIBERIAN GINSENG

This herb may safely be used to increase stamina in the face of undue demands and stress. These may be physical or mental – they are one to the body. Thus it is used for debility, exhaustion and depression, except where these are due to a specific medical reason that calls for defined treatment. It has a growing reputation for increasing all kinds of body resistance. However, the claims may be over-enthusiastic. The claims for circulatory effects come from excellent Russian research which has not yet been verified elsewhere.

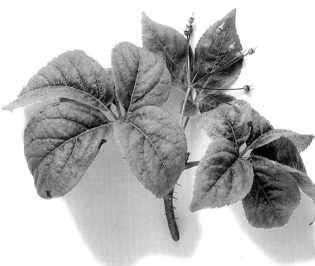

SIBERIAN GINSENG LEAVES AND FLOWERS

PART USED *Root*

COLLECTION *The roots are collected whilst the plant is dormant in the winter.*

CONSTITUENTS *The research so far indicates the pharmacologically important group to be triterpenoid saponins called eleutherosides.*

ACTIONS *Adaptogen, a circulatory stimulant, vasodilator*

PREPARATION AND DOSAGE

THIS HERB IS USUALLY AVAILABLE AS A TABLET OR POWDER, THE DOSAGE OF WHICH SHOULD BE 0.2–1G THREE TIMES A DAY OVER A PERIOD OF TIME.

COMBINATIONS

It is best used by itself, or with herbs that are specifically indicated for a person.

Ephedra sinica

PLANT FAMILY EPHEDRACEAE

EPHEDRA

The alkaloids present in Ephedra, or Ma Huang, have apparently opposite effects on the body. The overall action however is one of balance and benefit. It is used with great success in the treatment of asthma and associated conditions due to its power to relieve spasms in the bronchial tubes. It is thus used in bronchial asthma, bronchitis and whooping cough. It also reduces allergic reactions, giving it a role in the treatment of hayfever and other allergies. It may be used in the treatment of low blood pressure and circulatory insufficiency.

PART USED *Aerial stems*

COLLECTION *Gather the young branches in the Fall before the first frost, as the alkaloid content is then highest. They may be dried in the sun.*

CONSTITUENTS *More than 1.25% alkaloids which include ephedrine and norephedrine; tannins, saponin, flavone, essential oil*

ACTIONS *Vasodilator, hypertensive, circulatory stimulant, anti-allergic*

PREPARATION AND DOSAGE

DECOCTION

PUT 1–2 TEASPOONFULS OF THE DRIED HERB IN ONE CUP OF WATER, BRING IT TO THE BOIL AND SIMMER FOR 10–15 MINUTES. THIS SHOULD BE DRUNK THREE TIMES A DAY.

TINCTURE

TAKE 1–4ML OF THE TINCTURE THREE TIMES A DAY.

CAUTION

AVOID IN HIGH BLOOD PRESSURE OR ANXIETY.

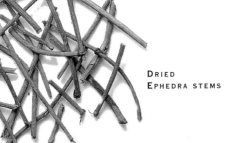

DRIED EPHEDRA STEMS

COMBINATIONS

Ephedra combines well with Lobelia and Thyme for asthmatic problems.

Equisetum arvense

PLANT FAMILY EQUISETACEAE

HORSETAIL

Horsetail is an excellent astringent for the genito-urinary system, reducing hemorrhage and healing wounds thanks to the high silica content. Whilst it acts as a mild diuretic, its toning and astringent actions make it invaluable in the treatment of incontinence and bed wetting in children. It is considered a specific in cases of inflammation or benign enlargement of the prostate gland. Externally it is a vulnerary (healing wounds). In some cases it has been found to ease the pain of rheumatism and stimulate the healing of chilblains.

HORSETAIL STEM AND LEAVES

PART USED
Dried aerial stems

COLLECTION *Collect in early summer. Cut the plants just above the ground, hang in bundles and dry in an airy place.*

CONSTITUENTS *Silicic acid (a source of silicon), saponin, flavone glycosides, organic acids, nicotine, palustrine*

ACTIONS *Astringent, diuretic, vulnerary*

PREPARATION AND DOSAGE

INFUSION

POUR A CUP OF BOILING WATER ONTO 2 TEASPOONFULS OF THE DRIED PLANT AND LET INFUSE FOR 15–20 MINUTES. THIS SHOULD BE DRUNK THREE TIMES A DAY.

BATH

A USEFUL BATH CAN BE MADE TO HELP IN RHEUMATIC PAIN AND CHILBLAINS. ALLOW 100G/3½OZ OF THE HERB TO STEEP IN HOT WATER FOR AN HOUR. ADD THIS TO THE BATH.

TINCTURE

TAKE 2–4ML OF THE TINCTURE THREE TIMES A DAY.

COMBINATIONS

Horsetail is often combined with Hydrangea in the treatment of prostate troubles.

Eryngium maritimum

PLANT FAMILY UMBELLIFERAE

SEA HOLLY

This most impressive plant of sandy shores is used in a whole range of urinary conditions. It is a diuretic in the herbal sense that it has an affinity for the system rather than being a strong remover of water from the body. It has most use in kidney stones and gravel, especially if there is an associated restriction of urine flow. It will ease colic due to urinary problems as well as reducing hemorrhage. It can help in cystitis, urethritis and enlarged and inflamed prostate glands.

PREPARATION AND DOSAGE

DECOCTION

PUT 1–2 TEASPOONFULS OF THE ROOT IN A CUP OF WATER, BRING TO THE BOIL AND SIMMER FOR 10 MINUTES. THIS SHOULD BE DRUNK THREE TIMES A DAY.

TINCTURE

TAKE 1–2ML OF THE TINCTURE THREE TIMES A DAY.

PART USED *Dried roots*

COLLECTION *The roots are unearthed from their shoreline habitat at the end of the flowering time.*

CONSTITUENTS *Saponins, coumarins, plant acids, flavonoids*

ACTIONS *Diuretic, anti-lithic*

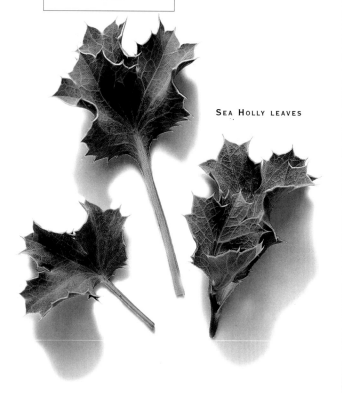

SEA HOLLY LEAVES

Eschscholzia california

PLANT FAMILY PAPAVERACEAE

CALIFORNIAN POPPY

Californian Poppy has the reputation of being a non-addictive alternative to the Opium Poppy, though it is less powerful. It has been used as a sedative and hypnotic for children, where there is over-excitability and sleeplessness. It can be used wherever an anti-spasmodic remedy is required. The Native North Americans used it for colic pains and it may be useful in the treatment of gall-bladder colic.

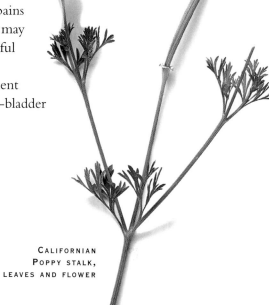

CALIFORNIAN POPPY STALK, LEAVES AND FLOWER

PART USED *Dried aerial parts*

COLLECTION *The aerial parts are collected at the time of flowering, which is between early summer and early Fall. They should be dried in the shade.*

CONSTITUENTS *Alkaloids similar to Opium Poppy, flavone glycosides*

ACTIONS *Sedative, hypnotic, anti-spasmodic, anodyne*

PREPARATION AND DOSAGE

INFUSION

POUR A CUP OF BOILING WATER ONTO 1–2 TEASPOONFULS OF THE DRIED HERB AND LEAVE TO INFUSE FOR 10 MINUTES. A CUP SHOULD BE DRUNK AT NIGHT TO PROMOTE RESTFUL SLEEP.

TINCTURE

TAKE 1–4ML OF THE TINCTURE AT NIGHT.

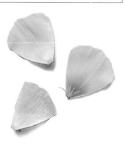

Euonymus atropurpureus

PLANT FAMILY CELASTRACEAE

WAHOO

Wahoo is one of the primary liver herbs. It acts to remove congestion from the liver, allowing the free flow of bile and so helping the digestive process. It may be used in the treatment of jaundice and gall-bladder problems such as inflammation and pain or congestion due to stones. It will relieve constipation where this is due to liver or gall-bladder problems. Through its normalizing action upon the liver it may help in a range of skin problems where there is a possible involvement of the liver.

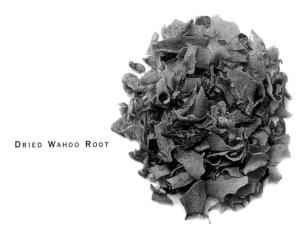

DRIED WAHOO ROOT

PREPARATION AND DOSAGE

DECOCTION

POUR A CUP OF WATER ONTO ½–1 TEASPOONFUL OF THE BARK. BRING TO THE BOIL AND LET INFUSE FOR 10–15 MINUTES. THIS SHOULD BE DRUNK THREE TIMES A DAY.

TINCTURE

TAKE 1–2ML OF THE TINCTURE THREE TIMES A DAY.

PART USED *Root bark*

COLLECTION *The bark is stripped off roots that have been unearthed in the Fall. Stem bark can be used as a substitute.*

CONSTITUENTS *Euonymol, euonysterol, atropurpurol, dulcitol, citrullol, fatty acids*

ACTIONS *Cholagogue, laxative, diuretic, circulatory stimulant, hepatic*

Eupatorium perfoliatum

PLANT FAMILY COMPOSITAE

BONESET

Boneset is perhaps the best remedy for the relief of the associated symptoms that accompany influenza. It will speedily relieve the aches and pains as well as aid the body in dealing with any fever that is present. Boneset may also be used to help clear the upper respiratory tract of mucous congestion. Its mild aperient activity will help clear the body of any build-up of waste and ease constipation. This remedy may safely be used in any fever and also as a general cleansing agent. It may provide symptomatic aid in the treatment of muscular rheumatism.

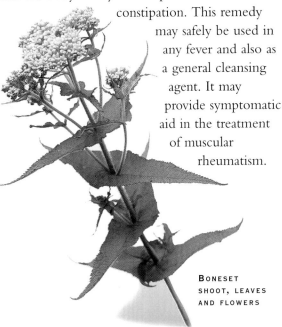

BONESET SHOOT, LEAVES AND FLOWERS

PART USED
Dried aerial parts

COLLECTION *Boneset should be collected as soon as the flowers open in late summer or early Fall.*

CONSTITUENTS *A bitter glycoside called eupatorin, volatile oil, gallic acid, a glucosidal tannin*

ACTIONS *Diaphoretic, aperient, tonic, anti-spasmodic, anti-catarrhal, bitter, diuretic, emetic*

PREPARATION AND DOSAGE

INFUSION

POUR A CUP OF BOILING WATER ONTO 1–2 TEASPOONFULS OF THE DRIED HERB AND LEAVE TO INFUSE FOR 10–15 MINUTES. THIS SHOULD BE DRUNK AS HOT AS POSSIBLE. DURING FEVERS OR FLU IT SHOULD BE DRUNK EVERY HALF HOUR.

TINCTURE

TAKE 2–4ML OF THE TINCTURE THREE TIMES A DAY.

COMBINATIONS
In the treatment of influenza it may be combined with Yarrow, Elder Flowers, Cayenne or Ginger.

Eupatorium purpureum

PLANT FAMILY COMPOSITAE

GRAVEL ROOT

Gravel Root is used primarily for kidney stones or gravel. In urinary infections such as cystitis and urethritis it may be used with benefit, whilst it can also play a useful role in a systemic treatment of rheumatism and gout.

PART USED
Rhizome and root

COLLECTION *The root and rhizome should be dug up in the Fall after the plant has stopped flowering. Wash thoroughly, slice and dry.*

CONSTITUENTS *Contains up to 0.07% of volatile oil, a yellow flavonoid called euparin, resin*

ACTIONS *Diuretic, anti-lithic, anti-rheumatic, tonic*

> ### PREPARATION AND DOSAGE
>
> #### DECOCTION
> PUT 1 TEASPOONFUL OF THE HERB IN A CUP OF WATER, BRING TO THE BOIL AND SIMMER FOR 10 MINUTES. THIS SHOULD BE DRUNK THREE TIMES A DAY.
>
> #### TINCTURE
> TAKE 1–2ML OF THE TINCTURE THREE TIMES A DAY.

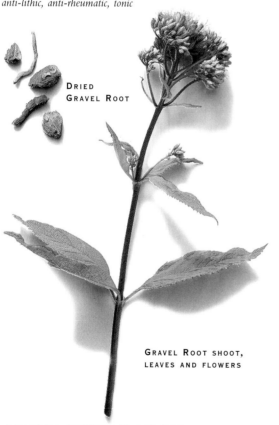

DRIED GRAVEL ROOT

GRAVEL ROOT SHOOT, LEAVES AND FLOWERS

COMBINATIONS
For kidney stones or gravel it combines well with Parsley Piert, Pellitory of the Wall or Hydrangea.

Euphorbia hirta

PLANT FAMILY EUPHORBIACEAE

PILL-BEARING SPURGE

Pill-bearing Spurge has a relaxing effect upon the smooth muscles of the lungs and acts with great benefit in conditions such as asthma and bronchitis. It will also relieve spasms in the larynx, helping nervous coughs. It will help to relieve upper respiratory catarrh. This herb has a specific action of destroying the organisms that cause amebic infections in the intestines.

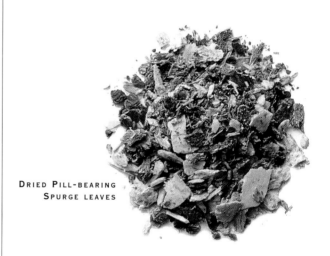

DRIED PILL-BEARING SPURGE LEAVES

PART USED *Aerial parts*

COLLECTION *Gather the aerial parts whilst Pill-bearing Spurge is in flower.*

CONSTITUENTS *Glycoside, alkaloids, sterols, tannins, phorbic acid*

ACTIONS *Anti-asthmatic, expectorant, anti-spasmodic*

> ### PREPARATION AND DOSAGE
>
> #### INFUSION
> POUR A CUP OF BOILING WATER ONTO ½–1 TEASPOONFUL OF THE DRIED LEAVES AND LET INFUSE FOR 10–15 MINUTES. THIS SHOULD BE DRUNK THREE TIMES A DAY.
>
> #### TINCTURE
> TAKE 1–2ML OF THE TINCTURE THREE TIMES A DAY.

COMBINATIONS
For the treatment of asthmatic conditions it will combine well with Grindelia and Lobelia.

Euphrasia officinalis

PLANT FAMILY SCROPHULARIACEAE

EYEBRIGHT

Eyebright is an excellent remedy for the problems of mucous membranes. The combination of anti-inflammatory and astringent properties makes it relevant in many conditions. Used internally it is a powerful anti-catarrhal and thus may be used in nasal catarrh, sinusitis and other congestive states. It is best known for its use in conditions of the eye, where it is helpful in acute or chronic inflammations, stinging and weeping eyes as well as over-sensitivity to light. Used as a compress and taken internally it is used in conjunctivitis and blepharitis.

PREPARATION AND DOSAGE

INFUSION

POUR A CUP OF BOILING WATER ONTO 1 TEASPOONFUL OF THE DRIED HERB AND LEAVE TO INFUSE FOR 5–10 MINUTES. THIS SHOULD BE DRUNK THREE TIMES A DAY.

COMPRESS

PLACE A TEASPOONFUL OF THE DRIED HERB IN 500ML/1PT OF WATER AND BOIL FOR 10 MINUTES, LET COOL SLIGHTLY. MOISTEN A COMPRESS (COTTON WOOL, GAUZE OR MUSLIN) IN THE LUKEWARM LIQUID, WRING OUT SLIGHTLY AND PLACE OVER THE EYES. LEAVE THE COMPRESS IN PLACE FOR 15 MINUTES. REPEAT SEVERAL TIMES A DAY.

TINCTURE

TAKE 1–4ML OF THE TINCTURE THREE TIMES A DAY.

DRIED EYEBRIGHT

PART USED
Dried aerial parts

COLLECTION Gather the whole plant in bloom in late summer or Fall and dry it in an airy place.

CONSTITUENTS Glycosides including aucubin, tannins, resins, volatile oil

ACTIONS Anti-catarrhal, astringent, anti-inflammatory, tonic

COMBINATIONS
In catarrhal conditions it combines well with Golden Rod, Elder Flower or Golden Seal. In allergic conditions where the eyes are affected it may be combined with Ephedra. As an eye lotion it mixes with Golden Seal and distilled Witch Hazel.

Filipendula ulmaria

PLANT FAMILY ROSACEAE

MEADOWSWEET

Meadowsweet is one of the best digestive remedies available and as such will be indicated in most conditions, if they are approached holistically. It acts to protect and soothe the mucous membranes of the digestive tract, reducing excess acidity and easing nausea. It is used in the treatment of heartburn, hyperacidity, gastric and peptic ulceration. Its gentle astringency is useful in treating diarrhea in children. The presence of aspirin-like chemicals explains Meadowsweet's action in reducing fever and relieving the pain of rheumatism in muscles and joints.

MEADOWSWEET SHOOTS, LEAVES AND FLOWERS

PART USED Aerial parts

COLLECTION The fully opened flowers and leaves are picked at the time of flowering, which is between early summer and late summer. They should be dried gently at a temperature not exceeding 40°C/104°F.

CONSTITUENTS Essential oil with salicylic acid compounds called spiraeine and gaultherin; salicylic acid, tannin, citric acid

ACTIONS Anti-rheumatic, anti-inflammatory, stomachic, anti-emetic, astringent, aromatic

PREPARATION AND DOSAGE

INFUSION

POUR A CUP OF BOILING WATER ONTO 1–2 TEASPOONFULS OF THE DRIED HERB AND LEAVE TO INFUSE FOR 10–15 MINUTES. THIS SHOULD BE DRUNK THREE TIMES A DAY OR AS NEEDED.

TINCTURE

TAKE 1–4ML OF THE TINCTURE THREE TIMES A DAY.

Foeniculum vulgare

PLANT FAMILY UMBELLIFERAE

FENNEL

Fennel is an excellent stomach and intestinal remedy which relieves flatulence and colic whilst also stimulating the digestion and appetite. It is similar to Aniseed in its calming effect on bronchitis and coughs. It may be used to flavour cough remedies. Fennel will increase the flow of milk in nursing mothers. Externally the oil eases muscular and rheumatic pains. The infusion may be used to treat conjunctivitis and inflammation of the eyelids (blepharitis) as a compress.

PREPARATION AND DOSAGE

INFUSION

POUR A CUP OF BOILING WATER ONTO 1–2 TEASPOONFULS OF SLIGHTLY CRUSHED SEEDS AND LEAVE TO INFUSE FOR 10 MINUTES. THIS SHOULD BE DRUNK THREE TIMES A DAY. TO EASE FLATULENCE, TAKE A CUP HALF AN HOUR BEFORE MEALS.

TINCTURE

TAKE 2–4ML OF THE TINCTURE THREE TIMES A DAY.

PART USED *Seeds*

COLLECTION *Harvest the seeds when ripe and split in the Fall. Cut the brown umbel off. Comb the seeds to clean them. Dry [slightly] in the shade.*

CONSTITUENTS *Up to 6% volatile oil which includes anethole and fenchone; fatty oil 10%*

ACTIONS *Carminative, aromatic, anti-spasmodic, stimulant, galactogogue, rubefacient, expectorant, anti-emetic, diaphoretic, hepatic*

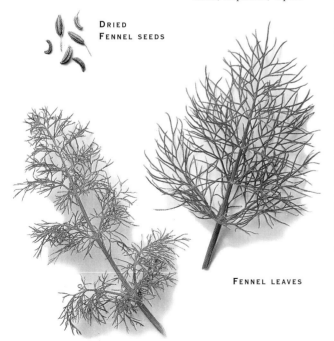

DRIED FENNEL SEEDS

FENNEL LEAVES

Fucus vesiculosus

PLANT FAMILY FUCACEAE

BLADDERWRACK

Bladderwrack, or Kelp, has proved most useful in the treatment of underactive thyroid glands and goitre. Through the regulation of thyroid function there is an improvement in all the associated symptoms. Where obesity is associated with thyroid trouble, this herb may be very helpful in reducing the excess weight. It has a reputation in helping the relief of rheumatism and rheumatoid arthritis, both used internally and as an external application upon inflamed joints.

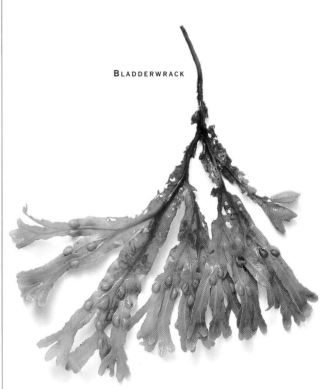

BLADDERWRACK

PART USED *Whole plant, which is a common seaweed*

COLLECTION *The entire plant is gathered from rocks along the seashore in early summer and dried in the sun.*

CONSTITUENTS *It is rich in algin and mannitol, carotene and zeaxanthin. Iodine and bromine are present.*

ACTIONS *Anti-hypothyroid, anti-rheumatic, alterative*

PREPARATION AND DOSAGE

IT MAY USEFULLY BE TAKEN IN TABLET FORM AS A DIETARY SUPPLEMENT OR AS AN INFUSION BY POURING A CUP OF BOILING WATER ONTO 2–3 TEASPOONFULS OF THE DRIED HERB AND LEAVING IT TO STEEP FOR 10 MINUTES. THIS SHOULD BE DRUNK THREE TIMES A DAY.

FUMITORY

Fumaria officinalis

PLANT FAMILY FUMARIACEAE

Fumitory has a long history of use in the treatment of skin problems such as eczema and acne. Its action is probably due to a general cleansing mediated via the kidneys and liver. Fumitory may also be used as an eyewash to ease conjunctivitis.

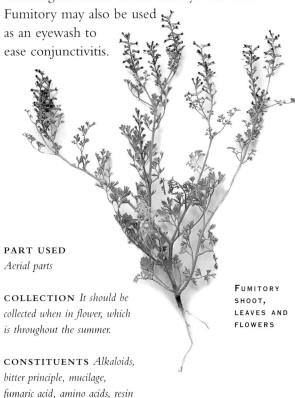

PART USED
Aerial parts

COLLECTION *It should be collected when in flower, which is throughout the summer.*

CONSTITUENTS *Alkaloids, bitter principle, mucilage, fumaric acid, amino acids, resin*

ACTIONS *Diuretic, laxative, alterative, cholagogue, hepatic, tonic*

FUMITORY SHOOT, LEAVES AND FLOWERS

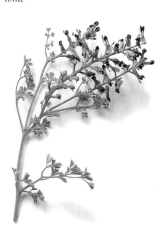

PREPARATION AND DOSAGE

INFUSION

POUR A CUP OF BOILING WATER ONTO 1–2 TEASPOONFULS OF THE DRIED HERB AND LET INFUSE FOR 10–15 MINUTES. THIS SHOULD BE DRUNK FREELY, BUT FOR SKIN PROBLEMS IT SHOULD BE DRUNK AT LEAST THREE TIMES A DAY.

TINCTURE

TAKE 1–2ML OF THE TINCTURE THREE TIMES A DAY.

COMBINATIONS
It may usefully be combined with Burdock, Cleavers or Figwort.

GOAT'S RUE

Galega officinalis

PLANT FAMILY PAPILIONACEAE

Goat's Rue is one of many herbal remedies with the action of reducing blood sugar levels. Its use is thus indicated in the treatment of diabetes mellitus. This must not replace insulin therapy, however, and should occur under professional supervision. It is also a powerful galactogogue, stimulating the production and flow of milk. It has been shown to increase milk output by up to 50% in some cases. It may also stimulate the development of the mammary glands.

PREPARATION AND DOSAGE

INFUSION

POUR A CUP OF BOILING WATER ONTO 1 TEASPOONFUL OF THE DRIED LEAVES AND LET INFUSE FOR 10–15 MINUTES. THIS SHOULD BE DRUNK TWICE A DAY.

TINCTURE

TAKE 1–2ML OF THE TINCTURE THREE TIMES A DAY.

PART USED
Dried aerial parts

COLLECTION *The stalks with the leaves and flowers are gathered at the time of flowering, which is between mid-summer and late summer. Dry in the shade.*

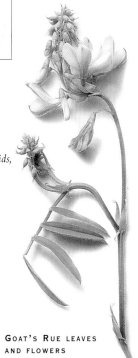

CONSTITUENTS *Alkaloids, saponins, flavone glycosides, bitters, tannin*

ACTIONS *Reduces blood sugar, galactogogue, diuretic, diaphoretic*

GOAT'S RUE LEAVES AND FLOWERS

Galium aparine

PLANT FAMILY RUBIACEAE

CLEAVERS

Cleavers, also known as Goosegrass and Clives, is a very valuable plant and is perhaps the best tonic to the lymphatic system available. As a lymphatic tonic with alterative and diuretic actions it may be used in a wide range of problems where the lymphatic system is involved. Thus it would be used in swollen glands (lymphadenitis) anywhere in the body and especially in tonsillitis and in adenoid trouble. It is widely used in skin conditions, especially in the dry varieties such as psoriasis. It will be useful in the treatment of cystitis and other urinary conditions where there is pain and may be combined with demulcents for this. There is a long tradition for the use of Cleavers in the treatment of ulcers and tumours, which may be the result of the lymphatic drainage.

CLEAVERS SHOOTS, LEAVES AND FLOWERS

PART USED *Dried aerial parts and the fresh expressed juice*

COLLECTION *The plant should be gathered before flowering and dried in the shade.*

CONSTITUENTS *Glycoside asperuloside, gallotannic acid, citric acid*

ACTIONS *Diuretic, alterative, anti-inflammatory, tonic, astringent, anti-neoplastic, hepatic, laxative, vulnerary*

> **PREPARATION AND DOSAGE**
>
> **INFUSION**
>
> POUR A CUP OF BOILING WATER ONTO 2–3 TEASPOONFULS OF THE DRIED HERB AND LEAVE TO INFUSE FOR 10–15 MINUTES. THIS SHOULD BE DRUNK THREE TIMES A DAY.
>
> **TINCTURE**
>
> TAKE 2–4ML OF THE TINCTURE THREE TIMES A DAY.

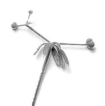

COMBINATIONS

For the lymphatic system it will work well with Poke Root, Echinacea and Marigold. For skin conditions it is best combined with Yellow Dock and Burdock.

Gaultheria procumbens

PLANT FAMILY ERICACEAE

WINTERGREEN

Wintergreen is largely used for its oil, which is naturally rich in methyl salicylate. This chemical is the basis of the aspirin group and explains much of the activity of Wintergreen in reducing pain and inflammation in acute rheumatism. It is most commonly used externally as a liniment for the treatment of chronic forms of muscular and skeletal troubles like lumbago and sciatica. Internally the plant has been used for its diuretic and emmenagogic activity. It is reported to be a galactogogue.

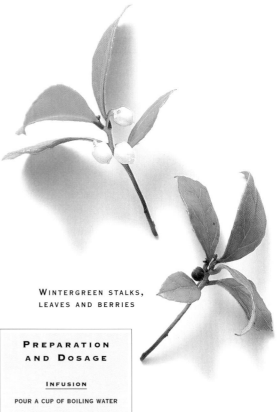

WINTERGREEN STALKS, LEAVES AND BERRIES

> **PREPARATION AND DOSAGE**
>
> **INFUSION**
>
> POUR A CUP OF BOILING WATER ONTO 1 TEASPOONFUL OF THE DRIED LEAVES AND LET INFUSE FOR 10–15 MINUTES. THIS SHOULD BE DRUNK THREE TIMES A DAY.
>
> **LINIMENTS & POULTICE**
>
> SEE SECTION ON 'PREPARATIONS' PAGE 31 FOR DETAILS.

PART USED *Leaves*

COLLECTION *The leaves can be gathered throughout the year but the summer is preferable. Dry in the shade.*

CONSTITUENTS *Volatile oil, which is largely salicylate*

ACTIONS *Anodyne, astringent, stimulant, diuretic, emmenagogue, galactogogue*

Gentiana lutea

PLANT FAMILY GENTIANACEAE

GENTIAN

Gentian is an excellent bitter which, as do all bitters, stimulates the appetite and digestion via a general stimulation of the digestive juices. Thus it promotes the production of saliva, gastric juices and bile. It also accelerates the emptying of the stomach. It is indicated wherever there is a lack of appetite and sluggishness of the digestive system. It may thus be used where the symptoms of sluggish digestion appear, these being dyspepsia and flatulence. Through the stimulation of the digestion it has a generally fortifying effect.

PART USED *Dried rhizome and root*

COLLECTION *The underground parts are dug up in the Fall, sliced and dried slowly.*

CONSTITUENTS *Bitter principles including gentiopicrin and amarogentine, pectin, tannin, mucilage, sugar*

ACTIONS *Bitter, gastric stimulant, sialagogue, cholagogue, anti-microbial, emmenagogue, hepatic, tonic*

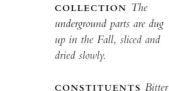

GENTIAN ROOT AND LEAVES

PREPARATION AND DOSAGE

DECOCTION

PUT ½ TEASPOONFUL OF THE SHREDDED ROOT IN A CUP OF WATER AND BOIL FOR 5 MINUTES. THIS SHOULD BE DRUNK WARM ABOUT 15–30 MINUTES BEFORE MEALS, OR AT ANY TIME WHEN ACUTE STOMACH PAINS RESULT FROM A FEELING OF FULLNESS.

TINCTURE

TAKE 1–4ML OF THE TINCTURE THREE TIMES A DAY ACCORDING TO THE ABOVE GUIDELINES.

COMBINATIONS

Gentian is often used with other digestives such as Ginger and Cardamon.

Geranium maculatum

PLANT FAMILY GERANIACEAE

AMERICAN CRANESBILL

American Cranesbill is an effective astringent used in diarrhea, dysentery and hemorrhoids. When bleeding accompanies duodenal or gastric ulceration this remedy is used in combination with other relevant herbs. Where blood is lost in the feces, this herb will help, though careful diagnosis is vital. It may be used when excessive blood loss during menstruation (menorrhagia) or a uterine hemorrhage (metrorrhagia) occur. As a douche it can be used in leucorrhea.

AMERICAN CRANESBILL LEAVES

PREPARATION AND DOSAGE

DECOCTION

PUT 1–2 TEASPOONFULS OF THE RHIZOME IN A CUP OF COLD WATER AND BRING TO THE BOIL. LET SIMMER FOR 10–15 MINUTES. THIS SHOULD BE DRUNK THREE TIMES A DAY.

TINCTURE

TAKE 2–4ML OF THE TINCTURE THREE TIMES A DAY.

PART USED *Rhizome*

COLLECTION *The rhizome is unearthed in early Fall and cut into pieces and dried.*

CONSTITUENTS *12–25% tannins, with the level being highest just before flowering*

ACTIONS *Astringent, anti-hemorrhagic, anti-inflammatory, vulnerary, anti-catarrhal*

COMBINATIONS

In peptic ulcers it may be used with Meadowsweet, Comfrey, Marshmallow or Agrimony. In leucorrhea it can be combined with Beth Root.

Geum urbanum

PLANT FAMILY ROSACEAE

AVENS

Its strong astringency combined with its digestive properties give Avens its role in many intestinal troubles, as in diarrhea, dysentery, mucous colitis and similar conditions. It may be used to settle nausea and to allay vomiting. Its astringency also explains its use in the treatment of gingivitis and sore throats as a mouthwash or gargle. It may also be used internally in feverish colds and in catarrhs. As a douche, Avens will be of value in leucorrhea.

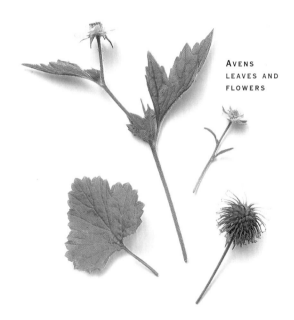

AVENS
LEAVES AND
FLOWERS

PREPARATION AND DOSAGE

DECOCTION

PLACE ONE TEASPOONFUL OF THE ROOT IN A CUP OF COLD WATER, BRING IT TO THE BOIL AND LET IT SIMMER FOR 5 MINUTES. TAKE ONE CUP THREE TIMES DAILY.

TINCTURE

TAKE 1–3ML OF THE TINCTURE THREE TIMES A DAY.

PART USED *Roots and aerial parts*

COLLECTION *The roots are collected in the spring when they are richest in volatile oils. The aerial parts are collected in mid-summer when the flowers are at their best.*

CONSTITUENTS *Essential oils with gein and eugenol, tannins, bitter principle, flavone, resin, organic acids*

ACTIONS *Astringent, styptic, diaphoretic, aromatic*

COMBINATIONS
It is often combined with Agrimony in the treatment of digestive troubles such as colitis.

Glechoma hederacea

PLANT FAMILY LABIATAE

GROUND IVY

Ground Ivy may be used to treat catarrhal conditions whether in the sinus region or in the chest. It will aid in the healing of coughs and bronchitis, but works better if combined with other remedies. Where the catarrh has built up in the middle ear and is causing noises (tinnitus), Ground Ivy can prove most beneficial. The astringency of the herb helps in the treatment of diarrhea and hemorrhoids. It may also be used to treat cystitis.

PREPARATION AND DOSAGE

INFUSION

POUR A CUP OF BOILING WATER ONTO 1 TEASPOONFUL OF THE DRIED LEAVES AND LET INFUSE FOR 10–15 MINUTES. THIS SHOULD BE DRUNK THREE TIMES A DAY.

TINCTURE

TAKE 1–4ML OF THE TINCTURE THREE TIMES A DAY.

PART USED *Aerial parts*

COLLECTION *The flowering stems should be collected between mid-spring and early summer.*

CONSTITUENTS *Bitter, tannin, volatile oil, resin, saponin*

ACTIONS *Anti-catarrhal, astringent, expectorant, diuretic, vulnerary, stimulant*

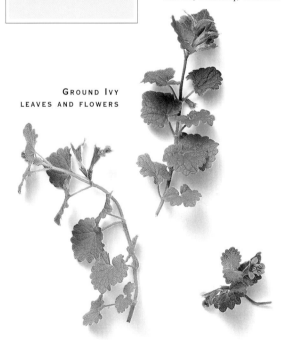

GROUND IVY
LEAVES AND FLOWERS

COMBINATIONS
For coughs it may be used with Coltsfoot, White Horehound and Elecampane. For sinus catarrh combine it with Golden Rod.

Glycyrrhiza glabra

PLANT FAMILY LEGUMINOSAE

LICORICE

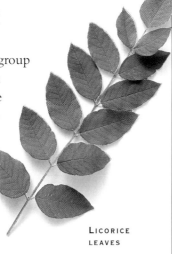

Licorice is one of a group of plants that has a marked effect upon the endocrine system. The glycosides present have a structure that is similar to the natural steroids of the body. The implications of this are discussed in the

LICORICE LEAVES

chapter on the glandular system. They explain the beneficial action that licorice has on the treatment of adrenal gland problems such as Addison's disease. It has a wide usage in bronchial problems such as catarrh, bronchitis and coughs in general. Licorice is used in allopathic medicine as a treatment for peptic ulceration, a similar use to its herbal use in gastritis and ulcers. It can be used in the relief of abdominal colic.

LICORICE ROOT

PART USED *Dried root*

COLLECTION *The roots are unearthed in the late Fall. Clean thoroughly and dry.*

CONSTITUENTS *Glycosides called glycyrrhizin and glycyrrhizinic acid, saponins, flavonoids, bitter, volatile oil, coumarins, asparagine, estrogenic substances*

ACTIONS *Expectorant, demulcent, anti-inflammatory, adrenal agent, anti-spasmodic, mild laxative, emollient, pectoral, tonic*

> **PREPARATION AND DOSAGE**
>
> **DECOCTION**
>
> PUT ½–1 TEASPOONFUL OF THE ROOT IN A CUP OF WATER, BRING TO THE BOIL AND SIMMER FOR 10–15 MINUTES. THIS SHOULD BE DRUNK THREE TIMES A DAY.
>
> **TINCTURE**
>
> TAKE 1–3ML OF THE TINCTURE THREE TIMES A DAY.

COMBINATIONS
For bronchitic conditions it is used with Coltsfoot or White Horehound. For gastric problems it may be combined with Marshmallow, Comfrey and Meadowsweet.

Gnaphalium uliginosum

PLANT FAMILY COMPOSITAE

CUDWEED

Cudweed may be used in all cases of upper respiratory catarrh or inflammatory conditions such as laryngitis, tonsillitis or quinsy. For these last conditions it may also be used as a gargle.

PART USED
Dried aerial parts

COLLECTION *The plant is collected in late summer when in flower and should be dried in the shade.*

CONSTITUENTS
Volatile oil

ACTIONS *Anti-catarrhal, astringent, antiseptic, anti-tussive*

> **PREPARATION AND DOSAGE**
>
> **INFUSION**
>
> POUR A CUP OF BOILING WATER ONTO 1–2 TEASPOONFULS OF THE DRIED HERB AND LEAVE TO INFUSE FOR 10 MINUTES. THIS SHOULD BE DRUNK THREE TIMES A DAY.
>
> **TINCTURE**
>
> TAKE 1–4ML OF THE TINCTURE THREE TIMES A DAY.

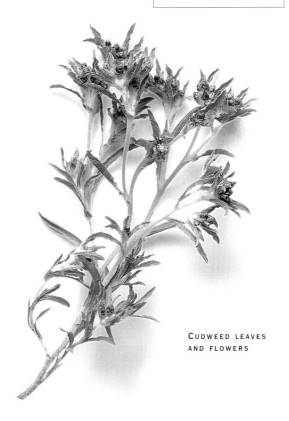

CUDWEED LEAVES AND FLOWERS

COMBINATIONS
For catarrh it may be used with Golden Rod.

Grindelia camporum

PLANT FAMILY COMPOSITAE

GRINDELIA

Grindelia acts to relax smooth muscles and heart muscles. This helps to explain its use in the treatment of asthmatic and bronchial conditions, especially where these are associated with a rapid heart beat and nervous response. It may be used in asthma, bronchitis, whooping cough and upper respiratory catarrh. Because of the relaxing effect on the heart and pulse rate, there may be a reduction in blood pressure. Externally the lotion is used in the dermatitis caused by poison ivy.

PART USED
Dried aerial parts

COLLECTION *The aerial parts are collected before the flower buds open. They are dried as soon as possible in the sun.*

CONSTITUENTS *Saponins, volatile oil, bitter alkaloids, resin, tannins*

ACTIONS *Anti-spasmodic, expectorant, hypotensive, tonic*

> **PREPARATION AND DOSAGE**
>
> **INFUSION**
>
> POUR A CUP OF BOILING WATER ONTO 1 TEASPOONFUL OF THE DRIED HERB AND LEAVE TO INFUSE FOR 10–15 MINUTES. THIS SHOULD BE DRUNK THREE TIMES A DAY.
>
> **TINCTURE**
>
> TAKE 1–2ML OF THE TINCTURE THREE TIMES A DAY.

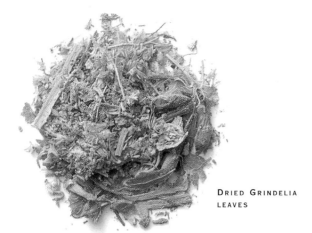

DRIED GRINDELIA LEAVES

COMBINATIONS
In the treatment of asthmatic conditions it may be used with Lobelia and Pill-bearing Spurge.

Guaiacum officinale

PLANT FAMILY ZYGOPHYLLACEAE

GUAIACUM

Guaiacum is a specific for rheumatic complaints. It is especially useful where there is much inflammation and pain present. It is thus used in chronic rheumatism and rheumatoid arthritis, particularly when an astringent is needed. It will aid in the treatment of gout and may be used as a preventative of recurrence in this disease.

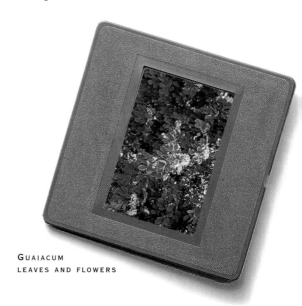

GUAIACUM LEAVES AND FLOWERS

PART USED
Heart-wood

COLLECTION *The resin of the wood exudes naturally and is often collected and used as such, otherwise the heart-wood itself is cut into small chips. The tree is found in South America and the Caribbean.*

CONSTITUENTS *Resin acids including guaiaconic, guaianetic and guaiacic acid; saponins, polyterpenoid, vanillin*

ACTIONS *Anti-rheumatic, anti-inflammatory, laxative, diaphoretic, diuretic, alterative*

> **PREPARATION AND DOSAGE**
>
> **DECOCTION**
>
> PUT 1 TEASPOONFUL OF THE WOOD CHIPS IN A CUP OF WATER, BRING TO THE BOIL AND SIMMER FOR 15–20 MINUTES. THIS SHOULD BE DRUNK THREE TIMES A DAY.

COMBINATIONS
It may be used together with Bogbean, Meadowsweet or Celery Seed.

Hagenia abyssinica

PLANT FAMILY **ROSACEAE**

KOUSSO

Kousso is an effective treatment for tapeworm. Its action is due to a potent natural chemical which has led to its inclusion in the poisons list in the UK.

PART USED *Flowers and unripe fruit*

COLLECTION *Flowers and fruits are collected from female plants in East Africa.*

CONSTITUENTS *Volatile oil, bitter principle, koso-toxin*

ACTIONS *Purgative, anthelmintic*

PREPARATION AND DOSAGE

THE DOSAGE LEVEL GIVEN FOR THIS HERB BY MRS GRIEVE IS 14G/½OZ OF THE HERB TO 500ML/1PT OF BOILING WATER. THIS SHOULD BE TAKEN IN 110ML/4FLOZ DOSES, REPEATED AT 2-HOURLY INTERVALS.

CAUTION

KOUSSO CONTAINS A POWERFUL NATURAL CHEMICAL AND IS LISTED AS A POISON IN THE UK AND ELSEWHERE.

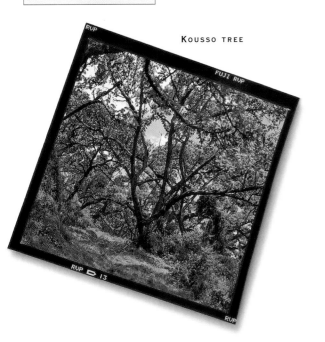

KOUSSO TREE

Hamamelis virginiana

PLANT FAMILY **HAMAMELIADACEAE**

WITCH HAZEL

This herb can be found in most households in the form of distilled Witch Hazel. It is the most applicable and easy-to-use astringent for common usage and may be used wherever there has been bleeding, either internally or externally. It is especially useful in the easing of hemorrhoids. It has a deserved reputation in the treatment of bruises and inflamed swellings, also for varicose veins. Witch Hazel will control diarrhea and aid in the easing of dysentery.

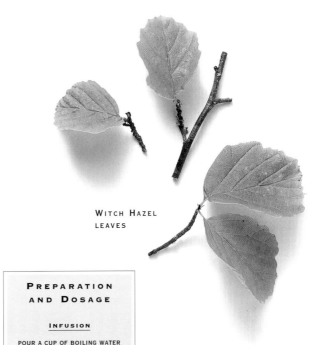

WITCH HAZEL LEAVES

PREPARATION AND DOSAGE

INFUSION

POUR A CUP OF BOILING WATER ONTO 1 TEASPOONFUL OF THE DRIED LEAVES AND LET INFUSE FOR 10–15 MINUTES. THIS SHOULD BE DRUNK THREE TIMES A DAY.

OINTMENT

WITCH HAZEL CAN BE MADE INTO AN EXCELLENT OINTMENT.

TINCTURE

TAKE 1–2ML OF THE TINCTURE THREE TIMES A DAY.

PART USED *Bark or leaves*

COLLECTION *The leaves should be gathered in early summer and mid-summer.*

CONSTITUENTS *Rich in tannin and gallic acid, bitters, traces of volatile oil*

ACTIONS *Astringent, anti-inflammatory, vulnerary*

COMBINATIONS

For the easing of hemorrhoids it will combine well with Pilewort.

Harpagophytum procumbens

PLANT FAMILY PEDALIACEAE

DEVIL'S CLAW

This valuable plant has been found effective in the treatment of some cases of arthritis. This action appears to be due to the presence of a glycoside called harpagoside that reduces inflammation in the joints. Unfortunately Devil's Claw is not always effective, but it is well worth considering in cases of arthritis where there is inflammation and pain. This plant also aids in liver and gall-bladder complaints.

PART USED *Rhizome*

COLLECTION *This plant grows in Namibia in very arid conditions. The roots are collected at the end of the rainy season.*

CONSTITUENTS
Harpagoside, harpagide, procumbine

ACTIONS
Anti-inflammatory, anodyne

> **PREPARATION AND DOSAGE**
>
> **DECOCTION**
>
> PUT ½–1 TEASPOONFUL OF THE RHIZOME INTO A CUP OF WATER, BRING TO THE BOIL AND SIMMER FOR 10–15 MINUTES. THIS SHOULD BE DRUNK THREE TIMES A DAY. IT SHOULD BE CONTINUED FOR AT LEAST ONE MONTH.
>
> **TINCTURE**
>
> TAKE 1–2ML OF THE TINCTURE THREE TIMES A DAY.

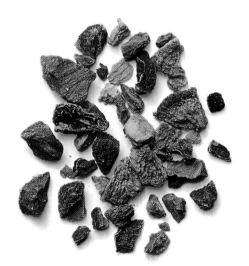

DRIED DEVIL'S CLAW

> **COMBINATIONS**
> It may be combined with Celery Seed, Bogbean or Meadowsweet in the treatment of arthritis.

Humulus lupulus

PLANT FAMILY CANNABINACEAE

HOPS

Hops have a marked relaxing effect upon the central nervous system. They are used extensively for the treatment of insomnia. They will ease tension and anxiety, and may be used where this tension leads to restlessness, headache and possibly indigestion. As an astringent with these relaxing properties they can be used in conditions such as mucous colitis. They should, however, be avoided where there is a marked degree of depression as this may be accentuated. Externally the antiseptic action is utilized for the treatment of ulcers.

HOP LEAVES AND FLOWERS

PART USED
Flower inflorescence

COLLECTION *The cones are gathered before they are fully ripe in late summer and early Fall. They should be dried with care in the shade.*

CONSTITUENTS *Lupulin, bitters, resin, volatile oil, tannin, estrogenic substance*

ACTIONS *Sedative, hypnotic, antiseptic, astringent, analgesic, bitter, nervine*

> **PREPARATION AND DOSAGE**
>
> **INFUSION**
>
> POUR A CUP OF BOILING WATER ONTO 1 TEASPOONFUL OF THE DRIED FLOWERS AND LET INFUSE FOR 10–15 MINUTES. A CUP SHOULD BE DRUNK AT NIGHT TO INDUCE SLEEP. THIS DOSE MAY BE STRENGTHENED IF NEEDED.
>
> **TINCTURE**
>
> TAKE 1–4ML OF THE TINCTURE THREE TIMES A DAY.

> **CAUTION**
> DO NOT USE IN CASES WITH MARKED DEPRESSION.

> **COMBINATIONS**
> For insomnia it can be combined with Valerian and Passion Flower.

Hydrangea arborescens

PLANT FAMILY SAXIFRAGACEAE

HYDRANGEA

Hydrangea's greatest use is in the treatment of inflamed or enlarged prostate glands. It may also be used for urinary stones or gravel associated with infections such as cystitis.

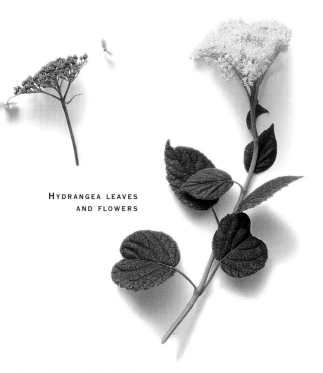

HYDRANGEA LEAVES
AND FLOWERS

**PREPARATION
AND DOSAGE**

DECOCTION

PUT 2 TEASPOONFULS OF THE
ROOT IN A CUP OF WATER, BRING
TO THE BOIL AND SIMMER FOR
10–15 MINUTES. THIS SHOULD BE
DRUNK THREE TIMES A DAY.

TINCTURE

TAKE 2–4ML OF THE TINCTURE
THREE TIMES A DAY.

PART USED *Dried roots
and rhizome*

COLLECTION *The roots
should be unearthed in the
Fall. Clean and slice whilst
still fresh as they become very
hard on drying.*

CONSTITUENTS
Glycosides, saponins, resins

ACTIONS *Diuretic,
anti-lithic, tonic*

COMBINATIONS
In kidney stones it is often combined with Parsley Piert,
Bearberry and Gravel Root. In prostate problems
it combines well with Horsetail.

Hydrastis canadensis

PLANT FAMILY RANUNCULACEAE

GOLDEN SEAL

Golden Seal owes most of its specific uses to the powerful tonic qualities shown towards the mucous membranes of the body. It is thus of service in all digestive problems. All catarrhal states benefit from Golden Seal, especially upper respiratory tract catarrh. The tonic and astringency contribute to its use in uterine conditions. Externally it is used for eczema, ringworm, pruritis, earache and conjunctivitis.

CAUTION

AS GOLDEN SEAL STIMULATES THE
INVOLUNTARY MUSCLES OF THE UTERUS,
IT SHOULD BE AVOIDED DURING PREGNANCY.

PART USED
Root and rhizome

COLLECTION *Unearth root
and rhizome from three-year-
old plants in the Fall, after the
ripening of the seeds.*

CONSTITUENTS *5% of the
root consists of the alkaloids
hydrastine, berberine and
canadine; traces of essential
oil, resin, fatty oil*

**PREPARATION
AND DOSAGE**

INFUSION

POUR A CUP OF BOILING WATER
ONTO ½–1 TEASPOONFUL OF THE
POWDERED HERB AND LEAVE TO
INFUSE FOR 10–15 MINUTES.
THIS SHOULD BE DRUNK
THREE TIMES A DAY.

TINCTURE

TAKE 2–4ML OF THE TINCTURE
THREE TIMES A DAY.

GOLDEN SEAL
ROOT AND RHIZOME

ACTIONS *Tonic, astringent,
anti-catarrhal, laxative,
oxytocic, bitter, alterative,
anti-bilious, cholagogue,
emmenagogue, expectorant,
hepatic, pectoral, vulnerary*

COMBINATIONS
In stomach conditions it combines well with
Meadowsweet and Chamomile. In uterine hemorrhage it
is best combined with Beth Root. Externally as a
wash for irritation and itching it combines well with
distilled Witch Hazel. As ear drops it may be
combined with Mullein.

103

Hypericum perforatum

PLANT FAMILY HYPERICACEAE

ST JOHN'S WORT

Taken internally, St John's Wort has a sedative and pain-reducing effect, which gives it a place in the treatment of neuralgia, anxiety, tension and similar problems. It is especially regarded as a herb to use where there are menopausal changes triggering irritability and anxiety. It is recommended in the treatment of depression, but may be slow in action and should be taken for at least one month. In addition to neuralgic pain, it will ease fibrositis, sciatica and rheumatic pain. Externally it is a valuable healing and anti-inflammatory remedy. As a lotion it will speed the healing of wounds and bruises, varicose veins and mild burns. The oil is especially useful for the healing of sunburn.

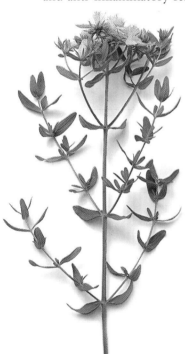

ST JOHN'S WORT
SHOOT, LEAVES AND
FLOWERS

PART USED *Aerial parts*

COLLECTION *The entire plant above ground should be collected when in flower and dried as quickly as possible.*

CONSTITUENTS *Glycosides including rutin; volatile oil, tannin, resin, pectin*

ACTIONS *Anti-inflammatory, astringent, vulnerary, sedative, analgesic*

PREPARATION AND DOSAGE

INFUSION

POUR A CUP OF BOILING WATER ONTO 1–2 TEASPOONFULS OF THE DRIED HERB AND LEAVE TO INFUSE FOR 10–15 MINUTES. THIS SHOULD BE DRUNK THREE TIMES A DAY.

EXTERNAL USE

SEE THE CHAPTER ON THE SKIN.

TINCTURE

TAKE 1–4ML OF THE TINCTURE THREE TIMES A DAY.

Hyssopus officinalis

PLANT FAMILY LABIATAE

HYSSOP

Hyssop has an interesting range of uses which are largely attributable to the anti-spasmodic actions of the volatile oil. It is used in coughs, bronchitis and chronic catarrh. Its diaphoretic properties explain its use in the common cold. As a nervine it may be used in anxiety states, hysteria and petit mal (a form of epilepsy).

HYSSOP SHOOTS,
LEAVES AND FLOWERS

PREPARATION AND DOSAGE

INFUSION

POUR A CUP OF BOILING WATER ONTO 1–2 TEASPOONFULS OF THE DRIED HERB AND LEAVE TO INFUSE FOR 10–15 MINUTES. THIS SHOULD BE DRUNK THREE TIMES A DAY.

TINCTURE

TAKE 1–4ML OF THE TINCTURE THREE TIMES A DAY.

PART USED *Dried aerial parts*

COLLECTION *Collect the flowering tops in late summer.*

CONSTITUENTS *Up to 1% volatile oil, flavonoid glycosides, diosmin, tannin*

ACTIONS *Anti-spasmodic, expectorant, diaphoretic, sedative, carminative, anti-catarrhal, aromatic, hepatic pectoral, tonic, vulnerary*

COMBINATIONS

It may be combined with White Horehound and Coltsfoot in the treatment of coughs and bronchitis. For the common cold it may be mixed with Boneset, Elder Flower and Peppermint.

Inula helenium

PLANT FAMILY COMPOSITAE

ELECAMPANE

Elecampane is a specific for irritating bronchial coughs, especially in children. It may be used wherever there is copious catarrh formed, for example, in bronchitis or emphysema. The mucilage has a relaxing effect accompanied by the stimulation of the essential oils. In this way expectoration is accompanied by a soothing action, which in this herb is combined with an anti-bacterial effect. It may be used in asthma and bronchitic asthma. Elecampane has been used in the treatment of tuberculosis. The bitter principle makes it useful also to stimulate digestion and appetite.

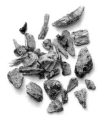

DRIED
ELECAMPANE ROOT

PART USED *Rhizome*

COLLECTION *The rhizome should be unearthed between early Fall and mid-Fall. The large pieces should be cut before drying in the sun or artificially at a temperature of 50–70°C/ 122–158°F.*

CONSTITUENTS
40% inulin, essential oil called helenin, mucilage, triterpenes, bitter principle

ACTIONS *Expectorant, anti-tussive, diaphoretic, stomachic, anti-microbial, astringent, anti-catarrhal, emollient, hepatic, pectoral, tonic, vulnerary*

PREPARATION AND DOSAGE

INFUSION

POUR A CUP OF COLD WATER ONTO 1 TEASPOONFUL OF THE SHREDDED ROOT. LET STAND FOR 8 TO 10 HOURS. HEAT UP AND TAKE VERY HOT THREE TIMES A DAY.

TINCTURE

TAKE 1–2ML OF THE TINCTURE THREE TIMES A DAY.

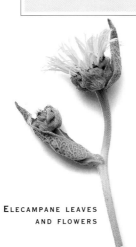

ELECAMPANE LEAVES
AND FLOWERS

COMBINATIONS
Elecampane combines well with White Horehound, Coltsfoot, Pleurisy Root and Yarrow for respiratory problems.

Iris versicolor

PLANT FAMILY IRIDACEAE

BLUE FLAG

This useful remedy has a wide application in the treatment of skin diseases, apparently aiding the skin by working through the liver, the main detoxifying organ of the body. It may be used in skin eruptions such as eczema, spots and blemishes. For the more chronic skin problems, such as eczema and psoriasis, it is valuable as part of a wider treatment. It may be used with value where there is constipation associated with liver problems or biliousness.

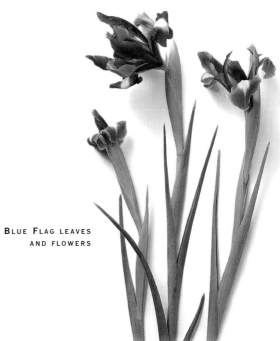

BLUE FLAG LEAVES
AND FLOWERS

PREPARATION AND DOSAGE

DECOCTION

PUT ½–1 TEASPOONFUL OF DRIED HERB INTO A CUP OF WATER AND BRING TO THE BOIL. LET IT SIMMER FOR 10–15 MINUTES. THIS SHOULD BE DRUNK THREE TIMES A DAY.

TINCTURE

TAKE 2–4ML OF THE TINCTURE THREE TIMES A DAY.

PART USED *Rhizome*

COLLECTION *The rhizome is best collected in the Fall.*

CONSTITUENTS
Oleoresin, salicylic acid, alkaloid, tannin

ACTIONS *Cholagogue, alterative, laxative, diuretic, anti-inflammatory, hepatic, sialagogue*

COMBINATIONS
Blue Flag combines well with Echinacea or Burdock and Yellow Dock.

Jateorhiza palmata

PLANT FAMILY MENISPERMACEAE

CALUMBA

Calumba is an excellent digestive remedy that tones the whole tract, stimulating it gently but having no astringent properties. It may be used whenever debility occurs that is connected with some digestive involvement.

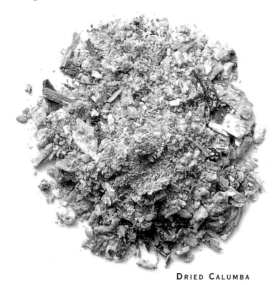

DRIED CALUMBA

PART USED *Root*

COLLECTION *This root is collected from a climbing plant indigenous to the forests of Mozambique and Madagascar.*

CONSTITUENTS *Alkaloids including calumbamine, jateor-rhizine, palmatine and bitter glycosides*

ACTIONS *Bitter tonic, digestive stimulant, sialagogue*

PREPARATION AND DOSAGE

DECOCTION

PUT 1–2 TEASPOONFULS OF THE ROOT IN A CUP OF COLD WATER AND BRING TO THE BOIL. LET IT INFUSE FOR 10 MINUTES AND DRINK A CUP HALF AN HOUR BEFORE MEALS.

TINCTURE

TAKE 1–4ML OF THE TINCTURE THREE TIMES A DAY.

Juniperus communis

PLANT FAMILY CUPRESSACEAE

JUNIPER

Juniper berries make an excellent antiseptic in conditions such as cystitis. The essential oil present is quite stimulating to the kidney nephrons and so this herb should be avoided in kidney disease. The bitter action aids digestion and eases flatulent colic. It is used in rheumatism and arthritis. Externally it eases pain in the joints or muscles.

JUNIPER BERRIES

PART USED *Dried ripe berries*

COLLECTION *Collect the ripe, unshrivelled berries in the Fall and dry slowly in the shade.*

CONSTITUENTS *Rich in essential oil which contains monoterpenes and sesquiterpenes; invert sugar, flavone glycosides, resin, tannin, organic acids*

ACTIONS *Diuretic, carminative, anti-rheumatic, anti-microbial, emmenagogue, stimulant*

PREPARATION AND DOSAGE

INFUSION

POUR A CUP OF BOILING WATER ONTO 1 TEASPOONFUL OF LIGHTLY CRUSHED BERRIES AND LEAVE TO INFUSE FOR 20 MINUTES. A CUP SHOULD BE DRUNK NIGHT AND MORNING. FOR THE TREATMENT OF CHRONIC RHEUMATISM, THIS TREATMENT SHOULD BE CONTINUED FOR 4–6 WEEKS IN THE SPRING AND FALL.

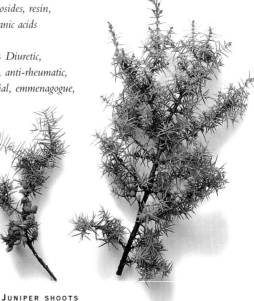

JUNIPER SHOOTS AND LEAVES

CAUTION

DUE TO THEIR ACTION ON THE KIDNEYS, JUNIPER BERRIES SHOULD BE AVOIDED IN ANY KIDNEY DISEASE. THEY SHOULD ALSO BE AVOIDED IN PREGNANCY.

Krameria triandra

PLANT FAMILY KRAMERIACEAE

RHATANY

Rhatany is a powerful astringent that was retained in the official pharmacopeia until recently. It may be used wherever an astringent is indicated, that is, in diarrhea, hemorrhoids, hemorrhages or as a styptic. Rhatany is often found in herbal toothpastes and powders as it is especially good for bleeding gums. It can be used as a snuff with Blood Root to treat nasal polyps.

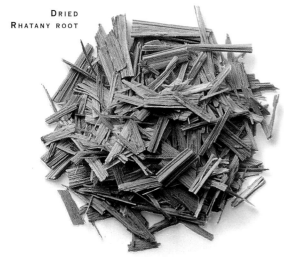

DRIED
RHATANY ROOT

PART USED *Root*

COLLECTION *The root of this shrub is collected in Peru.*

CONSTITUENTS *Up to 9% of a tannin called rhatanhia-tannic acid*

ACTIONS *Astringent*

PREPARATION AND DOSAGE

DECOCTION

PUT 1–2 TEASPOONFULS OF THE ROOT IN A CUP OF WATER, BRING TO THE BOIL AND SIMMER GENTLY FOR 10–15 MINUTES. THIS SHOULD BE DRUNK THREE TIMES A DAY.

TINCTURE

TAKE 1–4ML OF THE TINCTURE THREE TIMES A DAY.

Lactuca virosa

PLANT FAMILY COMPOSITAE

WILD LETTUCE

The latex of the Wild Lettuce was at one time sold as 'Lettuce Opium', naming the use of this herb quite well! It is a valuable remedy for use in insomnia, restlessness and excitability (especially in children) and other manifestations of an over-active nervous system. As an anti-spasmodic it can be used as part of a holistic treatment of whooping cough and dry irritated coughs in general. It will relieve colic pains in the guts and uterus and so may be used in painful periods. It will ease muscular pains related to rheumatism. It has been used as an anaphrodisiac.

PREPARATION AND DOSAGE

INFUSION

POUR A CUP OF BOILING WATER ONTO 1–2 TEASPOONFULS OF THE LEAVES AND LET INFUSE FOR 10–15 MINUTES. THIS SHOULD BE DRUNK THREE TIMES A DAY.

TINCTURE

TAKE 2–4ML OF THE TINCTURE THREE TIMES A DAY.

PART USED *Dried leaves*

COLLECTION *The leaves should be gathered in early summer and mid-summer.*

CONSTITUENTS *Latex containing lactucin, lactucone, lactupicrin, lactucic acid; alkaloids, triterpenes*

ACTIONS *Sedative, anodyne, hypnotic, anti-spasmodic, nervine*

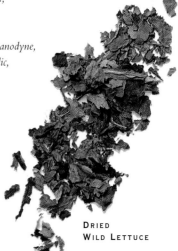

DRIED
WILD LETTUCE

COMBINATIONS
For irritable coughs it may be used with Wild Cherry Bark. For insomnia it combines with Valerian and Pasque Flower.

Lavandula angustifolia

PLANT FAMILY LABIATAE

LAVENDER

This is an effective herb for headaches, especially when they are related to stress. Lavender can be quite effective in the clearing of depression, especially if used in conjunction with other remedies. As a gentle strengthening tonic of the nervous system it may be used in states of nervous debility and exhaustion. It can be used to soothe and promote natural sleep. Externally the oil may be used as a stimulating liniment to help ease the aches and pains of rheumatism.

LAVENDER LEAVES

PART USED *Flowers*

COLLECTION *The flowers should be gathered just before opening between early summer and early Fall. They should be dried gently at a temperature not above 35°C/95°F.*

CONSTITUENTS *The fresh flowers contain up to 0.5% of volatile oil that contains among other constituents linalyl acetate, linalol, geraniol, cineole, limonene and sesquiterpenes.*

ACTIONS *Carminative, anti-spasmodic, anti-depressant, rubefacient, anti-emetic, nervine*

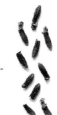

DRIED LAVENDER FLOWERS

PREPARATION AND DOSAGE

INFUSION

TO TAKE INTERNALLY, POUR A CUP OF BOILING WATER ONTO 1 TEASPOONFUL OF THE DRIED HERB AND LEAVE TO INFUSE FOR 10 MINUTES. THIS CAN BE DRUNK THREE TIMES A DAY.

EXTERNAL USE

THE OIL SHOULD NOT BE TAKEN INTERNALLY BUT CAN BE INHALED, RUBBED ON THE SKIN OR USED IN BATHS.

COMBINATIONS

For depression it will combine well with Rosemary, Kola or Skullcap. For headaches it may be used with Lady's Slipper or Valerian.

Leonurus cardiaca

PLANT FAMILY LABIATAE

MOTHERWORT

The names of this plant show its range of uses. 'Motherwort' shows its relevance to menstrual and uterine conditions whilst 'cardiaca' indicates its use in heart and circulation treatments. It is valuable in the stimulation of delayed or suppressed menstruation, especially where there is anxiety or tension involved. It is a useful relaxing tonic for aiding menopausal changes. It may be used to ease false labour pains. It is an excellent tonic for the heart, strengthening without straining. It is a specific for over-rapid heart beat where this is brought about by anxiety and other such causes. It may be used in all heart conditions that are associated with anxiety and tension.

PART USED *Aerial parts*

COLLECTION *The stalks should be gathered at the time of flowering, which is between early summer and early Fall.*

CONSTITUENTS *Bitter glycosides including leonurin and leonuridine; alkaloids including leonuinine and stachydrene; volatile oil, tannin*

ACTIONS *Sedative, emmenagogue, anti-spasmodic, cardiac tonic, hepatic, nervine*

PREPARATION AND DOSAGE

INFUSION

POUR A CUP OF BOILING WATER ONTO 1–2 TEASPOONFULS OF THE DRIED HERB AND LEAVE TO INFUSE FOR 10–15 MINUTES. THIS SHOULD BE DRUNK THREE TIMES A DAY OR AS NEEDED.

TINCTURE

TAKE 1–4ML OF THE TINCTURE THREE TIMES A DAY.

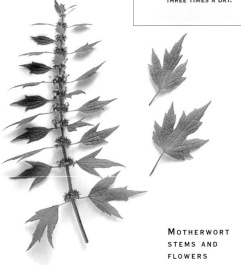

MOTHERWORT STEMS AND FLOWERS

Linum usitatissimum

PLANT FAMILY LINACEAE

FLAX

Flax may be used in all pulmonary infections, especially in bronchitis with much catarrh formed. It is often used as a poultice in pleurisy and other pulmonary conditions. As a poultice it can be used for boils and carbuncles, shingles and psoriasis. As a purgative it relieves constipation.

PART USED *Ripe seeds*

COLLECTION *The seed pods are gathered when fully ripe in early Fall.*

CONSTITUENTS *30–40% of fixed oil which includes linoleic, linolenic and oleic acids; mucilage, protein, the glycoside linamarin*

ACTIONS *Demulcent, anti-tussive, laxative, emollient, vulnerary*

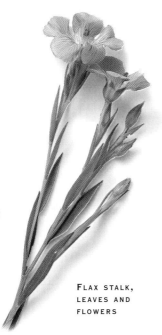

FLAX STALK, LEAVES AND FLOWERS

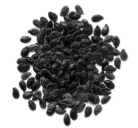

FLAX SEEDS

PREPARATION AND DOSAGE

INFUSION

POUR A CUP OF BOILING WATER ONTO 2–3 TEASPOONFULS OF THE DRIED HERB AND LEAVE TO INFUSE FOR 10–15 MINUTES. THIS SHOULD BE DRUNK MORNING AND EVENING.

POULTICE

FOR MAKING A POULTICE SEE THE SECTION ON 'PREPARATIONS'.

TINCTURE

TAKE 2–6ML OF THE TINCTURE THREE TIMES A DAY.

COMBINATIONS

As a poultice for the chest it combines well with Mustard. For boils, swellings and inflammations it combines with Marshmallow Root and Slippery Elm.

Lobaria pulmonaria

PLANT FAMILY STICTACEAE

LUNGWORT MOSS

This lichen has properties which have been recognized in European herbal medicine for many generations. It may be safely used wherever a soothing expectorant is called for. It may be used in all varieties of bronchitis and especially where there is an asthmatic tendency. It may also be used in children's coughs with much benefit.

PREPARATION AND DOSAGE

INFUSION

POUR A CUP OF BOILING WATER ONTO 1 TEASPOONFUL OF THE DRIED LICHEN AND LEAVE TO INFUSE FOR 10 MINUTES. THIS SHOULD BE DRUNK THREE TIMES A DAY.

TINCTURE

TAKE 1–2ML OF THE TINCTURE THREE TIMES A DAY.

PART USED *Dried lichen*

COLLECTION *This lichen grows on Oak Bark and more rarely on heather stems or mossy rocks.*

CONSTITUENTS *A well-analysed herb containing arabitol, gyrophoric acid, stictic acid, thelephoric acid, ergosterol, fugosterol; palmitic, oleic and linoleic acids*

ACTIONS *Expectorant, demulcent, pectoral*

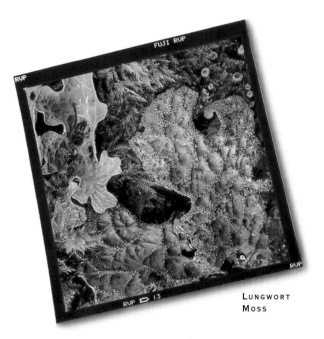

LUNGWORT MOSS

COMBINATIONS

Lungwort Moss is often used in combination with Coltsfoot and White Horehound.

Lobelia inflata

PLANT FAMILY CAMPANULACEAE

LOBELIA

Lobelia is one of the most useful systemic relaxants available to us. It has a general depressant action on the central and autonomic nervous system and on neuro-muscular action. It may be used in many conditions in combination with other herbs to further their effectiveness if relaxation is needed. Its primary specific use is in bronchitic asthma and bronchitis. An analysis of the action of the alkaloids present reveals apparently paradoxical effects. Lobeline is a powerful respiratory stimulant, whilst isolobelanine is an emetic and respiratory relaxant, which will stimulate catarrhal secretion and expectoration.

> **CAUTION**
> EMETIC AT
> HIGH DOSE

PART USED
Aerial parts

COLLECTION *Collect the entire plant above ground and seed pods at the end of the flowering time, between late summer and early Fall.*

CONSTITUENTS
Alkaloids including lobeline, lobelidine, lobelanine, isolobelanine; bitter glycosides, volatile oil, resin, gum substances

ACTIONS *Respiratory stimulant, anti-asthmatic, anti-spasmodic, expectorant, emetic, nervine, sedative*

LOBELIA
LEAVES AND
FLOWERS

> **PREPARATION
> AND DOSAGE**
>
> **INFUSION**
>
> POUR A CUP OF BOILING WATER
> ONTO ¼–½ TEASPOONFUL OF THE
> DRIED LEAVES AND LET INFUSE
> FOR 10–15 MINUTES. THIS
> SHOULD BE DRUNK
> THREE TIMES A DAY.
>
> **TINCTURE**
>
> TAKE ½–1ML OF THE TINCTURE
> THREE TIMES A DAY.

> **COMBINATIONS**
> It will combine well with Cayenne, Grindelia,
> Pill-bearing Spurge, Sundew and Ephedra
> in the treatment of asthma.

Lycopus europaeus

PLANT FAMILY LABIATAE

BUGLEWEED

Bugleweed, or Water Horehound, is a specific for over-active thyroid glands, especially where the symptoms include tightness of breathing, palpitation and shaking. It may safely be used where palpitations occur that are of nervous origin. Bugleweed will aid the weak heart where there is associated build-up of water in the body. As a sedative cough reliever it will ease irritating coughs, especially when they are of nervous origin.

PART USED *Aerial parts*

COLLECTION *It should be collected just before the buds open.*

CONSTITUENTS *Flavone glycosides, volatile oil, tannins*

ACTIONS *Cardioactive diuretic, peripheral vasoconstrictor, astringent, sedative, thyrocine antagonist, anti-tussive, nervine, tonic*

> **PREPARATION
> AND DOSAGE**
>
> **INFUSION**
>
> POUR A CUP OF BOILING WATER
> ONTO 1 TEASPOONFUL OF THE
> DRIED HERB AND LET INFUSE FOR
> 10–15 MINUTES. THIS SHOULD BE
> DRUNK THREE TIMES A DAY.
>
> **TINCTURE**
>
> TAKE 1–2ML OF THE TINCTURE
> THREE TIMES A DAY.

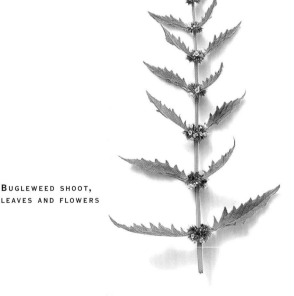

BUGLEWEED SHOOT,
LEAVES AND FLOWERS

> **COMBINATIONS**
> Bugleweed may be used with nervines such as
> Skullcap or Valerian.

Mahonia aquifolium

PLANT FAMILY BERBERIDACEAE

MOUNTAIN GRAPE

Mountain Grape, or Oregon Mountain Grape, is similar in action to both Golden Seal and Barberry. It finds its main use in the treatment of chronic and scaly skin conditions such as psoriasis and eczema. As skin problems of this sort are due to systemic causes within the body, the tonic activity of Mountain Grape on the liver and gall-bladder may explain its potency. It can be used in stomach and gall-bladder conditions, especially where there is associated nausea and vomiting. As a laxative it may safely be used in chronic constipation.

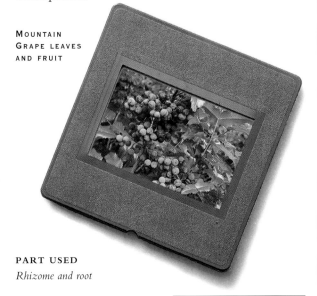

MOUNTAIN GRAPE LEAVES AND FRUIT

PART USED
Rhizome and root

COLLECTION *The underground parts are collected in the Fall, carefully cleaned, cut into slices and dried.*

CONSTITUENTS
Alkaloids including berberine, oxyacanthine and berbamine

ACTIONS *Alterative, cholagogue, laxative, anti-emetic, anti-catarrhal, tonic, hepatic*

> **PREPARATION AND DOSAGE**
>
> **DECOCTION**
>
> PUT 1–2 TEASPOONFULS OF THE ROOT IN A CUP OF WATER, BRING TO THE BOIL AND SIMMER FOR 10–15 MINUTES. THIS SHOULD BE DRUNK THREE TIMES A DAY.
>
> **TINCTURE**
>
> TAKE 1–4ML OF THE TINCTURE THREE TIMES A DAY.

> **COMBINATIONS**
> For skin problems it will combine well with Burdock Root, Yellow Dock and Cleavers. For gall-bladder problems it may be used with Black Root and Fringetree Bark.

Malva sylvestris

PLANT FAMILY MALVACEAE

MALLOW

Mallow may be used in very similar ways to Marshmallow, to which it is generally inferior. Internally it may be used to aid recovery from gastritis and stomach ulcers, laryngitis and pharyngitis, upper respiratory catarrh and bronchitis. Externally it may be used as an addition to bath water or as a compress against abscesses, boils and minor burns.

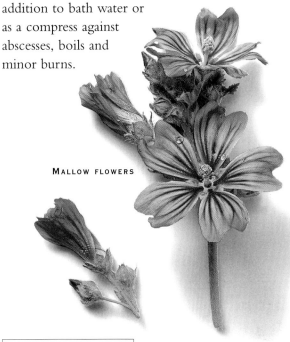

MALLOW FLOWERS

> **PREPARATION AND DOSAGE**
>
> **INFUSION**
>
> FOR INTERNAL USE, POUR A CUP OF BOILING WATER ONTO 2 TEASPOONFULS OF THE DRIED HERB AND LEAVE TO INFUSE FOR 10–15 MINUTES. THIS SHOULD BE DRUNK THREE TIMES A DAY.
>
> **DECOCTION**
>
> FOR EXTERNAL USE, PUT 1 TEASPOONFUL OF THE HERB IN A CUP OF WATER, BRING TO THE BOIL AND SIMMER GENTLY FOR 10–15 MINUTES. THIS DECOCTION CAN BE USED FOR A COMPRESS.
>
> **TINCTURE**
>
> TAKE 2–4ML OF THE TINCTURE THREE TIMES A DAY.

PART USED
Flowers and leaves

COLLECTION *The flowers and leaves are collected and dried with care between mid-summer and early Fall.*

CONSTITUENTS *Mucilage, essential oil, traces of tannin*

ACTIONS *Demulcent, anti-inflammatory, expectorant, astringent, emollient*

Marrubium vulgare

PLANT FAMILY LABIATAE

WHITE HOREHOUND

White Horehound is a valuable plant in the treatment of bronchitis where there is a non-productive cough. It combines the action of relaxing the smooth muscles of the bronchus whilst promoting mucus production and thus expectoration. It is used with benefit in the treatment of whooping cough. The bitter action stimulates the flow and secretion of bile from the gall-bladder and thus aids digestion. White Horehound is used externally to promote the healing of wounds.

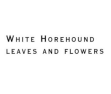

WHITE HOREHOUND
LEAVES AND FLOWERS

PART USED *Dried leaves and flowering tops*

COLLECTION *White Horehound is gathered whilst the herb is blossoming between early summer and early Fall. It is dried in the shade at a temperature not greater than 35°C/95°F.*

CONSTITUENTS *Sesquiterpene bitters including marrubin; essential oil, mucilage, tannins*

ACTIONS *Expectorant, anti-spasmodic, bitter digestive, vulnerary, diaphoretic, pectoral, stimulant*

PREPARATION AND DOSAGE

INFUSION

POUR A CUP OF BOILING WATER ONTO ½–1 TEASPOONFUL OF THE DRIED HERB AND LEAVE TO INFUSE FOR 10–15 MINUTES. THIS SHOULD BE DRUNK THREE TIMES A DAY.

TINCTURE

TAKE 1–2ML OF THE TINCTURE THREE TIMES A DAY.

COMBINATIONS
It combines well with Coltsfoot, Lobelia and Mullein.

Marsdenia condurango

PLANT FAMILY ASCLEPIADACEAE

CONDURANGO

This bitter may be used in a whole range of digestive and stomach problems. It is best known for its appetite-stimulating actions, common to all bitters. However, in addition it will relax the nerves of the stomach, making it of use in the settling of indigestion where this is affected by nervous tension and anxiety. The combination described in the section on the Digestive System gives this herb a role in the treatment of anorexia nervosa.

PART USED *Dried bark*

COLLECTION *Strips (or quills) of bark are collected from trees in Ecuador and other South American countries.*

CONSTITUENTS *Glycosides, resin, tannin, fixed oil*

ACTIONS *Bitter, stomach sedative, tonic*

PREPARATION AND DOSAGE

INFUSION

POUR A CUP OF BOILING WATER ONTO 1–2 TEASPOONFULS OF THE POWDERED BARK AND LEAVE TO INFUSE FOR 10–15 MINUTES. THIS SHOULD BE DRUNK THREE TIMES A DAY.

TINCTURE

TAKE 1–2ML OF THE TINCTURE THREE TIMES A DAY.

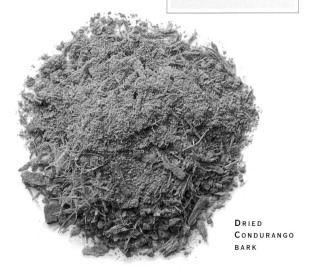

DRIED
CONDURANGO
BARK

COMBINATIONS
It will combine well with many bitters, carminatives and nervines depending upon the specific condition and individual.

Melissa officinalis

PLANT FAMILY LABIATAE

BALM

Balm is an excellent carminative herb that relieves spasms in the digestive tract and is used in flatulent dyspepsia. Because of its anti-depressive properties, it is primarily indicated where there is dyspepsia associated with anxiety or depression, as the gently sedative oils relieve tension and stress reactions, thus acting to lighten depression. Balm has a tonic effect on the heart and circulatory system, thus lowering blood pressure. It can be used in feverish conditions such as flu.

BALM
SHOOT
AND
LEAVES

PART USED *Dried aerial parts, or fresh in season*

COLLECTION *The leaves may be harvested two or three times a year between early summer and early Fall. They are gathered by cutting off the young shoots when they are approximately 30cm/12in long. They should be dried in the shade at a temperature not above 35°C/95°F.*

CONSTITUENTS *Rich in essential oil containing citral, citronellal, geraniol and linalol; bitter principles, flavones, resin*

ACTIONS *Carminative, anti-spasmodic, anti-depressive, diaphoretic, hypotensive, anti-emetic, aromatic, hepatic, nervine, tonic*

PREPARATION AND DOSAGE

INFUSION

POUR A CUP OF BOILING WATER ONTO 2–3 TEASPOONFULS OF THE DRIED HERB OR 4–6 FRESH LEAVES AND LEAVE TO INFUSE FOR 10–15 MINUTES, WELL COVERED UNTIL DRUNK. A CUP OF THIS TEA SHOULD BE TAKEN IN THE MORNING AND THE EVENING, OR WHEN NEEDED.

TINCTURE

TAKE 2–6ML OF THE TINCTURE THREE TIMES A DAY.

COMBINATIONS

In digestive troubles it may be combined with Hops, Chamomile or Meadowsweet. For stress and tension it will combine with Lavender and Lime Blossom.

Mentha x piperita

PLANT FAMILY LABIATAE

PEPPERMINT

Peppermint is one of the best carminative agents available. It has a relaxing effect on the visceral muscles, anti-flatulent properties and stimulates bile and digestive juice secretion, and so can relieve intestinal colic, flatulent dyspepsia and other associated conditions. The volatile oil acts as a mild anesthetic to the stomach wall, which helps to relieve the vomiting of pregnancy and travel sickness. Peppermint plays a role in the treatment of ulcerative colitis and Crohn's disease. It is most valuable in the treatment of fevers and especially colds and flu. As an inhalant it can be used as a temporary treatment for nasal catarrh. Where migraine headaches are associated with the digestion, this herb may be used. As a nervine it eases anxiety and tension. In painful periods it relieves the pain and eases tension. Externally it relieves itching and inflammations.

PEPPERMINT
LEAVES AND
FLOWERS

PART USED *Aerial parts*

COLLECTION *The aerial parts are collected just before the flowers open.*

CONSTITUENTS *Up to 2% volatile oil containing menthol, menthone and jasmone; tannins, bitter principle*

ACTIONS *Carminative, anti-spasmodic, aromatic, diaphoretic, anti-emetic, nervine, analgesic, anti-catarrhal, anti-microbial, emmenagogue, rubefacient, stimulant*

PREPARATION AND DOSAGE

INFUSION

POUR A CUP OF BOILING WATER ONTO A HEAPED TEASPOON OF THE DRIED HERB AND LEAVE TO INFUSE FOR 10 MINUTES. THIS SHOULD BE DRUNK AS OFTEN AS DESIRED.

TINCTURE

TAKE 1–2ML OF THE TINCTURE THREE TIMES A DAY.

COMBINATIONS

For colds and influenza it may be used with Boneset, Elder Flowers and Yarrow.

113

Mentha pulegium

PLANT FAMILY LABIATAE

PENNYROYAL

With its richly aromatic volatile oil, Pennyroyal will ease flatulence and abdominal colic due to wind. It will relax spasmodic pain and ease anxiety. However, its main use is as an emmenagogue to stimulate the menstrual process and to strengthen uterine contractions. As it has been used in large doses as an abortifacient, it should be avoided during pregnancy. The oil should also be avoided as it can act far too strongly.

PART USED *Aerial parts*

COLLECTION *The stems should be gathered just before flowering in mid-summer.*

CONSTITUENTS *Volatile oil, tannin, flavone glycosides*

ACTIONS *Carminative, diaphoretic, stimulant, emmenagogue, aromatic*

CAUTION

AVOID DURING PREGNANCY.

PREPARATION AND DOSAGE

INFUSION

POUR A CUP OF BOILING WATER ONTO 1–2 TEASPOONFULS OF THE DRIED LEAVES AND LET INFUSE FOR 10–15 MINUTES. THIS SHOULD BE DRUNK THREE TIMES A DAY.

TINCTURE

TAKE 1–2ML OF THE TINCTURE THREE TIMES A DAY.

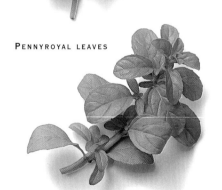

PENNYROYAL LEAVES

Menyanthes trifoliata

PLANT FAMILY MENYANTHACEAE

BOGBEAN

Bogbean, or Buckbean, is a most useful herb for the treatment of rheumatism, arthritis, and rheumatoid arthritis. It has a stimulating effect upon the walls of the colon which will act as an aperient, but it should not be used to help rheumatism where there is any colitis or diarrhea. It has a marked stimulating action on the digestive juices and on bile-flow and so will aid in debilitated states that are due to sluggish digestion, indigestion and problems of the liver and gall-bladder.

PART USED *Leaves*

COLLECTION *The leaves are best collected between late spring and mid-summer. They may be dried in the sun or under moderate heat.*

BOGBEAN SHOOTS AND LEAVES

CONSTITUENTS *Bitter glycosides, alkaloids, saponin, essential oil, flavonoids, pectin*

ACTIONS *Bitter, diuretic, cholagogue, anti-rheumatic, alterative, anti-inflammatory, hepatic, tonic*

PREPARATION AND DOSAGE

INFUSION

POUR A CUP OF BOILING WATER ONTO 1–2 TEASPOONFULS OF THE DRIED HERB AND LEAVE TO INFUSE FOR 10–15 MINUTES. THIS SHOULD BE DRUNK THREE TIMES A DAY.

TINCTURE

TAKE 1–4ML OF THE TINCTURE THREE TIMES A DAY.

COMBINATIONS

For the treatment of rheumatic conditions it will combine well with Black Cohosh and Celery Seed.

Mitchella repens

PLANT FAMILY RUBIACEAE

SQUAW VINE

Squaw Vine is one of the herbs brought to us via the Native North Americans. It is among the best remedies for preparing the uterus and whole body for childbirth. For this purpose it should be taken for some weeks before the child is due, thus ensuring a safe and wonderful birth for both. It may also be used for the relief of painful periods (dysmenorrhea). As an astringent it has been used in the treatment of colitis, especially if there is much mucus.

PART USED *Aerial parts*

COLLECTION *Being an evergreen herb, it may be found all year round in the forest and woodland habitat it likes. It is best collected in flower between mid-spring and early summer.*

CONSTITUENTS
Saponins, mucilage

ACTIONS *Parturient, emmenagogue, diuretic, astringent, tonic, oxytocic*

PREPARATION AND DOSAGE

INFUSION

POUR A CUP OF BOILING WATER ONTO 1 TEASPOONFUL OF THE HERB AND LET INFUSE FOR 10–15 MINUTES. THIS SHOULD BE DRUNK THREE TIMES A DAY.

TINCTURE

TAKE 1–2ML OF THE TINCTURE THREE TIMES A DAY.

DRIED SQUAW VINE

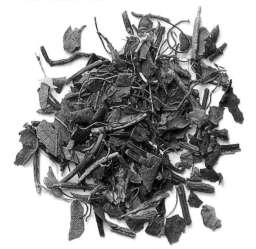

COMBINATIONS

As parturient to prepare for childbirth it may be used with Raspberry Leaves. For dysmenorrhea it could be combined with Cramp Bark and Pasque Flower.

Myrica cerifera

PLANT FAMILY MYRICACEAE

BAYBERRY

As a circulatory stimulant Bayberry plays a role in many conditions when they are approached in a holistic way. Due to its specific actions it is a valuable astringent in diarrhea and dysentery. It is indicated in mucous colitis. As a gargle it helps sore throats and as a douche it helps in leucorrhea. It may be used in the treatment of colds.

BAYBERRY LEAVES

PART USED
Bark of root

COLLECTION *The root should be unearthed in spring or Fall and its bark pared off and dried.*

CONSTITUENTS *Tannins, resin, volatile oil*

ACTIONS *Astringent, circulatory stimulant, diaphoretic, tonic*

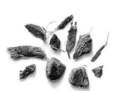

DRIED BAYBERRY BARK

PREPARATION AND DOSAGE

DECOCTION

PUT 1 TEASPOONFUL OF THE BARK INTO A CUP OF COLD WATER AND BRING TO THE BOIL. LEAVE FOR 10–15 MINUTES. THIS SHOULD BE DRUNK THREE TIMES A DAY.

TINCTURE

TAKE 1–3ML OF THE TINCTURE THREE TIMES A DAY.

COMBINATIONS

As a digestive astringent it may be used with Comfrey Root and Agrimony.

Myroxylon balsamum

PLANT FAMILY LEGUMINOSAE

BALSAM OF TOLU

This balsam works mainly on the respiratory mucous membranes. It is often used as an expectorant in cough mixtures in the form of a syrup or tincture.

PART USED *A liquid balsam is collected from the bark of live trees in the Andes and air-dried into a brittle resin.*

CONSTITUENTS *80% resin, which is rich in cinnamic acid and benzoic acid, plus a little vanillin*

ACTIONS *Antiseptic, expectorant, pectoral*

PREPARATION AND DOSAGE

THIS HERB IS RARELY ENCOUNTERED BY ITSELF TODAY. IT MAY BE USED AS AN INHALANT BY PUTTING ABOUT A TEASPOONFUL OF THE BALSAM INTO A STEAM BATH. THE INTERNAL DOSAGE IS ½–1G TAKEN THREE TIMES A DAY.

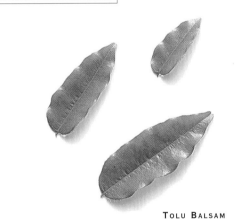

TOLU BALSAM
TREE LEAVES

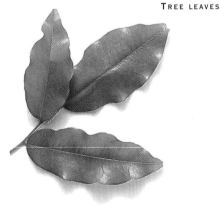

Nepeta cataria

PLANT FAMILY LABIATAE

CATNIP

Catnip is one of our traditional cold and flu remedies. It is a powerful diaphoretic used in any feverish condition, especially in bronchitis. As a carminative with anti-spasmodic properties, Catnip eases any stomach upsets, dyspepsia, flatulence and colic. It is a perfect remedy for the treatment of diarrhea in children. Its sedative action on the nerves adds to its generally relaxing properties.

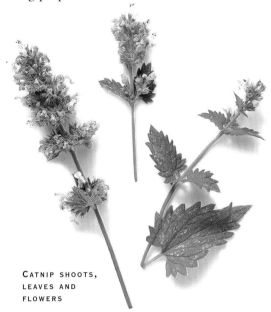

CATNIP SHOOTS,
LEAVES AND
FLOWERS

PART USED *Leaves and flowering tops*

COLLECTION *The leaves and flowering tops are collected between early summer and early Fall.*

CONSTITUENTS *Volatile oils including citronellol, geraniol and citral; bitter principle, tannins*

ACTIONS *Carminative, anti-spasmodic, diaphoretic, sedative, astringent*

PREPARATION AND DOSAGE

INFUSION

POUR A CUP OF BOILING WATER ONTO 2 TEASPOONFULS OF THE DRIED HERB AND LEAVE TO INFUSE FOR 10–15 MINUTES. THIS SHOULD BE DRUNK THREE TIMES A DAY.

TINCTURE

TAKE 2–4ML OF THE TINCTURE THREE TIMES A DAY.

COMBINATIONS
May be used with Boneset, Elder, Yarrow or Cayenne in colds.

Origanum vulgare

PLANT FAMILY LABIATAE

WILD MARJORAM

Marjoram is a widely used herb in folk remedies and cooking. As a stimulating diaphoretic it is often used in the treatment of colds and flu, its use here being similar to that of Hyssop. The antiseptic properties give it a use in the treatment of mouth conditions, as a mouthwash for inflammations of the mouth and throat. It may also be used externally for infected cuts and wounds. The infusion is used in coughs and whooping cough. Headaches, especially when due to tension, may be relieved by a tea of Marjoram or by rubbing the forehead and temples with oil. The oil may also be used for rubbing into areas of muscular and rheumatic pain. A lotion may be made which will soothe stings and bites.

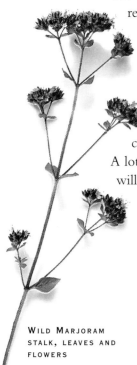

WILD MARJORAM
STALK, LEAVES AND
FLOWERS

PART USED *Aerial parts*

COLLECTION *The herb is gathered as soon as it flowers, avoiding the larger, thicker stalks.*

CONSTITUENTS *Essential oil with thymol, carvacrol; acids, tannin, bitter principle*

ACTIONS *Stimulant, diaphoretic, anti-microbial, expectorant, emmenagogue, rubefacient*

**PREPARATION
AND DOSAGE**

INFUSION

FOR INTERNAL USE, POUR A CUP
OF BOILING WATER ONTO
1 TEASPOONFUL OF THE HERB AND
LET INFUSE FOR 10–15 MINUTES.
THIS SHOULD BE DRUNK
THREE TIMES A DAY.

MOUTHWASH

THIS IS MADE BY POURING
500ML/1PT OF BOILING WATER
ONTO 2 TABLESPOONFULS OF THE
HERB. IT IS THEN LEFT
TO STAND IN A COVERED
CONTAINER FOR 10 MINUTES.
A GARGLE IS MADE FROM THIS
WHENEVER NEEDED BY REHEATING
IT. GARGLE FOR 5–10 MINUTES,
THREE TO FOUR TIMES A DAY.

TINCTURE

TAKE 1–2ML OF THE TINCTURE
THREE TIMES A DAY.

Packera aurea

PLANT FAMILY COMPOSITAE

LIFE ROOT

As a uterine tonic Life Root may be used safely wherever strengthening and aid are called for. It is especially useful in cases of menopausal disturbances of any kind. Where there is delayed or suppressed menstruation, Life Root may be used. For leucorrhea it can be used as a douche. It also has a reputation as a general tonic for debilitated states and conditions such as tuberculosis.

PART USED
Dried aerial parts

COLLECTION *The herb should be collected just before the small flowers open in the summer.*

CONSTITUENTS
Alkaloids including senecifoline, senecine, resins

ACTIONS *Uterine tonic, diuretic, expectorant, emmenagogue*

**PREPARATION
AND DOSAGE**

INFUSION

POUR A CUP OF BOILING WATER
ONTO 1–3 TEASPOONFULS OF
THE DRIED HERB AND LEAVE TO
INFUSE FOR 10–15 MINUTES.
THIS SHOULD BE DRUNK
THREE TIMES A DAY.

TINCTURE

TAKE 1–4ML OF THE TINCTURE
THREE TIMES A DAY.

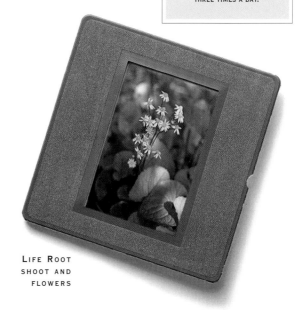

LIFE ROOT
SHOOT AND
FLOWERS

COMBINATIONS
For menopausal problems it may usefully be combined with St John's Wort, Oats or Pasque Flower.

Panax ginseng

PLANT FAMILY ARALIACEAE

GINSENG

Ginseng has an ancient history and as such has accumulated much folklore about its actions and uses. Many of the claims that surround it are inflated but it is clear that this is a unique plant. It enables people to attain their physical peak, generally increasing vitality and physical performance. Specifically it will raise lowered blood pressure to a normal

GINSENG ROOT

level. It affects depression, especially where this is due to debility and exhaustion. It can be used in general for exhaustion states and weakness. It has a reputation as an aphrodisiac. Ocasionally the use of this herb may produce headaches.

PART USED *Root*

COLLECTION *Ginseng is cultivated in China, Korea and northeast America.*

CONSTITUENTS *Steroidal glycosides called panaxosides; sterols, vitamins of D group*

ACTIONS *Anti-depressive, nervine, stimulant, tonic*

PREPARATION AND DOSAGE

THE ROOT IS OFTEN CHEWED OR A DECOCTION MAY BE MADE. PUT ½ TEASPOONFUL OF THE POWDERED ROOT IN A CUP OF WATER, BRING TO THE BOIL AND SIMMER GENTLY FOR 10 MINUTES. THIS SHOULD BE DRUNK THREE TIMES A DAY.

Papaver rhoeas

PLANT FAMILY PAPAVERACEAE

RED POPPY

This beautiful wayside herb does not have the potent activity of its relative the Opium Poppy. It may be used to soothe irritable coughs and in cases of respiratory catarrh. The petals are often added to herbal teas and pot-pourries to add colour.

PART USED *Petals*

COLLECTION *The petals should be collected on a dry morning after the dew has dried in the months of mid-summer and late summer. Dry carefully.*

CONSTITUENTS *Tannin, mucilage, traces of alkaloids*

ACTIONS *Mild sedative, expectorant*

PREPARATION AND DOSAGE

INFUSION

POUR A CUP OF BOILING WATER ONTO 1–2 TEASPOONFULS OF THE DRIED PETALS AND LEAVE TO INFUSE FOR 10–15 MINUTES. THIS SHOULD BE DRUNK THREE TIMES A DAY.

TINCTURE

TAKE 2–4ML OF THE TINCTURE THREE TIMES A DAY.

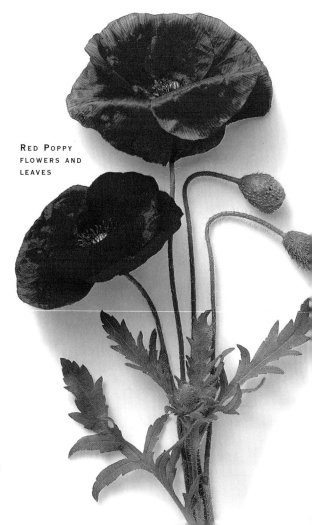

RED POPPY FLOWERS AND LEAVES

Parietaria diffusa

PLANT FAMILY URTICACEAE

PELLITORY OF THE WALL

Pellitory of the Wall may be used in the treatment of any inflammation of the urinary system and especially where soothing is needed. It may be used with benefit in cystitis and pyelitis and is a good general diuretic, which is used to relieve water retention due to kidney-based causes. It has a valuable role to play in the treatment of kidney stone or gravel.

**PELLITORY OF THE WALL
SHOOTS, LEAVES AND FLOWERS**

PART USED *Aerial parts*

COLLECTION *The parts above ground are collected between early summer and early Fall.*

CONSTITUENTS *Bitter principle, tannin*

ACTIONS *Diuretic, demulcent, anti-lithic, laxative*

PREPARATION AND DOSAGE

INFUSION

POUR A CUP OF BOILING WATER ONTO 1–2 TEASPOONFULS OF THE DRIED HERB AND LEAVE TO INFUSE FOR 10–15 MINUTES. THIS SHOULD BE DRUNK THREE TIMES A DAY.

TINCTURE

TAKE 2–4ML OF THE TINCTURE THREE TIMES A DAY.

COMBINATIONS
It combines well with Parsley Piert, Buchu, Bearberry or Juniper.

Passiflora incarnata

PLANT FAMILY PASSIFLORACEAE

PASSION FLOWER

Passion Flower is the herb of choice for treating intransigent insomnia. It aids the transition into a restful sleep without any 'narcotic' hangover. It may be used wherever an anti-spasmodic is required; for example, in Parkinson's disease, seizures and hysteria. It can be very effective in nerve pain such as neuralgia and the viral infection of nerves called shingles. It may be used in asthma where there is much spasmodic activity, especially when there is associated tension.

PART USED *Dried leaves*

COLLECTION *If the foliage alone is to be collected, this should happen just before the flowers bloom, between late spring and mid-summer. The foliage may be collected with the fruit after flowering. It should be dried in the shade.*

CONSTITUENTS *Alkaloids including harmine, harman, harmol and passiflorine; flavone glycosides, sterols*

ACTIONS *Sedative, hypnotic, anti-spasmodic, anodyne, nervine*

PREPARATION AND DOSAGE

INFUSION

POUR A CUP OF BOILING WATER ONTO 1 TEASPOONFUL OF THE DRIED HERB AND LET INFUSE FOR 15 MINUTES. DRINK A CUP IN THE EVENING FOR SLEEPLESSNESS, AND A CUP TWICE A DAY FOR THE EASING OF OTHER CONDITIONS.

TINCTURE

TAKE 1–4ML OF THE TINCTURE AND USE THE SAME WAY AS THE INFUSION.

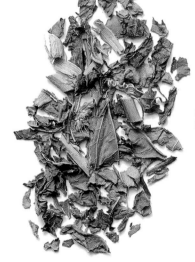

DRIED PASSION FLOWER

COMBINATIONS
For insomnia it will combine well with Valerian, Hops and Jamaican Dogwood.

Petasites hybridus

PLANT FAMILY COMPOSITAE

BUTTERBUR

Butterbur is a useful relaxant to muscles, used in conditions such as intestinal colic, asthma or dysmenorrhea (painful periods). It not only eases spasms in muscles, but has a pain-relieving effect too. It can also be used for fevers. The fresh leaves can be used externally as a wound dressing.

PART USED
Rhizome or leaves

COLLECTION *The rhizomes are collected in the summer, the leaves throughout the growing season.*

CONSTITUENTS *Essential oil, mucilage, bitter glycosides, tannin*

ACTIONS *Anti-spasmodic, diuretic, diaphoretic*

> ### PREPARATION AND DOSAGE
>
> #### DECOCTION
> PUT 1 TEASPOONFUL OF THE ROOT IN A CUP OF WATER, BRING TO THE BOIL AND SIMMER FOR 10–15 MINUTES. THIS SHOULD BE DRUNK THREE TIMES A DAY.
>
> #### TINCTURE
> TAKE 1–2ML OF THE TINCTURE THREE TIMES A DAY.

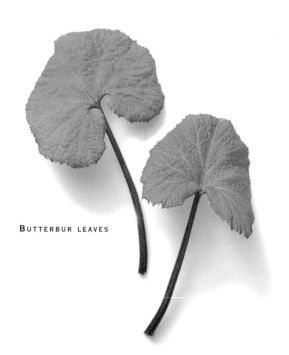

BUTTERBUR LEAVES

Petroselinum crispum

PLANT FAMILY UMBELLIFERAE

PARSLEY

The fresh herb, so widely used in cookery, is one of our richest sources of vitamin C. Medicinally, Parsley has three main areas of usage. Firstly, it is an effective diuretic, helping the body to get rid of excess water, and so may be used wherever such an effect is desired. Remember, however, that the cause of the problem must be sought and treated – do not just treat the symptoms. The second area of use is as an emmenagogue stimulating the menstrual process. It is advisable not to use parsley in medicinal dosage during pregnancy as there may be excessive stimulation of the womb. The third use is as a carminative, easing flatulence and the colic pains that may accompany it.

PARSLEY LEAVES

PARSLEY SEEDS

PART USED *Tap root, leaves and seeds*

COLLECTION *The root is collected in the Fall from two-year-old plants. The leaves can be used any time during the growing season.*

CONSTITUENTS *Essential oil including apiol and myristicin, vitamin C, glycoside apiin, starch*

ACTIONS *Diuretic, expectorant, emmenagogue, carminative, supposed aphrodisiac, tonic*

> ### PREPARATION AND DOSAGE
>
> #### INFUSION
> POUR A CUP OF BOILING WATER ONTO 1–2 TEASPOONFULS OF THE DRIED HERB AND LEAVE TO INFUSE FOR 5–10 MINUTES IN A CLOSED CONTAINER. THIS SHOULD BE DRUNK THREE TIMES A DAY.
>
> #### TINCTURE
> TAKE 2–4ML OF THE TINCTURE THREE TIMES A DAY.

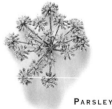

PARSLEY FLOWERS

> ### CAUTION
> DO NOT USE DURING PREGNANCY IN MEDICINAL DOSAGE.

Peumus boldo

PLANT FAMILY MONIMIACEAE

BOLDO

Boldo is a specific for gall-bladder problems like stones or inflammations. It is also used when there is visceral pain due to other problems in the liver or gall-bladder. Boldo has mild urinary demulcent and antiseptic properties and so would be used in cystitis.

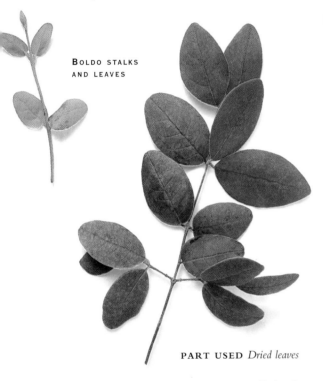

BOLDO STALKS AND LEAVES

PART USED *Dried leaves*

COLLECTION *Gather the evergreen leaves at any time. Dry them carefully in shade not over 40°C/104°F.*

CONSTITUENTS *2% volatile oils, the alkaloid boldine, glycosides, resins and tannin*

ACTIONS *Cholagogue, hepatic, diuretic, sedative, tonic*

PREPARATION AND DOSAGE

INFUSION

POUR A CUP OF BOILING WATER ONTO 1 TEASPOONFUL OF THE DRIED LEAVES AND LET INFUSE FOR 10–15 MINUTES. THIS SHOULD BE DRUNK THREE TIMES A DAY.

TINCTURE

TAKE 1–2ML OF THE TINCTURE THREE TIMES A DAY.

COMBINATIONS
When treating gall-bladder or liver problems, it combines well with Fringetree Bark and Mountain Grape.

Phytolacca americana

PLANT FAMILY PHYTOLACCACEAE

POKE ROOT

Poke Root has a wide range of uses and is a valuable addition to many holistic treatments. It may be seen primarily as a remedy for use in infections of the upper respiratory tract, removing catarrh and aiding the cleansing of the lymphatic glands. It may be used for catarrh, tonsillitis, laryngitis, swollen glands (adenitis), mumps, etc. It will be found of value in lymphatic problems elsewhere in the body and especially where it is long-standing. Care must be taken with this herb as in large doses it is powerfully emetic and purgative. Externally, as a lotion or ointment, it may be used to rid the skin of scabies and other pests.

PREPARATION AND DOSAGE

DECOCTION

ONLY SMALL AMOUNTS OF THIS HERB SHOULD BE USED. PUT ¼ TEASPOONFUL OF THE ROOT IN A CUP OF WATER, BRING TO THE BOIL AND SIMMER GENTLY FOR 10–15 MINUTES. THIS SHOULD BE DRUNK THREE TIMES A DAY.

TINCTURE

TAKE 0.1–0.5ML OF THE TINCTURE THREE TIMES A DAY.

PART USED *Root*

COLLECTION *The root should be unearthed in the late Fall or spring. Clean it and split lengthwise before drying.*

CONSTITUENTS *Tripterpenoid saponins, alkaloid, resins, phytolaccic acid, tannin, formic acid*

ACTIONS *Anti-rheumatic, stimulant, anti-catarrhal, purgative, emetic, tonic*

POKE ROOT LEAVES AND FLOWERS

CAUTION
IN LARGE DOSAGE POKE ROOT IS A POWERFUL EMETIC AND PURGATIVE.

COMBINATIONS
For lymphatic problems it may be used with Cleavers and Blue Flag.

Picrasma excelsor

PLANT FAMILY SIMARUBACEAE

QUASSIA

Quassia is an excellent remedy in dyspeptic conditions due to lack of tone. As with all bitters, it stimulates the production of saliva and digestive juices and so increases the appetite. It may safely be used in all cases of lack of appetite such as anorexia nervosa and digestive sluggishness. It is used in the expulsion of threadworms, both as an enema and an infusion. Externally as a lotion it may be used against lice infestations.

PREPARATION AND DOSAGE

COLD INFUSION

½–1 TEASPOONFUL OF WOOD IS PUT IN A CUP OF COLD WATER AND LEFT TO STEEP OVERNIGHT. THIS SHOULD BE DRUNK THREE TIMES A DAY.

ENEMA

MAKE A COLD INFUSION WITH ONE PART QUASSIA TO 20 PARTS WATER.

TINCTURE

TAKE ½–1ML OF THE TINCTURE THREE TIMES A DAY.

PART USED *Chips or raspings of stem wood, free of bark*

COLLECTION *Raspings of the wood are collected after felling the tree.*

CONSTITUENTS *Bitter glycosides, alkaloids*

ACTIONS *Bitter tonic, sialagogue, anthelmintic*

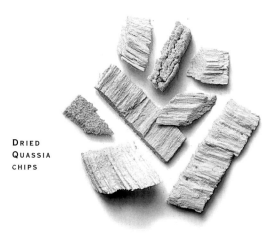

DRIED QUASSIA CHIPS

Pilosella officinarum

PLANT FAMILY COMPOSITAE

MOUSE EAR

Mouse Ear, or Hawkweed, named after the shape of the leaf, is one of the ancient traditional herbs of England and Wales. It is used for respiratory problems where there is a lot of mucus being formed, with soreness and possibly even the coughing of blood. It is considered a specific in cases of whooping cough. It may also be found beneficial in bronchitis or bronchitic asthma. Externally it may be used as a poultice to aid wound-healing or specifically to treat hernias and fractures.

MOUSE EAR LEAVES AND FLOWERS

PART USED *Aerial parts*

COLLECTION *Mouse Ear should be collected when in flower between late spring and early summer.*

CONSTITUENTS *The coumarin umbelliferone, flavones and flavonoids, caffeic acid, chlorogenic acid*

ACTIONS *Anti-spasmodic, expectorant, anti-catarrhal, astringent, sialagogue, vulnerary, pectoral*

PREPARATION AND DOSAGE

INFUSION

POUR A CUP OF BOILING WATER ONTO 1–2 TEASPOONFULS OF THE DRIED HERB AND LEAVE TO INFUSE FOR 10–15 MINUTES. THIS SHOULD BE DRUNK THREE TIMES A DAY OR AS NEEDED.

TINCTURE

TAKE 1–4ML OF THE TINCTURE THREE TIMES A DAY.

COMBINATIONS

In dyspepsia it may be used with Meadowsweet, Marshmallow Root and Hops.

COMBINATIONS

For whooping cough it may be used with Sundew, White Horehound, Mullein or Coltsfoot.

Pimento dioica

PLANT FAMILY MYRTACEAE

ALLSPICE

Allspice can be used freely wherever a pleasant carminative is called for. It will ease flatulence and dyspeptic pain. It may be applied as a compress in cases of rheumatism and neuralgia. It is primarily used as a spice in the food industry.

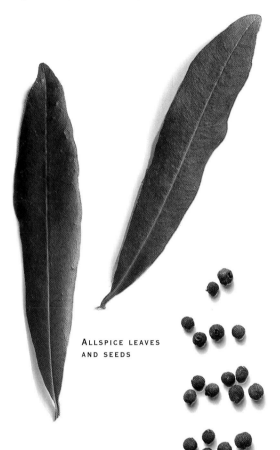

ALLSPICE LEAVES
AND SEEDS

PART USED *Berries*

COLLECTION *The berries are picked whilst still green, as they lose their aroma on ripening. On gentle drying they become reddish-brown.*

ACTIONS *Carminative, digestive stimulant, aromatic, rubifacient*

PREPARATION AND DOSAGE

INFUSION

THE DRIED BERRIES SHOULD BE GENTLY BRUISED JUST BEFORE USE TO RELEASE THE VOLATILE OILS. POUR ONE CUP OF BOILING WATER OVER 1 TEASPOONFUL OF THE BERRIES AND LET STAND FOR 5–10 MINUTES. DRINK WARM TO EASE SYMPTOMS OF ABDOMINAL DISTRESS, AS NEEDED.

COMBINATIONS
Allspice may be used as a flavouring agent for herbal combinations that might verge on the nauseating.

Pimpinella anisum

PLANT FAMILY UMBELLIFERAE

ANISEED

The volatile oil in Aniseed provides the basis for its internal use to ease griping, intestinal colic and flatulence. It also has a marked expectorant and anti-spasmodic action and may be used in bronchitis, in tracheitis where there is persistent irritable coughing, and in whooping cough. Externally, the oil may be used in an ointment base for the treatment of scabies. The oil by itself will help in the control of lice.

PART USED *Seeds*

COLLECTION *The ripe dry fruits should be gathered between mid-summer and early Fall.*

CONSTITUENTS *Up to 6% volatile oils, which include anethole, 30% fatty oils, choline*

ACTIONS *Expectorant, anti-spasmodic, carminative, parasiticide, aromatic, anti-microbial, galactagogue, pectoral, tonic*

PREPARATION AND DOSAGE

INFUSION

THE SEEDS SHOULD BE GENTLY CRUSHED JUST BEFORE USE TO RELEASE THE VOLATILE OILS. POUR ONE CUP OF BOILING WATER OVER 1–2 TEASPOONFULS OF THE SEEDS AND LET IT STAND COVERED FOR 5–10 MINUTES. TAKE ONE CUP THREE TIMES DAILY. TO TREAT FLATULENCE, THE TEA SHOULD BE DRUNK SLOWLY BEFORE MEALS.

OIL

ONE DROP OF THE OIL MAY BE TAKEN INTERNALLY BY MIXING IT INTO ½ TEASPOONFUL OF HONEY.

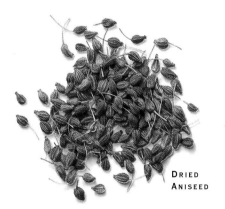

DRIED
ANISEED

COMBINATIONS
For flatulent colic mix Aniseed with equal amounts of Fennel and Caraway. For bronchitis it combines well with Coltsfoot, White Horehound and Lobelia.

Pinus sylvestris

PLANT FAMILY PINACEAE

SCOTS PINE

The Scots Pine may be used in cases of bronchitis, sinusitis or upper respiratory catarrh, both as an inhalant and internally. It may also be helpful in asthma. The stimulating action gives the herb a role in the internal treatment of rheumatism and arthritis. There is a tradition of adding a preparation of the twigs to bath water to ease fatigue, nervous debility and sleeplessness, as well as aiding the healing of cuts and soothing skin irritations.

SCOTS PINE
NEEDLES

PART USED *Needles and young buds*

COLLECTION *The needles and young buds are best collected with the twigs in the spring as young shoots. Other species can be used such as Pinus pinaster, Pinus pinea and Pinus nigra.*

CONSTITUENTS *Tannin, resin, essential oil, terpenes, pinipricin*

ACTIONS *Antiseptic, anti-catarrhal, stimulant, tonic*

PREPARATION AND DOSAGE

INFUSION

POUR A CUP OF BOILING WATER ONTO ½ TEASPOONFUL OF THE DRIED LEAVES AND LET INFUSE FOR 10–15 MINUTES. THIS SHOULD BE DRUNK THREE TIMES A DAY.

INHALANT

BRING 2–3 HANDFULS OF THE TWIGS TO THE BOIL IN 2L/4PT OF WATER, SIMMER FOR 5 MINUTES AND THEN USE AS AN INHALANT BY COVERING THE HEAD WITH A TOWEL AND INHALING THE STEAM FOR 15 MINUTES. THIS SHOULD BE REPEATED OFTEN.

BATH

LEAVE 3 HANDFULS OF TWIGS TO STAND IN 750ML/1½PT OF WATER FOR HALF AN HOUR, THEN BRING TO THE BOIL, SIMMER FOR 10 MINUTES, STRAIN AND ADD TO THE HOT BATH.

TINCTURE

TAKE 1–2ML OF THE TINCTURE THREE TIMES A DAY.

Piscidia piscipula

PLANT FAMILY LEGUMINOSAE

JAMAICAN DOGWOOD

Jamaican Dogwood is a powerful sedative, used in its West Indian homeland as a fish poison. Whilst not being poisonous to humans, the given dosage level should not be exceeded. It is a powerful remedy for the treatment of painful conditions such as neuralgia and migraine. It can also be used in the relief of ovarian and uterine pain. Its main use is perhaps in insomnia, where this is due to nervous tension and pain.

PART USED *Stem bark*

COLLECTION *The bark is collected in vertical strips from trees growing in the Caribbean, Mexico and Texas.*

CONSTITUENTS *Glycosides including piscidin, jamaicin, icthyone; flavonoids, including sumatrol, lisetin, piscerythrone, piscidine, rotenone; resin alkaloid*

ACTIONS *Hypnotic, anodyne*

PREPARATION AND DOSAGE

DECOCTION

PUT 1–2 TEASPOONFULS OF THE BARK IN A CUP OF WATER, BRING TO THE BOIL AND SIMMER GENTLY FOR 10–15 MINUTES. THIS SHOULD BE DRUNK WHEN NEEDED.

TINCTURE

TAKE 1–4ML OF THE TINCTURE THREE TIMES A DAY.

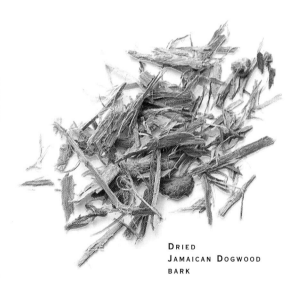

DRIED
JAMAICAN DOGWOOD
BARK

COMBINATIONS

For the easing of insomnia it is best combined with Hops and Valerian. For dysmenorrhea (painful periods) it may be used with Black Haw.

Plantago major

PLANT FAMILY PLANTAGINACEAE

GREATER PLANTAIN

Both the Greater Plantain and its close relative Ribwort Plantain have valuable healing properties. It acts as a gentle expectorant whilst also soothing inflamed and sore membranes, making it ideal for coughs and mild bronchitis. Its astringency aids in diarrhea, hemorrhoids and also in cystitis where there is bleeding.

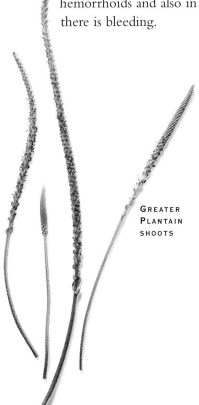

GREATER PLANTAIN SHOOTS

PART USED *Leaves or aerial parts*

COLLECTION *Gather during flowering throughout the summer. Dry as fast as possible as the leaves will discolour if dried improperly.*

CONSTITUENTS *Glycosides including aucubin, mucilage, chlorogenic acid and ursolic acid, silicic acid*

ACTIONS *Expectorant, demulcent, astringent, diuretic, emollient, vulnerary*

Polygala senega

PLANT FAMILY POLYGALACEAE

SENEGA

Senega, or Snake Root, comes to us from the Native North Americans. It was used by the Seneca tribe for snake bites. It has excellent expectorant effects which may be utilized in the treatment of bronchitic asthma, especially where there is some difficulty with expectoration. It has a general power of stimulating secretion, including saliva. It may be used as a mouthwash and gargle in the treatment of pharyngitis and laryngitis. If too much is taken it acts in a way that will irritate the lining of the gut and cause vomiting.

PART USED *Root and rhizome*

COLLECTION *The roots and rhizome are collected in early to mid-Fall*

CONSTITUENTS *5–6% saponins, fixed oil, mucilage, salicylic acid, resin*

ACTIONS *Expectorant, diaphoretic, sialogogue, emetic*

DRIED SENEGA ROOT

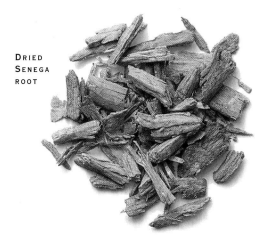

COMBINATIONS

For bronchitic conditions it may be used with Blood Root, White Horehound, Grindelia or Pill-bearing Spurge.

Polygonum bistorta

PLANT FAMILY POLYGONACEAE

BISTORT

Bistort is a powerful though soothing astringent that can be used widely whenever astringency is needed, especially in diarrhea and dysentery. It is considered a specific in childhood diarrhea and dysentery. It will add its astringency to any digestive remedy and may be used in mucous colitis. It can be used in nasal catarrh as an adjunct to other remedies. Externally it will make a useful mouthwash for inflamed conditions of the mouth or tongue, as a gargle for laryngitis or pharyngitis and as a douche for leucorrhea. It has been used as an ointment for hemorrhoids and anal fissures.

BISTORT LEAVES
AND FLOWER

PART USED
Root and rhizome

COLLECTION *Roots and rhizomes are dug up in the Fall from the moist pastures where Bistort thrives. The large roots should be cut longitudinally and dried in the sun.*

CONSTITUENTS *Between 15–20% tannins*

ACTIONS *Astringent, anti-catarrhal, demulcent, anti-inflammatory, vulnerary*

> ### PREPARATION AND DOSAGE
>
> #### DECOCTION
>
> POUR A CUP OF WATER ONTO 1 TEASPOONFUL OF THE DRIED HERB, BRING TO THE BOIL AND SIMMER FOR 10–15 MINUTES. THIS SHOULD BE DRUNK THREE TIMES A DAY. FOR EXTERNAL USE, THIS TEA CAN ALSO BE USED AS A MOUTHWASH OR GARGLE.
>
> #### TINCTURE
>
> TAKE 2–4ML OF THE TINCTURE THREE TIMES A DAY.

Populus gileadensis

PLANT FAMILY SALICACEAE

BALM OF GILEAD

As it soothes, disinfects and astringes the mucous membranes, Balm of Gilead is an excellent remedy for sore throats, coughs and laryngitis that is accompanied by loss of voice. It may be used in chronic bronchitis. Externally it can be used to ease inflammations due to rheumatism and arthritis, as well as for dry and scaly skin conditions such as psoriasis and dry eczema.

PART USED
Closed buds

COLLECTION *The leaf buds are collected while still closed during the winter.*

CONSTITUENTS
Oleo-resin, salicin

ACTIONS *Stimulating expectorant, antiseptic, anti-irritant, vulnerary, pectoral*

> ### PREPARATION AND DOSAGE
>
> #### INFUSION
>
> POUR ONE CUP OF BOILING WATER ONTO 2 TEASPOONFULS OF THE BUD AND LEAVE TO INFUSE FOR 10–15 MINUTES. THIS SHOULD BE DRUNK THREE TIMES A DAY OR MORE UNTIL EFFECTIVE.
>
> #### TINCTURE
>
> TAKE 1–2ML OF THE TINCTURE THREE TIMES A DAY.

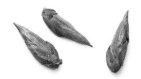

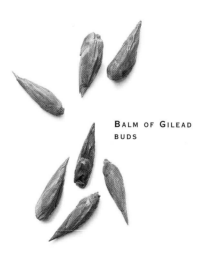

BALM OF GILEAD
BUDS

COMBINATIONS
Coltsfoot, Red Sage and White Horehound will combine well with it to enhance its actions on the respiratory system, whilst Chickweed will aid its strength in external applications.

Populus tremuloides

PLANT FAMILY SALICACEAE

WHITE POPLAR

White Poplar is an excellent remedy to use in the treatment of arthritis and rheumatism where there is much pain and swelling. Its use is quite similar to Black Willow. It is most effective when used in a broad therapeutic approach and not by itself. It is very helpful during the flare-ups of rheumatoid arthritis. As a cholagogue it can be used to stimulate digestion and especially stomach and liver functions, particularly where there is loss of appetite. In feverish colds and in infection such as cystitis it may be considered. As an astringent it can be used in the treatment of diarrhea.

PREPARATION AND DOSAGE

DECOCTION

PUT 1–2 TEASPOONFULS OF THE DRIED BARK IN A CUP OF WATER, BRING TO THE BOIL AND SIMMER FOR 10–15 MINUTES. THIS SHOULD BE DRUNK THREE TIMES A DAY. TO STIMULATE APPETITE, DRINK 30 MINUTES BEFORE MEALS.

TINCTURE

TAKE 2–4ML OF THE TINCTURE THREE TIMES A DAY.

PART USED *Bark*

COLLECTION *The bark should be collected in the spring, taking care not to ring-bark the tree and thus kill it.*

CONSTITUENTS *Glycosides, flavonoids, essential oil, tannin*

ACTIONS *Anti-inflammatory, astringent, antiseptic, anodyne, cholagogue*

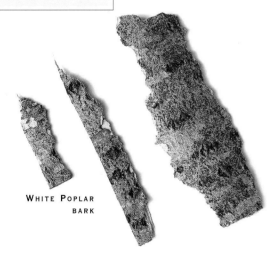

WHITE POPLAR
BARK

COMBINATIONS
In the treatment of rheumatoid arthritis it may be used with Black Cohosh, Bogbean and Celery. As a digestive stimulant it can be used with Balmony and Golden Seal.

Potentilla anserina

PLANT FAMILY ROSACEAE

SILVERWEED

Silverweed is an effective anti-catarrhal herb which may be used wherever there is an over-production of mucus. It is known primarily for its astringent action. For hemorrhoids it may be taken internally and also used as an effective compress. It is indicated in diarrhea, especially when accompanied by indigestion. Where inflammations of the mouth occur, such as gingivitis or apthous ulcers, a mouthwash of the infusion of Silverweed will be found effective. As a gargle it will relieve sore throats.

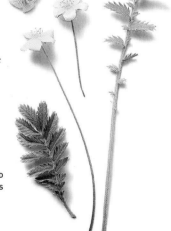

SILVERWEED
LEAVES AND FLOWERS

PREPARATION AND DOSAGE

INFUSION

POUR A CUP OF BOILING WATER ONTO 2 TEASPOONFULS OF THE DRIED HERB AND LEAVE TO INFUSE FOR 15 MINUTES. THIS SHOULD BE DRUNK THREE TIMES A DAY.

COMPRESS

BRING 1–2 TABLESPOONS OF CHOPPED SILVERWEED TO THE BOIL IN 500ML/1PT OF WATER. LET STAND FOR 20 MINUTES. MAKE A MOIST COMPRESS WITH THE LUKEWARM LIQUID. MOISTEN AGAIN AS SOON AS THE COMPRESS BEGINS TO DRY.

TINCTURE

TAKE 2–4ML OF THE TINCTURE THREE TIMES A DAY.

PART USED
Dried aerial parts

COLLECTION *Silverweed should be collected in the early summer, with all discoloured or insect-eaten leaves being rejected. It should be dried in the shade.*

CONSTITUENTS *Tannins, flavonoids, bitter principle, organic acids*

ACTIONS *Astringent, anti-catarrhal, diuretic, local anti-inflammatory*

Potentilla erecta

PLANT FAMILY ROSACEAE

TORMENTIL

Tormentil is a most useful astringent for use in cases of diarrhea, especially when it is acute or of nervous origin. It has often been used as part of the treatment of colitis, both the mucous and the ulcerative kind. Tormentil makes a good astringent gargle for the mucous membranes of the mouth and throat, where it may be used to help laryngitis, pharyngitis, bleeding gums, mouth ulcers and the like. As a lotion it is used externally to ease hemorrhoids. As an ointment, a lotion, compress or poultice, it will speed the healing of wounds and cuts.

PART USED *Rhizome*

COLLECTION *The rhizome is dug up in the Fall, cut into small pieces, washed and then dried.*

CONSTITUENTS *15% tannins, glycosides, red colouring matter*

ACTIONS *Astringent, vulnerary*

PREPARATION AND DOSAGE

DECOCTION

PUT 1–2 TEASPOONFULS OF THE DRIED RHIZOME IN A CUP OF WATER, BRING TO THE BOIL AND SIMMER GENTLY FOR 10–15 MINUTES. THIS SHOULD BE DRUNK THREE TIMES A DAY.

TINCTURE

TAKE 2–4ML OF THE TINCTURE THREE TIMES A DAY.

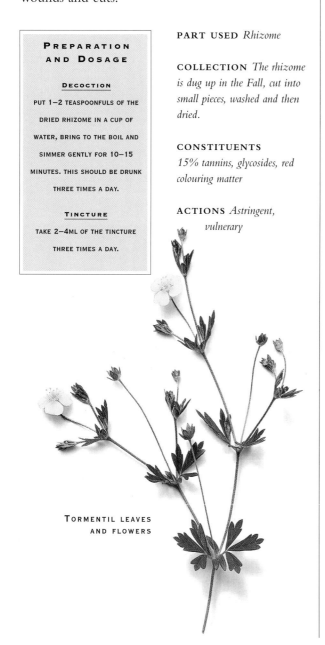

TORMENTIL LEAVES AND FLOWERS

Primula veris

PLANT FAMILY PRIMULACEAE

COWSLIP

Cowslip is an excellent, generally applicable, relaxing, sedative remedy. It will ease reactions to stress and tension, relaxing nervous excitement and facilitating restful sleep. It may be used with safety in bronchitis, colds, chills and coughs. Try it in nervous headaches and insomnia.

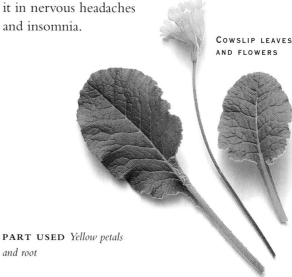

COWSLIP LEAVES AND FLOWERS

PART USED *Yellow petals and root*

COLLECTION *The flower corollae should be gathered, without the green calyx, between early spring and late spring. Dry quickly in the shade. The roots should be unearthed either before Cowslip flowers or in the Fall. Over-collecting has led to this plant becoming increasingly rare. Only pick if present in abundance and then only pick limited amounts.*

CONSTITUENTS *Up to 10% saponins, glycosides, essential oil, flavonoids*

ACTIONS *Sedative, anti-spasmodic, expectorant*

PREPARATION AND DOSAGE

DECOCTION FOR ROOT

PUT 1 TEASPOONFUL OF THE ROOT IN A CUP OF WATER, BRING TO THE BOIL AND SIMMER FOR 5 MINUTES. TAKE A CUP THREE TIMES A DAY.

TINCTURE

TAKE 2–4ML OF THE TINCTURE THREE TIMES A DAY.

COMBINATIONS

For stress-related problems it may be used with any of the relaxing nervines such as Lime Blossom or Skullcap. For coughs it may be used with Coltsfoot and Aniseed.

Prunella vulgaris

PLANT FAMILY LABIATAE

SELF-HEAL

As its name suggests, Self-Heal has a long tradition as a wound-healing herb. The fresh leaf may be used or a poultice or compress made to aid in the clean healing of cuts and wounds. As a gentle astringent it is used internally for diarrhea, hemorrhoids or mild hemorrhages. For sore throats it may be used as a gargle, sweetened with honey. For bleeding piles it may be used as an ointment or lotion. Self-Heal may be used as a spring tonic or as a general tonic in convalescence.

PREPARATION AND DOSAGE

INFUSION

POUR A CUP OF BOILING WATER ONTO 1–2 TEASPOONFULS OF THE DRIED HERB AND LEAVE TO INFUSE FOR 10 MINUTES. THIS SHOULD BE DRUNK THREE TIMES A DAY OR USED AS A GARGLE OR LOTION.

TINCTURE

TAKE 1–2ML OF THE TINCTURE THREE TIMES A DAY.

PART USED *Aerial parts*

COLLECTION *The young shoots and leaves are collected in early summer before flowering.*

CONSTITUENTS *Volatile oil, bitter principle, tannin*

ACTIONS *Astringent, vulnerary, tonic*

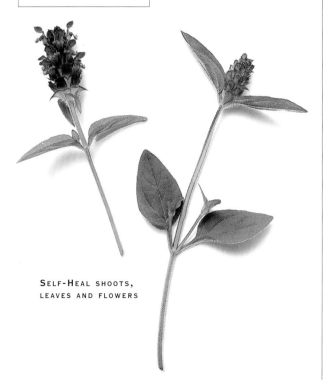

SELF-HEAL SHOOTS, LEAVES AND FLOWERS

Prunus persica

PLANT FAMILY ROSACEAE

PEACH

The leaves of this tree, which gives us that most pleasant fruit, the peach, provide a useful soothing demulcent to aid the digestive tract in conditions such as gastritis. It has a tradition of also being used in whooping cough and bronchitis.

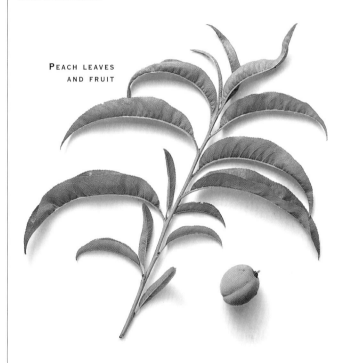

PEACH LEAVES AND FRUIT

PREPARATION AND DOSAGE

INFUSION

POUR A CUP OF BOILING WATER ONTO 1 TEASPOONFUL OF BARK OR 2 TEASPOONFULS OF THE LEAVES AND LET INFUSE FOR 10 MINUTES. THIS SHOULD BE DRUNK THREE TIMES A DAY.

PART USED
Leaves or bark

COLLECTION *The bark is collected in the spring by stripping it from young trees. The leaves are collected in early summer and mid-summer.*

CONSTITUENTS *The leaves contain a cyanogenic glycoside*

ACTIONS *Demulcent, sedative, diuretic, expectorant, anti-emetic*

Prunus serotina

PLANT FAMILY ROSACEAE

WILD CHERRY

Due to its powerful sedative action on the cough reflex, Wild Cherry bark finds its main use in the treatment of bronchitis and whooping cough. It can be used with other herbs in the control of asthma. It must be remembered, however, that the inhibition of a cough does not equate with the healing of a chest infection, which will still need to be treated. It may also be used as a bitter where digestion is sluggish. The cold infusion of the bark may be helpful as a wash in cases of inflammation of the eyes.

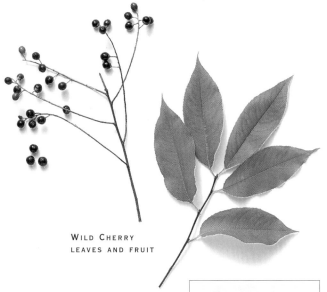

WILD CHERRY
LEAVES AND FRUIT

PART USED *Dried bark*

COLLECTION *The bark is gathered from young plants in the Fall, when it is most active. The outer bark is stripped off and the inner bark is carefully dried in the shade. It must be stored in an airtight container and protected from light.*

CONSTITUENTS *Cyanogenic glycosides including prunasin; volatile oil, coumarins, gallitannins, resin*

ACTIONS *Anti-tussive, expectorant, astringent, sedative, digestive bitter*

PREPARATION AND DOSAGE

INFUSION

POUR A CUP OF BOILING WATER ONTO 1 TEASPOONFUL OF THE DRIED BARK AND LEAVE TO INFUSE FOR 10–15 MINUTES. THIS SHOULD BE DRUNK THREE TIMES A DAY.

TINCTURE

TAKE 1–2ML OF THE TINCTURE THREE TIMES A DAY.

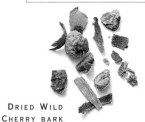

DRIED WILD
CHERRY BARK

Psychotria ipecacuanha

PLANT FAMILY RUBIACEAE

IPECACUANHA

Ipecacuanha is mainly used as an expectorant in bronchitis and conditions such as whooping cough. At higher doses it is a powerful emetic and as such is used in the treatment of poisoning. Care must be taken in the use of this herb. After an effective emetic dose has been given, large amounts of water should be taken as well. Ipecacuanha stimulates saliva production and helps expectoration through stimulation of mucous secretion and then its removal.

PREPARATION AND DOSAGE

INFUSION

ONLY A SMALL AMOUNT OF THE HERB SHOULD BE USED: 0.01–0.25G FOR AN INFUSION. POUR A CUP OF BOILING WATER ONTO A SMALL AMOUNT OF THE HERB (THE SIZE OF A PEA) AND LEAVE TO INFUSE FOR 5 MINUTES. DRINK THREE TIMES A DAY. FOR A POWERFUL EMETIC, 1–2G SHOULD BE USED, WHICH EQUALS ¼–½ TEASPOONFUL WHEN USED FOR AN INFUSION.

PART USED *Root and rhizome*

COLLECTION *The root of this small South American shrub is gathered throughout the year, although the Indians collect it when it is in flower during mid-winter and late winter.*

CONSTITUENTS *Alkaloids including emetine and cephaeline; the glycosidal tannins ipec-acuanhic acid and ipecacuanhin; ipecoside, starch, calcium oxalate*

ACTIONS *Expectorant, emetic, sialagogue, anti-protozoal*

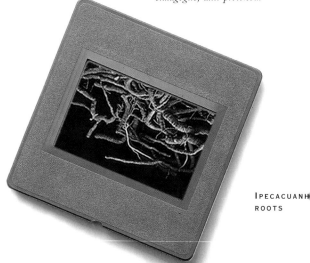

IPECACUANHA
ROOTS

COMBINATIONS
In bronchial conditions it combines well with White Horehound, Coltsfoot and Grindelia; in amebic dysentery, with American Cranesbill or Echinacea.

Pulmonaria officinalis

PLANT FAMILY BORAGINACEAE

LUNGWORT HERB

Lungwort has two broad areas of use. The one that provides its name is its use in the treatment of coughs and bronchitis, especially where associated with upper respiratory catarrh. The other broad area is that related to its astringency. This explains its use in the treating of diarrhea, especially in children, and in easing hemorrhoids. As with all plants, these two broad areas must be seen as part of the whole activity of the herb, acting as a unity. Externally this plant may be used to heal cuts and wounds.

PREPARATION AND DOSAGE

INFUSION

POUR A CUP OF BOILING WATER ONTO 1–2 TEASPOONFULS OF THE DRIED HERB AND LEAVE TO INFUSE FOR 10–15 MINUTES. THIS SHOULD BE DRUNK THREE TIMES A DAY.

TINCTURE

TAKE 1–4ML OF THE TINCTURE THREE TIMES A DAY.

PART USED *Leaves*

COLLECTION *The leaves should be gathered during and after flowering, between early spring and early Fall.*

CONSTITUENTS *Mucins, silicic acid, tannin, saponin, allantoin, quercetin, kaempferol, vitamin C*

ACTIONS *Demulcent, expectorant, astringent, vulnerary, pectoral*

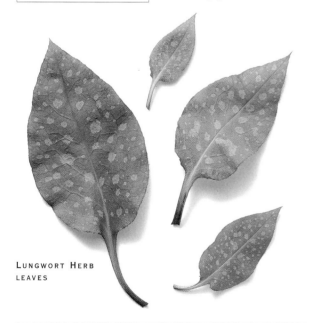

LUNGWORT HERB
LEAVES

COMBINATIONS
For lung conditions, this herb may be used with White Horehound, Coltsfoot or Lobelia.

Pulsatilla vulgaris

PLANT FAMILY RANUNCULACEAE

PASQUE FLOWER

Pasque Flower is an excellent relaxing nervine for use in problems relating to nervous tension and spasm in the reproductive system. It may be used with safety in the relief of dysmenorrhea, ovarian pain and painful conditions of the testes. It may be used to reduce tension reactions and headaches associated with them. It will help insomnia and general over-activity. The anti-bacterial actions give this herb a role in treating infections that affect the skin, especially boils. It is similarly useful in the treatment of respiratory infections and asthma. The oil or tincture will ease earache.

PASQUE FLOWER
SHOOTS AND LEAVES

CAUTION
DO NOT USE THE FRESH PLANT!

PART USED *Aerial parts*

COLLECTION *Gather the stalks at the time of flowering, in early spring or mid-spring.*

CONSTITUENTS *Glycosides, saponins, tannins, resin*

ACTIONS *Sedative, analgesic, anti-spasmodic, anti-microbial, emmenagogue, nervine*

PREPARATION AND DOSAGE

INFUSION

POUR A CUP OF BOILING WATER ONTO ½–1 TEASPOONFUL OF THE DRIED HERB AND LEAVE TO INFUSE FOR 10–15 MINUTES. THIS SHOULD BE DRUNK THREE TIMES A DAY OR WHEN NEEDED.

TINCTURE

TAKE 1–2ML OF THE TINCTURE THREE TIMES A DAY.

COMBINATIONS
For painful periods it will combine well with Cramp Bark. For skin conditions it will combine with Echinacea.

Punica granatum

PLANT FAMILY LYTHRACEAE

POMEGRANATE

Various parts of the Pomegranate can be used in medicine; however, the bark has marked anti-tapeworm activity. It can be rather strong and traumatic, associated as it often is with nausea and vomiting, since the treatment for tapeworm includes a regime of strict fasting followed by purging or enemas.

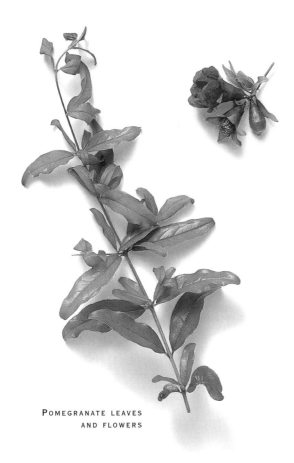

POMEGRANATE LEAVES
AND FLOWERS

PART USED *Bark*

COLLECTION *The bark of the stem or root is collected from the cultivated plant.*

CONSTITUENTS *Tannins, alkaloids*

ACTIONS *Anthelmintic*

PREPARATION
AND DOSAGE

DECOCTION

MRS GRIEVE GIVES A DOSAGE
OF 120G/4OZ OF BARK
TO 500ML/1PT OF WATER MADE
INTO A DECOCTION.
OF THIS, 15ML (½ FL OZ)
IS TAKEN.

Quercus robur

PLANT FAMILY FAGACEAE

OAK

Oak bark may be used wherever an effective astringent is called for, in diarrhea, dysentery or hemorrhoids, for example. As a gargle, the decoction can be used in tonsillitis, pharyngitis and laryngitis. It can be used as an enema for the treatment of hemorrhoids and as a douche for leucorrhea. It is primarily indicated for use in acute diarrhea, taken in frequent small doses.

PREPARATION
AND DOSAGE

DECOCTION

PUT 1 TEASPOONFUL OF THE BARK
IN A CUP OF WATER, BRING TO THE
BOIL AND SIMMER GENTLY FOR
10–15 MINUTES. THIS CAN BE
DRUNK THREE TIMES A DAY.

TINCTURE

TAKE 1–2ML OF THE TINCTURE
THREE TIMES A DAY.

PART USED *Bark*

COLLECTION *The young bark is carefully pared from the trunk or from branches which are not more than 10cm/4in thick. Take care to only take off patches, never to take a whole ring around the trunk, which would kill the tree. The bark is collected in mid-spring or late spring. It must be smooth and free from blemishes.*

CONSTITUENTS *Up to 20% tannin, gallic acid, ellagitannin*

ACTIONS *Astringent, anti-inflammatory, antiseptic*

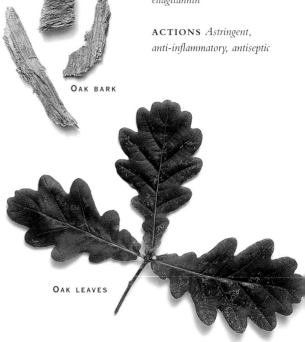

OAK BARK

OAK LEAVES

COMBINATIONS
It is often given with Ginger before meals.

Ranunculus ficaria

PLANT FAMILY RANUNCULACEAE

PILEWORT

As one would expect from the name, Pilewort, or Lesser Celandine, is almost a specific for the treatment of hemorrhoids or piles. For this use it can be taken internally or made into a very effective ointment. It may also be used wherever an astringent is called for.

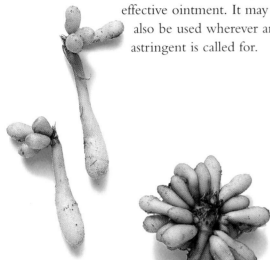

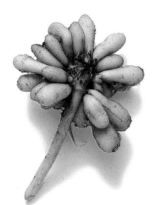

PILEWORT
ROOT

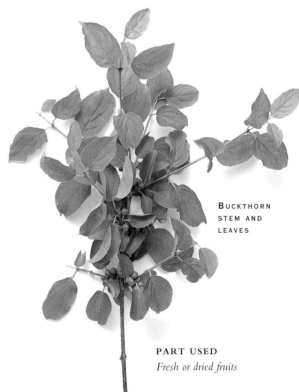

Rhamnus cathartica

PLANT FAMILY RHAMNACEAE

BUCKTHORN

Buckthorn is an effective and safe laxative, as indicated by its Latin name. Make sure that you follow dosage instructions carefully, as too much may cause an excessive reaction.

BUCKTHORN
STEM AND
LEAVES

PREPARATION AND DOSAGE

INFUSION

POUR A CUP OF BOILING WATER ONTO 1–2 TEASPOONFULS OF THE DRIED HERB AND LEAVE TO INFUSE FOR 10 MINUTES. THIS SHOULD BE DRUNK THREE TIMES A DAY.

OINTMENT

OINTMENT IS BEST MADE IN PETROLEUM JELLY AS DESCRIBED IN THE SECTION ON 'PREPARATIONS'.

TINCTURE

TAKE 2–4ML OF THE TINCTURE THREE TIMES A DAY.

PART USED *Root*

COLLECTION *The root should be unearthed during late spring and early summer.*

CONSTITUENTS *Anemonin, protoanemonin, tannin*

ACTIONS *Astringent*

PREPARATION AND DOSAGE

INFUSION

POUR A CUP OF BOILING WATER ONTO 2 TEASPOONFULS OF THE FRUIT AND LEAVE TO INFUSE FOR 10–15 MINUTES. THIS SHOULD BE DRUNK IN THE MORNING OR EVENING AS IT TAKES ABOUT 12 HOURS TO BE EFFECTIVE. THE SEEDS (ABOUT 10) MAY ALSO BE CHEWED BEFORE EATING IN THE MORNING. IF THE DOSE IS TOO HIGH, BUCKTHORN MIGHT CAUSE EXTREME DIARRHEA AND POSSIBLY VOMITING.

TINCTURE

TAKE 1–2ML OF THE TINCTURE NIGHT AND MORNING.

PART USED
Fresh or dried fruits

COLLECTION *The fruit should be collected in early Fall and mid-Fall.*

CONSTITUENTS
Anthraquinone derivates including rhamnocarthrin; vitamin C

ACTIONS *Laxative, diuretic, alterative*

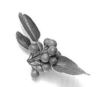

BUCKTHORN
FRUIT

COMBINATIONS

Pilewort combines well with Plantain, Marigold or Agrimony for the internal treatment of piles.

Rhamnus pushiana

PLANT FAMILY RHAMNACEAE

CASCARA SAGRADA

Cascara Sagrada may be used in chronic constipation as it encourages peristalsis and tones relaxed muscles of the digestive system.

PREPARATION AND DOSAGE

DECOCTION

PUT 1–2 TEASPOONFULS OF THE BARK IN A CUP OF WATER, BRING TO THE BOIL AND LEAVE TO INFUSE FOR 10 MINUTES. THIS SHOULD BE DRUNK AT BEDTIME.

TINCTURE

TAKE 1–2ML OF THE TINCTURE AT BEDTIME.

PART USED *Dried bark*

COLLECTION *The bark is stripped from the trunk of this western American tree in the spring and summer and left to age for a few years. Due to indiscriminate cutting by white settlers during the last century, the number of wild trees has been greatly reduced.*

CONSTITUENTS *Anthraquinones, tannin, volatile oil*

ACTIONS *Mild purgative, bitter tonic, hepatic, laxative*

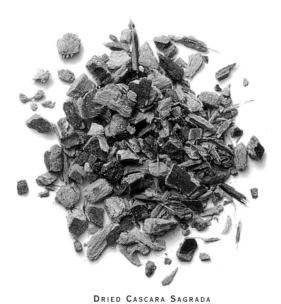

DRIED CASCARA SAGRADA

COMBINATIONS
Cascara Sagrada should be combined with aromatics and carminatives, for instance with Licorice.

Rheum palmatum

PLANT FAMILY POLYGONACEAE

RHUBARB ROOT

Rhubarb Root has a purgative action for use in the treatment of constipation, but also has an astringent effect following this. It therefore has a truly cleansing action upon the gut, removing debris and then astringing with antiseptic properties as well.
Note: Rhubarb Root may colour the urine yellow or red.

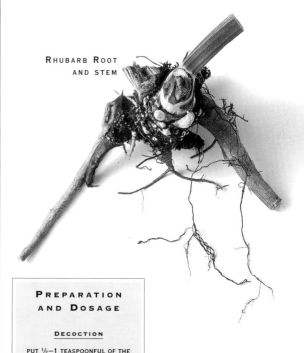

RHUBARB ROOT AND STEM

PREPARATION AND DOSAGE

DECOCTION

PUT ½–1 TEASPOONFUL OF THE ROOT IN A CUP OF WATER, BRING TO THE BOIL AND SIMMER GENTLY FOR 10 MINUTES. THIS SHOULD BE DRUNK MORNING AND EVENING.

TINCTURE

TAKE 1–2ML OF THE TINCTURE THREE TIMES A DAY.

PART USED *Rhizome of Rheum palmatum and other species, not the garden rhubarb*

COLLECTION *This root is collected in China and Turkey.*

CONSTITUENTS *Anthraquinones, tannins, bitter aromatic principle*

ACTIONS *Bitter stomachic, astringent, laxative*

COMBINATIONS
It should be combined with carminative herbs to relieve any griping that may occur.

134

Rhus aromatica

PLANT FAMILY ANACARDIACEAE

SWEET SUMACH

Sweet Sumach is a useful astringent that is especially indicated in the treatment of urinary incontinence for both the young and old alike. It may safely be used wherever an astringent is called for, such as in diarrhea or hemorrhage. This herb has a reputation for being able to reduce blood sugar. Its power in this direction is open to debate however.

PART USED *Root bark*

COLLECTION *Fruit is collected in the Fall.*

CONSTITUENTS *Tannin*

ACTIONS *Astringent*

PREPARATION AND DOSAGE

DECOCTION

PUT 1 TEASPOONFUL OF THE ROOT BARK IN A CUP OF WATER, BRING TO THE BOIL AND SIMMER FOR 10 MINUTES. THIS SHOULD BE DRUNK THREE TIMES A DAY.

TINCTURE

TAKE 1–2ML OF THE TINCTURE THREE TIMES A DAY.

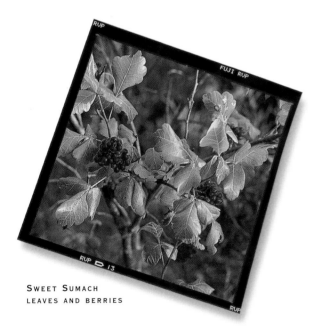

**SWEET SUMACH
LEAVES AND BERRIES**

COMBINATIONS
For the control of urinary incontinence it may be combined with Horsetail and Agrimony.

Rosa canina

PLANT FAMILY ROSACEAE

ROSEHIPS

Rosehips provide one of the best natural and freely available sources of vitamin C. They may be used wherever this vitamin is required. They will help the body's defences against infections and especially the development of colds. They make an excellent spring tonic and aid in general debility and exhaustion. They will help in cases of constipation and mild gall–bladder problems as well as conditions of the kidney and bladder.

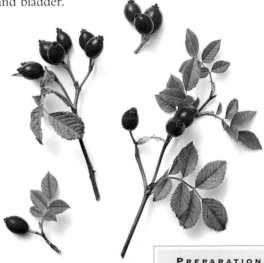

ROSEHIPS

PART USED *Fruit (hips) and seeds of the Dog Rose*

COLLECTION *The hips are collected in the Fall.*

CONSTITUENTS *Vitamin C, tannin, pectin, carotene, fruit acids, fatty oil*

ACTIONS *Nutrient, mild laxative, mild diuretic, mild astringent*

PREPARATION AND DOSAGE

THE DECOCTION OR SYRUP MAY BE TAKEN QUITE FREELY.

DECOCTION

PUT 2½ TEASPOONFULS OF THE CUT HIPS IN A CUP OF WATER, BRING TO THE BOIL AND SIMMER GENTLY FOR 10 MINUTES.

SYRUP

TO MAKE A SYRUP, FOLLOW THE GUIDELINES GIVEN IN THE CHAPTER ON 'PREPARATIONS'. FOR THIS OR ANY OTHER CULINARY PREPARATION, IT IS IMPORTANT TO REMOVE THE SEEDS FROM THE HIPS AS WELL AS THE FINE, BRITTLE HAIRS FOUND AT ONE END.

TINCTURE

TAKE 2–4ML OF THE TINCTURE THREE TIMES A DAY.

Rosmarinus officinalis

PLANT FAMILY LABIATAE

ROSEMARY

Rosemary acts as a circulatory and nervine stimulant, which in addition to the toning and calming effect on the digestion makes it a remedy that is used where psychological tension is present. This may show for instance as flatulent dyspepsia, headache or depression associated with debility. Externally it may be used to ease muscular pain, sciatica and neuralgia. It acts as a stimulant to the hair follicles and may be used in premature baldness. The oil is most effective here.

PART USED
Leaves and twigs

COLLECTION *Gather the leaves throughout the summer; they are at their best during flowering time.*

CONSTITUENTS *1% volatile oil including borneol, linalol, camphene, cineole and camphor; tannins, bitter principle, resins*

ACTIONS *Carminative, aromatic, anti-spasmodic, anti-depressive, rubefacient, parasiticide, anti-microbial, astringent, emmenagogue, nervine, stimulant*

> **PREPARATION AND DOSAGE**
>
> **INFUSION**
>
> POUR A CUP OF BOILING WATER ONTO 1–2 TEASPOONFULS OF THE DRIED HERB AND LEAVE TO INFUSE IN A COVERED CONTAINER FOR 10–15 MINUTES. THIS SHOULD BE DRUNK THREE TIMES A DAY.
>
> **TINCTURE**
>
> TAKE 1–2ML OF THE TINCTURE THREE TIMES A DAY.

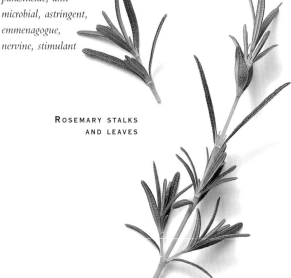

ROSEMARY STALKS AND LEAVES

COMBINATIONS
For depression it may be used with Skullcap, Kola and Oats.

Rubus idaeus

PLANT FAMILY ROSACEAE

RASPBERRY

Raspberry leaves have a long tradition of use in pregnancy to strengthen and tone the tissue of the womb, assisting contractions and checking any hemorrhage during labour. This action will occur if the herb is drunk regularly throughout pregnancy and also taken during labour. As an astringent it may be used in a wide range of cases, including diarrhea, leucorrhea and other loose conditions. It is valuable in the easing of mouth problems such as mouth ulcers, bleeding gums and inflammations. As a gargle it will help sore throats.

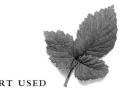

RASPBERRY LEAVES AND FRUIT

PART USED
Leaves and fruit

COLLECTION *The leaves may be collected throughout the growing season. Dry slowly in a well-ventilated area to ensure preservation of properties.*

CONSTITUENTS *Leaves: fruit sugar, volatile oil, pectin, citric acid, malic acid*

ACTIONS *Astringent, tonic, refrigerant, parturient, emmenagogue, febrifuge*

> **PREPARATION AND DOSAGE**
>
> **INFUSION**
>
> POUR A CUP OF BOILING WATER ONTO 2 TEASPOONFULS OF THE DRIED HERB AND LET INFUSE FOR 10–15 MINUTES. THIS MAY BE DRUNK FREELY.
>
> **TINCTURE**
>
> TAKE 2–4ML OF THE TINCTURE THREE TIMES A DAY.

COMBINATIONS
For the treatment of skin problems it will combine well with Burdock, Yellow Dock, Cleavers and Blue Flag.

Rumex crispus

PLANT FAMILY POLYGONACEAE

YELLOW DOCK

Yellow Dock is used extensively in the treatment of chronic skin complaints such as psoriasis. The anthraquinones present have a markedly cathartic action on the bowel, but in this herb they act in a mild way, possibly tempered by the tannin content. Thus it makes a valuable remedy for constipation, working as it does in a much wider way than simply stimulating the gut muscles. It promotes the flow of bile and has that somewhat obscure action of being a 'blood cleanser'. The action on the gall-bladder gives it a role in the treatment of jaundice when this is due to congestion.

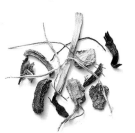

DRIED YELLOW
DOCK ROOT

PART USED *Root*

COLLECTION *The roots should be unearthed in late summer and mid-Fall. Clean well and split lengthways before drying.*

CONSTITUENTS *Anthraquinone glycosides, tannins*

ACTIONS *Alterative, cholagogue, hepatic, laxative, tonic*

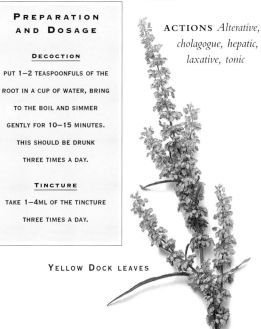

YELLOW DOCK LEAVES

PREPARATION AND DOSAGE

DECOCTION

PUT 1–2 TEASPOONFULS OF THE ROOT IN A CUP OF WATER, BRING TO THE BOIL AND SIMMER GENTLY FOR 10–15 MINUTES. THIS SHOULD BE DRUNK THREE TIMES A DAY.

TINCTURE

TAKE 1–4ML OF THE TINCTURE THREE TIMES A DAY.

COMBINATIONS

It will combine well with Dandelion, Burdock and Cleavers.

Ruta graveolens

PLANT FAMILY RUTACEAE

RUE

Rue is a herb with an ancient history. The genus name 'Ruta' comes from the Greek word 'reuo', to set free, showing its reputation as a freer from disease. Its main use is the regulation of menstrual periods, where it is used to bring on suppressed menses. The oil of Rue is a powerful abortifacient, therefore the plant is best avoided during pregnancy. The other area of usage is due to the plant's anti-spasmodic action. It may be used to relax smooth muscles, especially in the digestive system where it will ease griping and bowel tension. The easing of spasm gives it a role in the stopping of spasmodic coughs. It also increases peripheral circulation and lowers elevated blood pressure. If the fresh leaf is chewed, it will relieve tension headaches, ease palpitations and other anxiety problems.

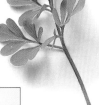

RUE LEAVES

CAUTION

AVOID DURING PREGNANCY.

PART USED
Dried aerial parts

COLLECTION *The herbs should be collected before the flowers open in the summer and dried in the shade.*

CONSTITUENTS *Essential oil, rutin, furanocoumarins, alkaloids, tannins*

ACTIONS *Anti-spasmodic, emmenagogue, anti-tussive, abortifacient, anthelmintic, anti-microbial, bitter, rubefacient, stimulant*

PREPARATION AND DOSAGE

INFUSION

POUR A CUP OF BOILING WATER ONTO 1–2 TEASPOONFULS OF THE DRIED HERB AND LEAVE TO INFUSE FOR 10–15 MINUTES. THIS SHOULD BE DRUNK THREE TIMES A DAY.

TINCTURE

TAKE 1–4ML OF THE TINCTURE THREE TIMES A DAY.

COMBINATIONS

For use in the regulation of periods it will combine well with False Unicorn Root and Life Root.

Salix nigra

PLANT FAMILY SALICACEAE

BLACK WILLOW

Black Willow is a safe natural source of aspirin-like chemicals, which helps to explain its reputation in the treatment of rheumatism and arthritis where there is much associated pain and inflammation. It may be used as part of a wider treatment for any connective tissue inflammation anywhere in the body, but it is especially useful in rheumatoid arthritis. It may also be used in fevers such as influenza.

PREPARATION AND DOSAGE

DECOCTION

POUR A CUP OF WATER ONTO 1–2 TEASPOONFULS OF THE BARK, BRING TO THE BOIL AND SIMMER FOR 10 MINUTES. THIS SHOULD BE DRUNK THREE TIMES A DAY.

TINCTURE

TAKE 2–4ML OF THE TINCTURE THREE TIMES A DAY.

PART USED Bark

COLLECTION The bark is collected in the spring when new growth starts.

CONSTITUENTS Salicin, tannin

ACTIONS Anti-inflammatory, anti-pyretic, analgesic, antiseptic, astringent, vulnerary

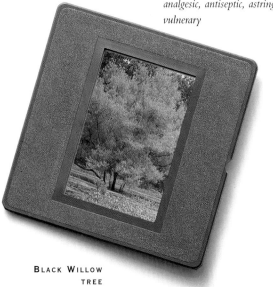

BLACK WILLOW
TREE

COMBINATIONS
It may be used with Black Cohosh, Celery Seed, Guaiacum and Bogbean in the treatment of rheumatoid arthritis.

Salvia officinalis

PLANT FAMILY LABIATEAE

RED SAGE

Red Sage is the classic remedy for inflammations of the mouth, gums, tongue, throat and tonsils, its volatile oils soothing the mucous membranes. It may be used internally and as a mouthwash, and as a gargle it will help laryngitis, pharyngitis, tonsillitis and quinsy. It is a valuable carminative used in dyspepsia. It reduces sweating when taken internally and may be used to reduce the production of breast milk. As a compress it promotes the healing of wounds. Red Sage stimulates the muscles of the uterus.

CAUTION
AVOID DURING PREGNANCY.

RED SAGE
LEAVES

PREPARATION AND DOSAGE

INFUSION

POUR A CUP OF BOILING WATER ONTO 1–2 TEASPOONFULS OF THE LEAVES AND LET INFUSE FOR 10 MINUTES. THIS SHOULD BE DRUNK THREE TIMES A DAY.

MOUTHWASH

PUT 2 TEASPOONFULS OF THE LEAVES IN 500ML/1PT OF WATER, BRING TO THE BOIL AND LET STAND, COVERED, FOR 15 MINUTES. GARGLE DEEPLY WITH THE HOT TEA FOR 5–10 MINUTES SEVERAL TIMES A DAY.

TINCTURE

TAKE 2–4ML OF THE TINCTURE THREE TIMES A DAY.

PART USED Leaves

COLLECTION Gather the leaves at the beginning of flowering in late spring or early summer. Dry in the shade or not above 35°C/95°F.

CONSTITUENTS Volatile oil including 30% thujone, 5% cineole, linalol, borneol, camphor, salvene and pinene; a bitter, tannins, triterpenoids, flavonoids, estrogenic substances, resin

ACTIONS Carminative, spasmolytic, astringent, anti-hidrotic, anti-catarrhal, anti-microbial, emmenagogue, febrifuge, stimulant

COMBINATIONS
As a gargle for throat conditions it combines well with Tormentil and Balm of Gilead. In dyspepsia it can be combined with Meadowsweet and Chamomile.

Sambucus nigra

PLANT FAMILY CAPRIFOLIACEAE

ELDER

The Elder tree is a veritable medicine chest by itself. The leaves are used primarily for bruises, sprains, wounds and chilblains. It has been reported that Elder Leaves may be useful in an ointment for tumours. Elder Flowers are ideal for the treatment of colds and influenza. They are indicated in any catarrhal inflammation of the upper respiratory tract such as hayfever and sinusitis. Catarrhal deafness responds well to Elder Flowers. Elder Berries have similar properties to the Flowers with the addition of their usefulness in rheumatism.

ELDER BERRIES
AND LEAVES

PART USED *Bark, flowers, berries, leaves*

COLLECTION *The flowers are collected in spring and early summer and dried as rapidly as possible in the shade. The bark and berries are best collected in late summer and early Fall.*

CONSTITUENTS *Flowers: Flavonoids including rutin, isoquercitrine and kampherol; the hydrocyanic glycoside sambunigrine; tannins, essential oil*
Berries: Invert sugar, fruit acids, tannin, vitamin C and P, anthrocyanic pigments, traces of essential oil

ACTIONS *Bark: purgative, emetic, diuretic*
Leaves: Externally emollient and vulnerary, internally as purgative, expectorant, diuretic and diaphoretic
Flowers: Diaphoretic, anti-catarrhal, pectoral
Berries: Diaphoretic, diuretic, laxative

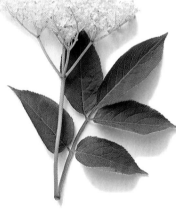

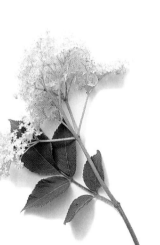

ELDER FLOWERS

COMBINATIONS

For colds and fevers it may be used with Peppermint, Yarrow or Hyssop. For influenza combine it with Boneset. For catarrhal states mix it with Golden Rod.

Sanguinaria canadensis

PLANT FAMILY PAPAVERACEAE

BLOOD ROOT

Blood root finds its main use in the treatment of bronchitis in any of its forms. Whilst the stimulating properties show in its power as an emetic and expectorant, it demonstrates a relaxing action on the bronchial muscles. It thus has a role in the treatment of asthma, croup and also laryngitis. It acts as a stimulant in cases of deficient peripheral circulation. It may be used as a snuff in the treatment of nasal polyps.

PART USED *Dried rhizome*

COLLECTION *The rhizome is unearthed in late spring to early summer or in Fall when the leaves have dried. It should be dried carefully in the shade.*

CONSTITUENTS *Alkaloids including sanguinarine, chelery-thrine, protopine and homoche-lidine; red resin, citric acid, malic acids*

ACTIONS *Expectorant, anti-spasmodic, emetic, cathartic, antiseptic, cardio-active, topical irritant, pectoral*

> ### PREPARATION AND DOSAGE
>
> #### DECOCTION
> PUT ½ TEASPOONFUL OF THE RHIZOME IN A CUP OF COLD WATER, BRING TO THE BOIL AND LEAVE TO INFUSE FOR 10 MINUTES. THIS SHOULD BE DRUNK THREE TIMES A DAY.
>
> #### TINCTURE
> TAKE 0.5–1ML OF THE TINCTURE THREE TIMES A DAY.

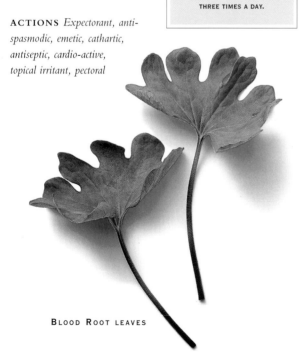

BLOOD ROOT LEAVES

COMBINATIONS
May be combined with Lobelia in bronchitic asthma. In pharyngitis it combines well with Red Sage and a pinch of Cayenne.

Saponaria officinalis

PLANT FAMILY CARYOPHYLLACEAE

SOAPWORT

Medicinally Soapwort can be used as an effective expectorant in bronchitis and dry coughs. It is also reported to have an effect upon gall-stones. In higher doses, Soapwort is a powerful laxative, but it can cause stomach upsets. Externally it may be used as a wash in skin problems such as eczema.

SOAPWORT SHOOT, LEAVES AND FLOWERS

PART USED *Rhizome and roots, aerial parts to a lesser extent*

COLLECTION *The root and rhizome are best dug up and dried between early to mid-Fall. The leaves are collected between mid-summer and late summer.*

CONSTITUENTS *Saponins*

ACTIONS *Expectorant, laxative, mild diuretic*

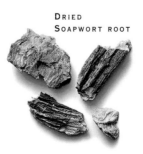

DRIED SOAPWORT ROOT

> ### PREPARATION AND DOSAGE
>
> #### DECOCTION
> THE BEST WAY TO MAKE A DECOCTION OF THIS ROOT IS TO SOAK 4 TABLESPOONS OF THE DRIED ROOT (OR 2 OF THE FINELY CUT FRESH ROOT) IN 1L/1¾PT OF COLD WATER FOR 5 HOURS. BRING THIS TO THE BOIL AND SIMMER FOR 10 MINUTES. THIS SHOULD BE DRUNK THREE TO FOUR TIMES A DAY.
>
> #### TINCTURE
> TAKE 1–2ML OF THE TINCTURE THREE TIMES A DAY.

Sassafras albidum

PLANT FAMILY LAURACEAE

SASSAFRAS

Sassafras is used primarily in skin problems such as eczema and psoriasis. As another aspect of its undoubted systemic activity, it may be used with benefit in the treatment of rheumatism and gout. As a diaphoretic it may be used in fevers and systemic infections. The plant has a disinfectant action and makes a valuable mouthwash and dentifrice. It acts as a specific to combat head lice and other body infestations.

DRIED
SASSAFRAS BARK

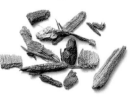

PART USED *Root bark*

COLLECTION *The root is unearthed to gather this herb, which grows over large areas of North America.*

CONSTITUENTS *Essential oil including safrole; sesamin, tannins, resin*

ACTIONS *Alterative, carminative, diaphoretic, diuretic*

PREPARATION AND DOSAGE

INFUSION

POUR A CUP OF BOILING WATER ONTO 1–2 TEASPOONFULS OF THE DRIED HERB AND LEAVE TO INFUSE FOR 10–15 MINUTES. THIS SHOULD BE DRUNK THREE TIMES A DAY.

OIL

THE OIL OF SASSAFRAS SHOULD BE USED FOR THE EXTERNAL TREATMENT OF LICE AND NEVER TAKEN INTERNALLY.

TINCTURE

TAKE 1–2ML OF THE TINCTURE THREE TIMES A DAY.

SASSAFRAS LEAVES

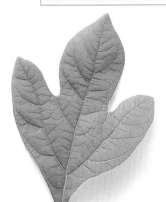

COMBINATIONS

For skin problems it may be used with Burdock, Nettles and Yellow Dock.

Scrophularia nodosa

PLANT FAMILY SCROPHULARIACEAE

FIGWORT

Figwort finds most use in the treatment of skin problems. It acts in a broad way to help the body function well, bringing about a state of inner cleanliness. It may be used for eczema, psoriasis and any skin condition where there is itching and irritation. Part of the cleansing occurs due to the purgative and diuretic actions. It may be used as a mild laxative in constipation. As a heart stimulant, Figwort should be avoided where there is any abnormally rapid heartbeat (tachycardia).

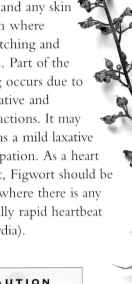

FIGWORT
SHOOT, LEAVES
AND FLOWERS

CAUTION
AVOID IN CASES OF ABNORMALLY RAPID HEARTBEAT.

PART USED *Aerial parts*

COLLECTION *The stalks and leaves are gathered during flowering between early summer and late summer.*

CONSTITUENTS *Saponins, cardioactive glycosides, flavonoids, resin, sugar, organic acids*

ACTIONS *Alterative, diuretic, mild purgative, heart stimulant*

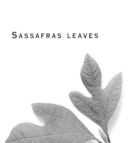

PREPARATION AND DOSAGE

INFUSION

POUR A CUP OF BOILING WATER ONTO 1–3 TEASPOONFULS OF THE DRIED LEAVES AND LET INFUSE FOR 10–15 MINUTES. THIS SHOULD BE DRUNK THREE TIMES A DAY.

TINCTURE

TAKE 2–4ML OF THE TINCTURE THREE TIMES A DAY.

COMBINATIONS

It will combine well with Yellow Dock and Burdock Root in the treatment of skin problems.

Scutellaria laterifolia

PLANT FAMILY LABIATAE

SKULLCAP

Skullcap is perhaps the most widely relevant nervine available to us in the materia medica. It relaxes states of nervous tension whilst at the same time renewing and revivifying the central nervous system. It has a specific use in the treatment of seizure and hysterical states as well as epilepsy. It may be used in all exhausted or depressed conditions. It can be used to ease pre-menstrual tension.

PART USED *Aerial parts*

COLLECTION *The whole of the aerial parts should be collected late in the flowering period during late summer and early Fall.*

CONSTITUENTS *Flavonoid glycoside including scutellarin and scutellarein; trace of volatile oil, bitter*

ACTIONS *Nervine tonic, sedative, anti-spasmodic, analgesic, hypnotic*

PREPARATION AND DOSAGE

INFUSION

POUR A CUP OF BOILING WATER ONTO 1–2 TEASPOONFULS OF THE DRIED HERB AND LEAVE TO INFUSE FOR 10–15 MINUTES. THIS SHOULD BE DRUNK THREE TIMES A DAY OR WHEN NEEDED.

TINCTURE

TAKE 2–4ML OF THE TINCTURE THREE TIMES A DAY.

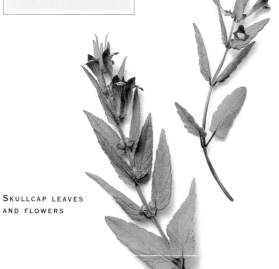

SKULLCAP LEAVES AND FLOWERS

COMBINATIONS
It combines well with Valerian.

Selenicereus grandiflorus

PLANT FAMILY CACTACEAE

NIGHT BLOOMING CEREUS

This is a very useful herb in the treatment of mild heart failure and its associated symptoms of water retention and breathlessness. It may also be of value in cases of heart palpitations related to nervousness. Night Blooming Cereus does not contain a cardiac glycoside and so would not replace such medications if they were necessary.

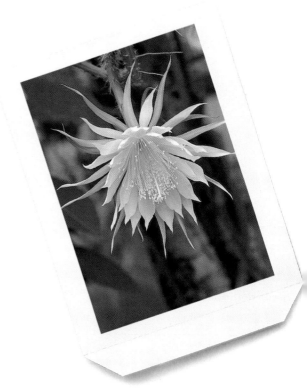

NIGHT BLOOMING CEREUS FLOWER

PART USED *Fresh stems*

COLLECTION *Succulent stems and flowers are collected when in bloom.*

CONSTITUENTS
Flavones, phenylalkylamines (eg hordenine), alkaloids (eg grandifoline)

ACTIONS *Cardio-tonic*

PREPARATION AND DOSAGE

TAKE 1.25–1.5 ML OF THE TINCTURE THREE TIMES A DAY.

142

RAGWORT

Senecio jacobaea

PLANT FAMILY COMPOSITAE

Ragwort is potentially poisonous to the liver and must on no occasion be taken internally. As a liniment, it provides a stimulating and warming preparation used externally on rheumatic muscles.

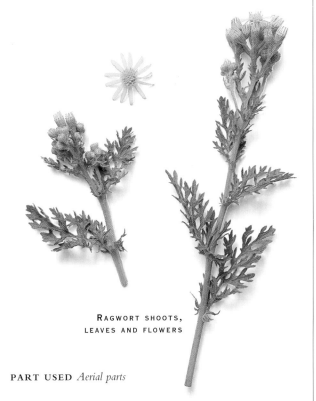

RAGWORT SHOOTS, LEAVES AND FLOWERS

PART USED *Aerial parts*

COLLECTION *This common plant is collected when in flower between early summer and early Fall.*

CONSTITUENTS *Essential oil, rutin, an alkaloid, mucilage*

ACTIONS *Rubefacient*

CAUTION
NEVER TAKE THIS PLANT INTERNALLY.

PREPARATION AND DOSAGE

POULTICE
THIS HERB MAY BE MADE INTO A POULTICE ACCORDING TO THE INSTRUCTIONS IN THE SECTION ON 'PREPARATIONS'.

SENNA

Senna alexandrina

PLANT FAMILY LEGUMINOSAE

Senna pods are used as a powerful cathartic in the treatment of constipation. It is vital to recognize, however, that the constipation is a result of something else and that this has to be sought and dealt with. See section on the Digestive System for more information.

PREPARATION AND DOSAGE

INFUSION
THE DRIED PODS SHOULD BE STEEPED IN WARM WATER FOR 6–12 HOURS. IF THEY ARE ALEXANDRIAN SENNA PODS USE 3–6 IN A CUP OF WATER; IF THEY ARE TINNEVELLY SENNA, USE 4–12 PODS. THESE NAMES ARE GIVEN TO TWO DIFFERENT SPECIES WHEN SOLD COMMERCIALLY.

TINCTURE
TAKE 2–7ML OF THE TINCTURE THREE TIMES A DAY.

PART USED
Dried fruit pods

COLLECTION *The pods are gathered during the winter in Egypt, Sudan, Jordan and India.*

CONSTITUENTS
Anthraquinones

ACTIONS *Laxative*

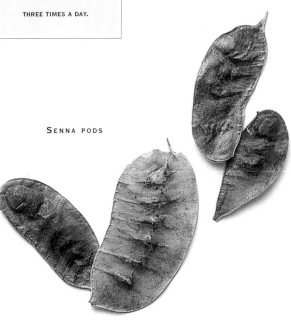

SENNA PODS

COMBINATIONS
It is best to combine Senna pods with aromatic, carminative herbs to increase palatability and reduce griping, for instance by using Cardamon, Ginger or Fennel.

Seronoa repens

PLANT FAMILY PALMAE

SAW PALMETTO

Saw Palmetto is a herb that acts to tone and strengthen the male reproductive system. It may be used with safety where a boost to the male sex hormones is required. It is a specific in cases of enlarged prostate glands. It will be of value in all infections of the gastro-urinary tract.

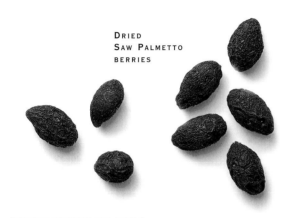

DRIED
SAW PALMETTO
BERRIES

PREPARATION AND DOSAGE

DECOCTION

PUT ½–1 TEASPOONFUL OF THE BERRIES IN A CUP OF WATER, BRING TO THE BOIL AND SIMMER GENTLY FOR 5 MINUTES. THIS SHOULD BE DRUNK THREE TIMES A DAY.

TINCTURE

TAKE 1–2ML OF THE TINCTURE THREE TIMES A DAY.

PART USED *Berries*

COLLECTION *The berries of this impressive palm are gathered from early Fall through until mid-winter.*

CONSTITUENTS *Volatile oil, steroids, dextrose, resins*

ACTIONS *Diuretic, urinary antiseptic, endocrine agent*

COMBINATIONS

For debility associated with the reproductive system it will combine well with Damiana and Kola.
For the treatment of enlarged prostate glands it may be used with Horsetail and Hydrangea.

Silybum marianum

PLANT FAMILY COMPOSITAE

MILK THISTLE

As the name of this herb shows, it is an excellent promoter of milk secretion and is perfectly safe to be used by all breastfeeding mothers. Milk Thistle can also be used to increase the secretion and flow of bile from the liver and gall-bladder and as such it may be used in all problems associated with the gall-bladder.

PREPARATION AND DOSAGE

INFUSION

POUR A CUP OF BOILING WATER ONTO 1 TEASPOONFUL OF THE DRIED HERB AND LEAVE TO INFUSE FOR 10–15 MINUTES. THIS SHOULD BE DRUNK THREE TIMES A DAY OR AS NEEDED.

TINCTURE

TAKE 1–2ML OF THE TINCTURE THREE TIMES A DAY.

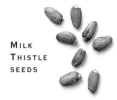

MILK
THISTLE
SEEDS

PART USED *Seeds*

COLLECTION *The mature achenes (seed heads) are cut and stored in a warm place. After a few days, tap the heads and collect the seeds.*

CONSTITUENTS *Flavones silybin, silydianin and silychristin, essential oil, bitter principle, mucilage*

ACTIONS *Cholagogue, galactogogue, demulcent*

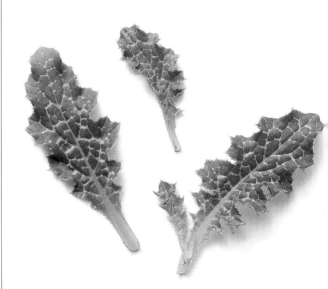

MILK THISTLE LEAVES

Smilax regelii

PLANT FAMILY LILIACEAE

SARSAPARILLA

Sarsaparilla is a widely applicable alterative. It may be used to aid proper functioning of the body as a whole and in the correction of such diffuse systemic problems as skin and rheumatic conditions. It is particularly useful in scaling skin conditions such as psoriasis, especially where there is much irritation. As part of a wider treatment for chronic rheumatism it should be considered and is especially useful for rheumatoid arthritis. It has been shown that Sarsaparilla contains chemicals with properties that aid testosterone activity in the body.

PART USED *Root and rhizome*

COLLECTION *The roots and rhizome can be unearthed throughout the year.*

CONSTITUENTS *Sapogenins, glycosides, essential oil, resin*

ACTIONS *Alterative, anti-rheumatic, diuretic, diaphoretic, tonic*

PREPARATION AND DOSAGE

DECOCTION

PUT 1–2 TEASPOONFULS OF THE ROOT IN A CUP OF WATER, BRING TO THE BOIL AND SIMMER FOR 10–15 MINUTES. THIS SHOULD BE DRUNK THREE TIMES A DAY.

TINCTURE

TAKE 1–2ML OF THE TINCTURE THREE TIMES A DAY.

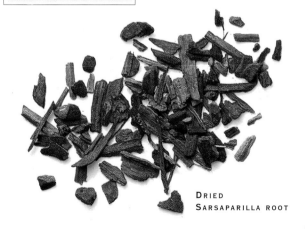

DRIED SARSAPARILLA ROOT

COMBINATIONS

For psoriasis it will combine well with Burdock, Yellow Dock and Cleavers.

Solanum dulcamara

PLANT FAMILY SOLANACEAE

BITTERSWEET

The primary use of the stems of Bittersweet is in the treatment of skin and rheumatic complaints, possibly indicating a similarity of origin of those illnesses, both being the result of systemic factors. Bittersweet may be used in psoriasis, eczema and pityriasis. Rheumatic and arthritic inflammations are eased as well as gradually improved. It may be used for diarrhea and dysentery, jaundice and hepatic disease. Ointments can be made from the stems and especially from the leaves and used for eczema, psoriasis and ulcers.

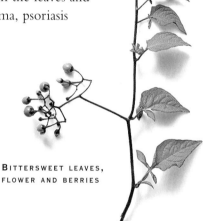

BITTERSWEET LEAVES, FLOWER AND BERRIES

CAUTION

AS THE BERRIES CONTAIN A MUCH HIGHER LEVEL OF ALKALOIDS, THEY MAY BE POISONOUS AND MUST BE AVOIDED.

PREPARATION AND DOSAGE

INFUSION

POUR A CUP OF BOILING WATER ONTO 1 TEASPOONFUL OF THE DRIED HERB AND LEAVE TO INFUSE FOR 10 MINUTES. THIS SHOULD BE DRUNK TWICE DAILY.

TINCTURE

TAKE 1–2ML OF THE TINCTURE THREE TIMES A DAY.

PART USED *Leaves and stems*

COLLECTION *The stems are collected in early Fall and mid-Fall, leaves in summer.*

CONSTITUENTS *Dulcamarin, tannin, gum, 1% alkaloids including solanidine*

ACTIONS *Diuretic, alterative, anti-rheumatic, expectorant, mild sedative*

Solidago virgauria

PLANT FAMILY COMPOSITAE

GOLDEN ROD

Golden Rod is perhaps the first plant to think of for upper respiratory catarrh, whether acute or chronic. It may be used in combination with other herbs in the treatment of influenza. The carminative properties reveal a role in the treatment of flatulent dyspepsia. As an anti-inflammatory urinary antiseptic, Golden Rod may be used in cystitis, urethritis and the like. It can be used to promote the healing of wounds. As a gargle it can be used in laryngitis and pharyngitis.

GOLDEN ROD LEAVES AND FLOWERS

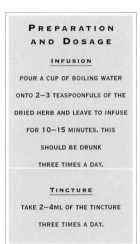

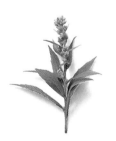

PREPARATION AND DOSAGE

INFUSION

POUR A CUP OF BOILING WATER ONTO 2–3 TEASPOONFULS OF THE DRIED HERB AND LEAVE TO INFUSE FOR 10–15 MINUTES. THIS SHOULD BE DRUNK THREE TIMES A DAY.

TINCTURE

TAKE 2–4ML OF THE TINCTURE THREE TIMES A DAY.

PART USED
Dried aerial parts

COLLECTION *Gather stalks at the time of flowering, which is between mid-summer and mid-Fall, preferably from plants not yet blooming. Dry in the shade or not above a temperature of 40°C/104°F.*

CONSTITUENTS *Saponins, essential oil, bitter principle, tannins, flavonoids*

ACTIONS *Anti-catarrhal, anti-inflammatory, antiseptic, diaphoretic, carminative, diuretic*

COMBINATIONS
For upper respiratory catarrh it may be used with Cudweed, Echinacea, Poke Root and Wild Indigo.

Stachys officinalis

PLANT FAMILY LABIATAE

WOOD BETONY

Wood Betony feeds and strengthens the central nervous system and also has a sedative action. It finds use in nervous debility associated with anxiety and tension. It will ease headaches and neuralgia when they are of nervous origin.

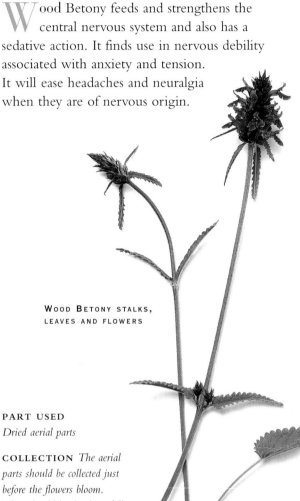

WOOD BETONY STALKS, LEAVES AND FLOWERS

PART USED
Dried aerial parts

COLLECTION *The aerial parts should be collected just before the flowers bloom. They should be dried carefully in the sun.*

CONSTITUENTS *Alkaloids including betonicine, stachydrene and trigonelline*

ACTIONS *Sedative, nervine tonic, bitter, aromatic, vulnerary*

PREPARATION AND DOSAGE

INFUSION

POUR A CUP OF BOILING WATER ONTO 1–2 TEASPOONFULS OF THE DRIED HERB AND LEAVE TO INFUSE FOR 10–15 MINUTES. THIS SHOULD BE DRUNK THREE TIMES A DAY.

TINCTURE

TAKE 2–6ML OF THE TINCTURE THREE TIMES A DAY.

COMBINATIONS
For the treatment of nervous headache it combines well with Skullcap.

Stachys palustris

PLANT FAMILY LABIATAE

WOUNDWORT

As its name implies, Woundwort is renowned in folklore as a wound-healer. Used as a vulnerary it is an equivalent of Comfrey in its effect on wounds. It may be used directly on the wound or as an ointment or compress. Internally it will ease cramps and some joint pains, and also relieve diarrhea and dysentery.

PREPARATION AND DOSAGE

INFUSION

POUR A CUP OF BOILING WATER ONTO 1 TEASPOONFUL OF THE DRIED HERB AND LEAVE TO INFUSE FOR 10–15 MINUTES. THIS SHOULD BE DRUNK THREE TIMES A DAY.

EXTERNAL USE

FOLLOW THE INSTRUCTIONS GIVEN IN THE SECTION ON 'PREPARATIONS'.

TINCTURE

TAKE 1–2ML OF THE TINCTURE THREE TIMES A DAY.

PART USED *Aerial parts*

COLLECTION *The herb is collected in mid-summer when coming into flower.*

CONSTITUENTS *Flavonoids, iridoids*

ACTIONS *Vulnerary, antiseptic, anti-spasmodic, astringent*

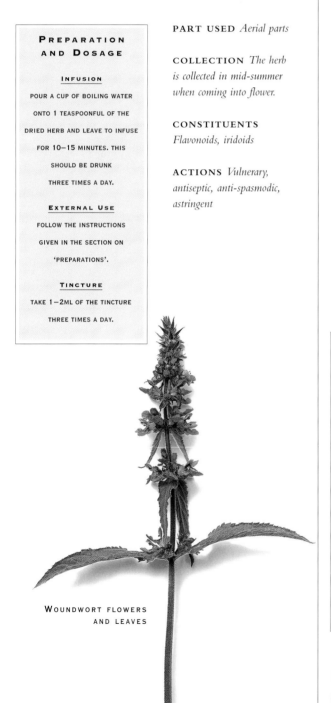

WOUNDWORT FLOWERS AND LEAVES

Stellaria media

PLANT FAMILY CARYOPHYLLACEAE

CHICKWEED

Chickweed finds its most common use as an external remedy for cuts, wounds and especially for itching and irritation. If eczema or psoriasis causes this sort of irritation, Chickweed may be used with benefit. Internally it has a reputation as a remedy for rheumatism.

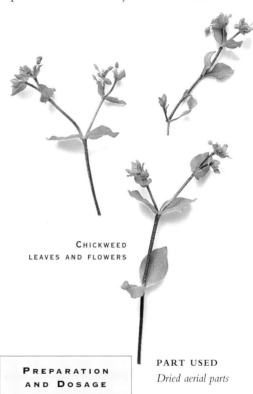

CHICKWEED LEAVES AND FLOWERS

PREPARATION AND DOSAGE

INFUSION

POUR A CUP OF BOILING WATER ONTO 2 TEASPOONFULS OF THE DRIED HERB AND LEAVE TO INFUSE FOR 5 MINUTES. THIS SHOULD BE DRUNK THREE TIMES A DAY.

EXTERNAL USE

TO EASE ITCHING, A STRONG INFUSION OF THE FRESH PLANT MAKES A USEFUL ADDITION TO BATH WATER. CHICKWEED MAY BE MADE INTO AN OINTMENT OR CAN BE USED AS A POULTICE.

PART USED *Dried aerial parts*

COLLECTION *This very common weed of gardens and fields can be collected all year round, although it is not abundant during the winter.*

CONSTITUENTS *Saponins*

ACTIONS *Anti-rheumatic, vulnerary, emollient*

COMBINATIONS

Chickweed makes an excellent ointment when combined with Marshmallow.

Stillingia sylvatica

PLANT FAMILY EUPHORBIACEAE

QUEEN'S DELIGHT

This North American herb finds a use in the treatment of chronic skin conditions such as eczema and psoriasis. The treatment must be spread over a long period of time however. These skin conditions can be due to a whole range of contributing factors. Queen's Delight is most useful where there is lymphatic involvement. Another area of application is in bronchitis and laryngitis, especially where it is accompanied by loss of voice. As an astringent it may be used in a number of conditions, especially hemorrhoids.

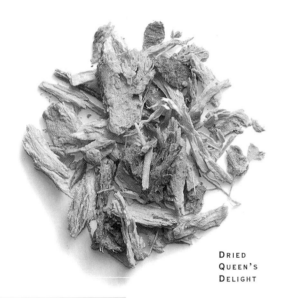

DRIED QUEEN'S DELIGHT

PREPARATION AND DOSAGE

DECOCTION

PUT ½−1 TEASPOONFUL OF THE DRIED ROOT IN A CUP OF WATER, BRING TO THE BOIL AND SIMMER GENTLY FOR 10−15 MINUTES. THIS SHOULD BE DRUNK THREE TIMES A DAY.

TINCTURE

TAKE 1−2ML OF THE TINCTURE THREE TIMES A DAY.

PART USED *Root*

COLLECTION *The root is unearthed after flowering has finished in mid-summer.*

CONSTITUENTS *Diterpenes, fixed and volatile oils, resins*

ACTIONS *Alterative, expectorant, diaphoretic, sialagogue, astringent, anti-spasmodic*

COMBINATIONS

For the treatment of skin problems it will combine well with Burdock, Yellow Dock, Cleavers and Blue Flag.

Symphytum officinale

PLANT FAMILY BORAGINACEAE

COMFREY

Comfrey is a powerful healing agent in gastric and duodenal ulcers, hiatus hernia and ulcerative colitis. Its astringency will help hemorrhages whenever they occur. It has been used with benefit in cases of bronchitis and irritable cough, where it will soothe and reduce irritation whilst helping expectoration. Comfrey may be used externally to speed wound-healing and guard against scar tissue developing incorrectly. It is excellent in chronic varicose ulcers.

CAUTION

TAKE CARE WITH VERY DEEP WOUNDS AS THE EXTERNAL APPLICATION OF COMFREY CAN LEAD TO TISSUE FORMING OVER THE WOUND BEFORE IT IS HEALED DEEPER DOWN, POSSIBLY LEADING TO ABSCESSES.

PART USED *Root and rhizome, leaf*

COLLECTION *Unearth the roots in the spring or Fall when the allantoin levels are highest. Split the roots down the middle and dry in moderate temperatures of about 40−60°C/ 104−140°F.*

CONSTITUENTS *Mucilage, gum, allantoin, tannin, alkaloids, resin, volatile oil*

ACTIONS *Vulnerary, demulcent, astringent, expectorant, emollient, pectoral, tonic*

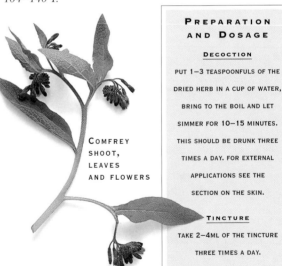

COMFREY SHOOT, LEAVES AND FLOWERS

PREPARATION AND DOSAGE

DECOCTION

PUT 1−3 TEASPOONFULS OF THE DRIED HERB IN A CUP OF WATER, BRING TO THE BOIL AND LET SIMMER FOR 10−15 MINUTES. THIS SHOULD BE DRUNK THREE TIMES A DAY. FOR EXTERNAL APPLICATIONS SEE THE SECTION ON THE SKIN.

TINCTURE

TAKE 2−4ML OF THE TINCTURE THREE TIMES A DAY.

COMBINATIONS

For gastric ulcers and inflammations it combines well with Marshmallow and Meadowsweet.
For chest and bronchial troubles use it with Coltsfoot, White Horehound or Elecampane.

Symplocarpus foetidus

PLANT FAMILY ARACEAE

SKUNK CABBAGE

Skunk Cabbage may be used whenever there is a tense or spasmodic condition in the lungs. It will act to relax and ease irritable coughs. It may be used in asthma, bronchitis and whooping cough. As a diaphoretic it will aid the body during fevers.

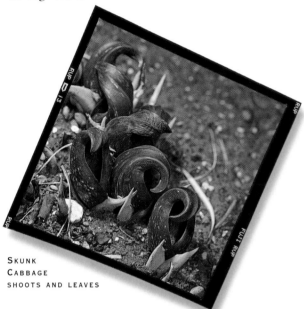

SKUNK
CABBAGE
SHOOTS AND LEAVES

PART USED
Root and rhizome

COLLECTION *The underground parts should be unearthed in the Fall or early spring. However, they should not be kept for more than one year as they deteriorate with age and drying.*

CONSTITUENTS *Volatile oil, resin, an acid principle*

ACTIONS *Anti-spasmodic, diaphoretic, expectorant*

COMBINATIONS
For the treatment of asthmatic conditions it may be used with Grindelia, Pill-bearing Spurge and Lobelia.

Syzygium aromaticum

PLANT FAMILY MYRTACEAE

CLOVES

Cloves may be used to allay nausea, vomiting and flatulence and to stimulate the digestive system. It is a powerful local antiseptic and mild anesthetic, which may be used externally in toothache.

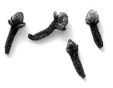

CLOVES

PART USED
Dried flowers and oil

COLLECTION *The flower buds are collected from this tree when their lower parts turn from green to purple. It grows all around the Indian Ocean.*

CONSTITUENTS *Up to 20% of volatile oil*

ACTIONS *Stimulant, carminative, aromatic, anti-emetic, anti-microbial*

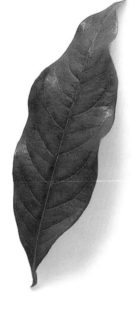

CLOVE LEAF
AND CLOVES

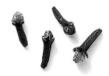

Syzygium cumini

PLANT FAMILY MYRTACEAE

JAMBUL

Jambul may be used in diarrhea or in any condition where a mild and effective astringent is called for. Its carminative properties, due to the volatile oil, make it ideal for conditions where diarrhea is associated with griping pain. Jambul has been used in orthodox medicine for the treatment of diabetes.

PART USED *Dried fruits*

COLLECTION *The fruit of this tree, which grows from India to Australia, is collected in the late summer.*

CONSTITUENTS
Volatile oil, fixed oil, resin containing ellagic acid, tannin

ACTIONS *Astringent, carminative, reputed hypoglycemic*

PREPARATION AND DOSAGE

INFUSION

POUR A CUP OF BOILING WATER ONTO 1–2 TEASPOONFULS OF THE DRIED FRUIT AND LEAVE TO INFUSE FOR 10–15 MINUTES. THIS SHOULD BE DRUNK THREE TIMES A DAY.

TINCTURE

TAKE 1–4ML OF THE TINCTURE THREE TIMES A DAY.

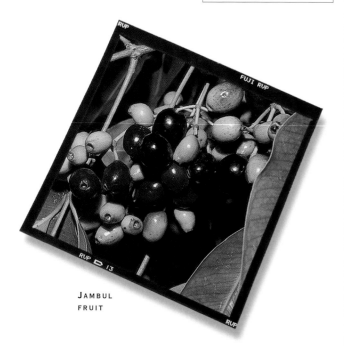

JAMBUL
FRUIT

Tanacetum parthenium

PLANT FAMILY COMPOSITAE

FEVERFEW

Feverfew has regained its deserved reputation as a primary remedy in the treatment of migraine headaches, especially those that are relieved by applying warmth to the head. It may also help arthritis when it is in the painfully active inflammatory stage. Dizziness and tinnitus may be eased, especially if it is used in conjunction with other remedies. Painful periods and sluggish menstrual flow will be relieved by Feverfew.

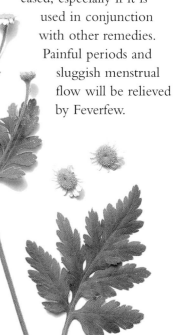

FEVERFEW LEAVES
AND FLOWERS

PREPARATION AND DOSAGE

IT IS BEST TO USE THE EQUIVALENT OF ONE FRESH LEAF ONE TO THREE TIMES A DAY. IT IS BEST USED FRESH OR FROZEN.

PART USED *Leaves*

COLLECTION *The leaves may be picked throughout the spring and summer, although just before flowering is best.*

CONSTITUENTS
Sesquiterpene lactones such as parthenolides, volatile oils

ACTIONS *Anti-inflammatory, vasodilatory, relaxant, digestive bitter, uterine stimulant*

CAUTION

FEVERFEW SHOULD NOT BE USED DURING PREGNANCY BECAUSE OF THE STIMULANT ACTION ON THE WOMB. THE FRESH LEAVES MAY CAUSE MOUTH ULCERS IN SENSITIVE PEOPLE.

Tanacetum vulgare

PLANT FAMILY COMPOSITAE

TANSY

Tansy is an effective remedy for use in ridding the digestive tract of infestations of worms. Whilst it is quite safe for this, its continued use over a period of time should be avoided as some of the constituents of the oil are quite dangerous in large dosage. The herb is effective against roundworm and threadworm and may be used in children as an enema. As a bitter it will stimulate the digestive process and ease dyspepsia, having all the actions of a bitter tonic. It may be used as an emmenagogue to stimulate menstruation, but must be avoided during pregnancy. Externally a lotion will be useful in cases of scabies.

CAUTION
AVOID DURING PREGNANCY.

PREPARATION AND DOSAGE

INFUSION
POUR A CUP OF BOILING WATER ONTO 1 TEASPOONFUL OF THE DRIED HERB AND LEAVE TO INFUSE FOR 10–15 MINUTES. THIS SHOULD BE DRUNK TWICE A DAY.

TINCTURE
TAKE 1–2ML OF THE TINCTURE THREE TIMES A DAY.

PART USED *Aerial parts*

COLLECTION *The leaves and flowers are collected during the flowering time between early summer and early Fall.*

CONSTITUENTS
Volatile oil containing thujone; bitter glycosides, sesquiterpene lactones, terpenoids, flavonoids, tannin

ACTIONS *Vermifuge, anthelmintic, digestive bitter, carminative, emmenagogue, stimulant*

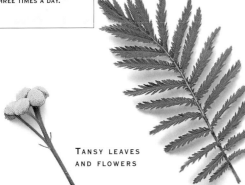

TANSY LEAVES AND FLOWERS

COMBINATIONS
For intestinal worms it may be used with Wormwood and a carminative such as Chamomile in conjunction with a purgative such as Senna.

Taraxacum officinale

PLANT FAMILY COMPOSITAE

DANDELION

Dandelion is a very powerful diuretic and one of the best natural sources of potassium. It thus makes an ideally balanced diuretic even in cases of water retention due to heart problems. As a cholagogue it may be used in inflammation and congestion of the liver and gall-bladder. It is specific in cases of congestive jaundice. As part of a wider treatment for muscular rheumatism it can be most effective.

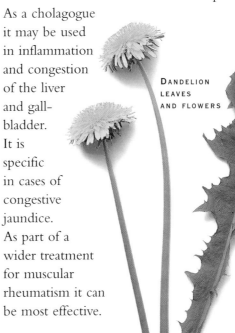

DANDELION LEAVES AND FLOWERS

PART USED *Root or leaf*

COLLECTION *The roots are best collected between early summer and late summer when they are at their bitterest. Split longitudinally before drying. The leaves may be collected at any time.*

CONSTITUENTS
Glycosides, triterpenoids, choline, up to 5% potassium

ACTIONS *Diuretic, cholagogue, anti-rheumatic, laxative, tonic, anti-bilious, hepatic*

PREPARATION AND DOSAGE

DECOCTION
PUT 2–3 TEASPOONFULS OF THE ROOT INTO ONE CUP OF WATER, BRING TO THE BOIL AND GENTLY SIMMER FOR 10–15 MINUTES. THIS SHOULD BE DRUNK THREE TIMES A DAY. THE LEAVES MAY BE EATEN RAW IN SALADS.

TINCTURE
TAKE 5–10ML OF THE TINCTURE THREE TIMES A DAY.

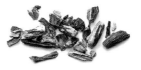

DRIED DANDELION ROOT

COMBINATIONS
For liver and gall-bladder problems it may be used with Couchgrass or Yarrow.

151

Teucrium scorodonia

PLANT FAMILY LABIATAE

WOOD SAGE

Wood Sage may be used for all infections of the upper respiratory tract, especially for colds and influenza. It may be used as a diaphoretic in all fevers. It can prove beneficial in some cases of rheumatism. There is a marked stimulation of gastric juices, thereby aiding digestion and relieving flatulent indigestion. Externally Wood Sage will speed the healing of wounds, boils and abscesses.

PREPARATION AND DOSAGE

INFUSION

POUR A CUP OF BOILING WATER ONTO 1–2 TEASPOONFULS OF THE DRIED HERB AND LEAVE TO INFUSE FOR 10 MINUTES. THIS SHOULD BE DRUNK THREE TIMES A DAY.

TINCTURE

TAKE 2–4ML OF THE TINCTURE THREE TIMES A DAY.

PART USED *Aerial parts*

COLLECTION *The herb should be gathered when in flower throughout the summer.*

CONSTITUENTS *Essential oil, bitter principle, tannin, polyphenols, flavonoids, saponins*

ACTIONS *Astringent, diaphoretic, carminative, vulnerary, anti-rheumatic, anti-microbial*

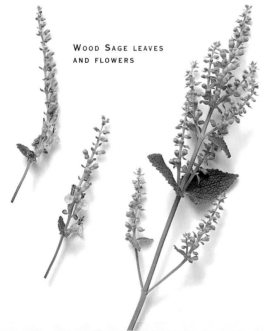

WOOD SAGE LEAVES AND FLOWERS

COMBINATIONS
In the treatment of colds and influenza it will combine well with Yarrow, Peppermint and Elder Flower. Used as a poultice or ointment it may be combined with Chickweed.

Thuja occidentalis

PLANT FAMILY CUPRESSACEAE

THUJA

Thuja's main action is due to its stimulating and alterative volatile oil. In bronchial catarrh Thuja combines expectoration with a systemic stimulation, which is beneficial if there is also heart weakness. It has a specific reflex action on the uterus and may help in delayed menstruation, but it should be avoided in pregnancy. Where urinary incontinence occurs due to loss of muscle tone, Thuja may be used. It has a role in the treatment of psoriasis and rheumatism. Externally it may be used to treat warts.

THUJA TWIG AND LEAVES

CAUTION
AVOID DURING PREGNANCY.

PART USED *Young twigs*

COLLECTION *The twigs of this evergreen conifer can be gathered all year round, but are best during the summer.*

CONSTITUENTS *1% volatile oil including thujone; flavonoid glycoside, mucilage, tannin*

ACTIONS *Expectorant, stimulant to smooth muscles, diuretic, astringent, alterative, anthelmintic, diaphoretic*

PREPARATION AND DOSAGE

INFUSION

POUR A CUP OF BOILING WATER ONTO 1 TEASPOONFUL OF THE DRIED HERB AND LEAVE TO INFUSE FOR 10–15 MINUTES. THIS SHOULD BE DRUNK THREE TIMES A DAY.

TINCTURE

TAKE 1–2ML OF THE TINCTURE THREE TIMES A DAY.

COMBINATIONS
When used in pulmonary conditions it may be combined with Senega, Grindelia or Lobelia.

Thymus vulgaris

PLANT FAMILY LABIATAE

THYME

With its high content of volatile oil, Thyme makes a good carminative for use in dyspepsia and sluggish digestion. This oil is also a strongly antiseptic substance, which explains many of Thyme's uses. It can be used externally as a lotion for infected wounds, but also internally for respiratory and digestive infections. It may be used as a gargle in laryngitis and tonsillitis, easing sore throats and soothing irritable coughs. It is an excellent cough remedy, producing expectoration and reducing unnecessary spasm. It may be used in bronchitis, whooping cough and asthma. As a gentle astringent it has found use in childhood diarrhea and bed wetting.

PART USED *Leaves and flowering tops*

COLLECTION *Collect the flowering stems between early summer and late summer on a dry sunny day. Strip the leaves off the dried stems.*

CONSTITUENTS *More than 1% volatile oil which includes thymol, carvacrol, cymol, linalol, borneol; bitter principles, tannin, flavonoids, triterpenoids*

ACTIONS *Carminative, anti-microbial, anti-spasmodic, expectorant, astringent, anthelmintic, anti-catarrhal, diaphoretic, tonic, vulnerary*

THYME LEAVES
AND FLOWERS

PREPARATION AND DOSAGE

INFUSION

POUR A CUP OF BOILING WATER ONTO 2 TEASPOONFULS OF THE DRIED HERB AND LET INFUSE FOR 10 MINUTES. THIS SHOULD BE DRUNK THREE TIMES A DAY.

TINCTURE

TAKE 2–4ML OF THE TINCTURE THREE TIMES A DAY.

COMBINATIONS

For asthmatic problems it will combine well with Lobelia and Ephedra, adding its anti-microbial effect. For whooping cough use it with Wild Cherry and Sundew.

Tilia x vulgaris

PLANT FAMILY TILIACEAE

LIME BLOSSOM

Lime Blossom, or Linden, is well known as a relaxing remedy for use in nervous tension. It has a reputation as a prophylactic against the development of arteriosclerosis and hypertension. It is considered to be a specific in the treatment of raised blood pressure associated with arteriosclerosis and nervous tension. Its relaxing action combined with a general effect upon the circulatory system give Lime Blossom a role in the treatment of some forms of migraine. The diaphoresis combined with the relaxation explains its value in feverish colds and flu.

PART USED *Dried flowers*

COLLECTION *Gather the flowers immediately after flowering in mid-summer on a dry day. Dry carefully in the shade.*

CONSTITUENTS *Essential oil containing farnesol; mucilage, flavonoids, hesperidin, coumarin fraxoside, vanillin*

ACTIONS *Nervine, anti-spasmodic, diaphoretic, diuretic, mild astringent, tonic*

PREPARATION AND DOSAGE

INFUSION

POUR A CUP OF BOILING WATER ONTO 1 TEASPOONFUL OF THE BLOSSOM AND LEAVE TO INFUSE FOR 10 MINUTES. THIS SHOULD BE DRUNK THREE TIMES A DAY. FOR A DIAPHORETIC EFFECT IN FEVER, USE 2–3 TEASPOONFULS.

TINCTURE

TAKE 1–2ML OF THE TINCTURE THREE TIMES A DAY.

DRIED LIME
BLOSSOM

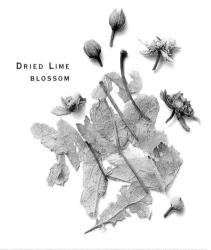

COMBINATIONS

In raised blood pressure it may be used with Hawthorn and Mistletoe, with Hops in nervous tension and with Elder Flower in the common cold.

Trifolium pratense

PLANT FAMILY PAPILIONACEAE

RED CLOVER

Red Clover is one of the most useful remedies for children with skin problems. It may be used with complete safety in any case of childhood eczema. It may also be of value in other chronic skin conditions such as psoriasis. Whilst being most useful with children it can also be of value for adults. The expectorant and anti-spasmodic action give this remedy a role in the treatment of coughs and bronchitis, but especially in whooping cough. As an alterative it is indicated in a wide range of problems when approached in a holistic sense. There is some evidence to suggest an anti-neoplastic action in animals.

RED CLOVER STALKS
LEAVES AND FLOWERS

PART USED *Flower heads*

COLLECTION *The flower heads are gathered between late spring and early Fall.*

CONSTITUENTS *Phenolic glycosides, flavonoids, coumarins, cyanogenic glycosides*

ACTIONS *Alterative, expectorant, anti-spasmodic, nervine, sedative, tonic*

PREPARATION AND DOSAGE

INFUSION

POUR A CUP OF BOILING WATER ONTO 1–3 TEASPOONFULS OF THE DRIED HERB AND LEAVE TO INFUSE FOR 10–15 MINUTES. THIS SHOULD BE DRUNK THREE TIMES A DAY.

TINCTURE

TAKE 2–6ML OF THE TINCTURE THREE TIMES A DAY.

COMBINATIONS

For skin problems it combines well with
Yellow Dock and Nettles.

Trigonella foenum-graecum

PLANT FAMILY PAPILIONACEAE

FENUGREEK

Fenugreek is a herb that has an ancient history. It has great use in local healing and reducing inflammation for conditions such as wounds, boils, sores, fistulas and tumours. It can be taken to help bronchitis and gargled to ease sore throats. Its bitterness explains its role in soothing disturbed digestion. It is a strong stimulator of milk production in mothers, for which it is perfectly safe, and has a reputation of stimulating development of the breasts.

PART USED *Seeds*

COLLECTION *The seeds are collected in the Fall.*

CONSTITUENTS *Steroidal saponins including diosgenin, alkaloid, 30% mucilage, bitter principle, volatile and fixed oil*

ACTIONS *Expectorant, demulcent, tonic, galactogogue, emmenagogue, emollient, vulnerary*

PREPARATION AND DOSAGE

POULTICE

FOR EXTERNAL USE, THE SEEDS SHOULD BE PULVERIZED TO MAKE A POULTICE.

DECOCTION

TO INCREASE MILK PRODUCTION, GENTLY SIMMER 1 ½ TEASPOON-FULS OF THE SEEDS IN A CUP OF WATER FOR 10 MINUTES. DRINK A CUP THREE TIMES A DAY. TO MAKE A MORE PLEASANT DRINK, ADD 1 TEASPOONFUL OF ANISEED TO THIS MIXTURE.

TINCTURE

TAKE 1–2ML OF THE TINCTURE THREE TIMES A DAY.

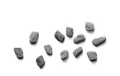
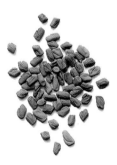

FENUGREEK SEEDS

Trillium erectum

PLANT FAMILY LILIACEAE

BETH ROOT

Beth Root is a plant that contains a natural precursor of the female sex hormones, which the body may use if it needs to or otherwise leaves unused, an example of the normalizing power of some herbs. Whilst this remedy is an excellent tonic for the uterus, its associated astringent power explains its use for bleeding and hemorrhage. It may be used where there is excessive blood flow during a period (menorrhagia) or where there is blood loss between periods (metrorrhagia). It is considered to be a specific for excessive blood loss associated with menopausal changes. It may be used in leucorrhea as a douche and as a poultice or ointment for the treatment of external ulcers. Its astringency can be utilized where there is a hemorrhage anywhere in the body, as long as the cause of the blood loss is treated as well.

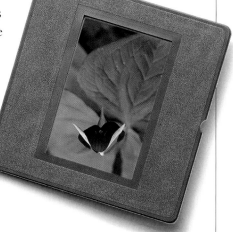

BETH ROOT
LEAVES AND
FLOWER

PART USED
Dried rhizome or root

COLLECTION *The root and rhizome should be unearthed in late summer or early Fall.*

CONSTITUENTS *Steroidal saponins, steroidal glycosides, tannins, fixed oil*

ACTIONS *Uterine tonic, astringent, expectorant, emmenagogue, oxytocic*

PREPARATION AND DOSAGE

DECOCTION

POUR A CUP OF WATER ONTO 1–2 TEASPOONFULS OF THE DRIED HERB AND SIMMER FOR 10 MINUTES. THIS SHOULD BE DRUNK THREE TIMES A DAY.

TINCTURE

TAKE 1–4ML OF THE TINCTURE THREE TIMES A DAY.

COMBINATIONS
For excessive menstruation it may be combined with Periwinkle or American Cranesbill.

Tropaeolum majus

PLANT FAMILY TROPAEOLACEAE

NASTURTIUM

Nasturtium is quite a powerful anti-microbial, especially when used as a local remedy for the treatment of bacterial infection. Internally it can be used with benefit in any bacterial infection but it is especially indicated for respiratory infections such as bronchitis. It has been found to be beneficial in influenza and the common cold. Some herbalists report it to be indicated in infections of the female reproductive organs.

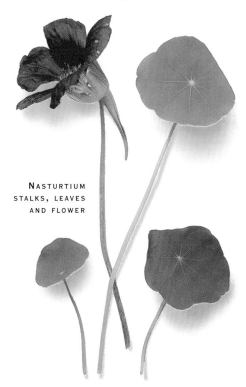

NASTURTIUM
STALKS, LEAVES
AND FLOWER

PART USED *Aerial parts*

COLLECTION *The leaves and flowers should be collected between mid-summer and mid-Fall.*

CONSTITUENTS
Glucosilinates, unknown anti-bacterial substance, vitamin C

ACTIONS *Anti-microbial*

PREPARATION AND DOSAGE

NASTURTIUM IS MOST EFFECTIVE WHEN FRESH. USE IT EXTERNALLY AS A POULTICE OR COMPRESS.

INFUSION

POUR A CUP OF BOILING WATER ON 1–2 TEASPOONFULS OF THE FRESH LEAVES AND LET INFUSE FOR 10–15 MINUTES. THIS SHOULD BE DRUNK THREE TIMES A DAY.

TINCTURE

TAKE 1–4ML OF THE TINCTURE THREE TIMES A DAY.

Turnera diffusa var. *aphrodisiaca*

PLANT FAMILY TURNERACEAE

DAMIANA

Damiana is an excellent strengthening remedy for the nervous system. It has an ancient reputation as an aphrodisiac. While this may or may not be true, it has a definite tonic action on the central nervous and the hormonal system. The pharmacology of the plant suggests that the alkaloids could have a testosterone-like action (testosterone is a male hormone). As a useful anti-depressant, Damiana is considered to be a specific in cases of anxiety and depression where there is a sexual factor. It may be used to strengthen the male sexual system.

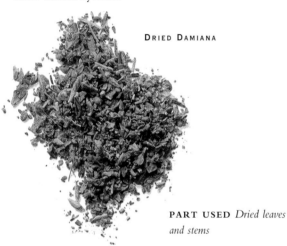

DRIED DAMIANA

PART USED *Dried leaves and stems*

COLLECTION *The leaves and stems are gathered at the time of flowering.*

CONSTITUENTS *Essential oil that includes pinene, cineol, cymol, arbutin, cymene, cadinene and copaenen; alkaloids, bitter, flavonoid, cyanogenic glycoside, tannins, resin*

ACTIONS *Nerve tonic, anti-depressant, urinary antiseptic, laxative*

PREPARATION AND DOSAGE

INFUSION

POUR A CUP OF BOILING WATER ONTO 1 TEASPOONFUL OF THE DRIED LEAVES AND LET INFUSE FOR 10–15 MINUTES. THIS SHOULD BE DRUNK THREE TIMES A DAY.

TINCTURE

TAKE 1–2ML OF THE TINCTURE THREE TIMES A DAY.

COMBINATIONS

As a nerve tonic it is often used with Oats. Depending on the situation it combines well with Kola or Skullcap.

Tussilago farfara

PLANT FAMILY COMPOSITAE

COLTSFOOT

Coltsfoot combines a soothing expectorant effect with an anti-spasmodic action. There are useful levels of zinc in the leaves. This mineral has been shown to have marked anti-inflammatory effects. Coltsfoot may be used in chronic or acute bronchitis, irritating coughs, whooping coughs and asthma. Its soothing expectorant action gives Coltsfoot a role in most respiratory conditions, including the chronic state of emphysema. As a mild diuretic it has been used in cystitis. The fresh bruised leaves can be applied to boils, abscesses and suppurating ulcers.

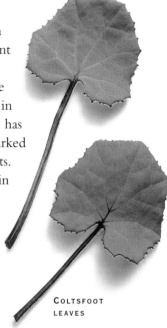

COLTSFOOT LEAVES

PART USED *Dried flowers and leaves*

COLLECTION *The flowers should be gathered before they have fully bloomed (end of late winter to mid-spring) and dried carefully in the shade. The leaves are best collected between late spring and early summer. They should be chopped up before they are dried and stored. The fresh leaves can be used until Fall.*

CONSTITUENTS
*Flowers: Mucin, flavonoids rutin and carotene, taraxan-thin, arnidiol and faradiol, tannin, essential oil
Leaves: Mucin, abundant tannin, glycosidal bitter principle, inulin, sitosterol, zinc*

ACTIONS *Expectorant, anti-tussive, demulcent, anti-catarrhal, diuretic, emollient, pectoral, tonic*

PREPARATION AND DOSAGE

INFUSION

POUR A CUP OF BOILING WATER ONTO 1–2 TEASPOONFULS OF THE DRIED FLOWERS OR LEAVES AND LET INFUSE FOR 10 MINUTES. THIS SHOULD BE DRUNK THREE TIMES A DAY, AS HOT AS POSSIBLE.

TINCTURE

TAKE 2–4ML OF THE TINCTURE THREE TIMES A DAY.

COMBINATIONS

In the treatment of coughs it may be used with White Horehound and Mullein.

Ulmus rubra

PLANT FAMILY ULMACEAE

SLIPPERY ELM

Slippery Elm bark is a soothing nutritive demulcent which is perfectly suited for sensitive or inflamed mucous membrane linings in the digestive system. It may be used in gastritis, gastric or duodenal ulcer, enteritis, colitis and the like. It is often used as a food during convalescence as it is gentle and easily assimilated. In diarrhea it will soothe and astringe at the same time. Externally it makes an excellent poultice for use in cases of boils, abscesses or ulcers.

PART USED *Inner bark*

COLLECTION *The bark is stripped from the trunk and large branches in the spring. In commercial use this usually leads to the tree dying, as a large part of the bark is stripped. Ten-year-old bark is recommended.*

CONSTITUENTS *Mucilage, tannin*

ACTIONS *Demulcent, emollient, nutrient, astringent, vulnerary*

PREPARATION AND DOSAGE

DECOCTION

USE 1 PART OF THE POWDERED BARK TO 8 PARTS OF WATER. MIX THE POWDER IN A LITTLE WATER INITIALLY TO ENSURE IT WILL MIX. BRING TO THE BOIL AND SIMMER GENTLY FOR 10–15 MINUTES. DRINK HALF A CUP THREE TIMES A DAY.

POULTICE

MIX THE COARSE POWDERED BARK WITH ENOUGH BOILING WATER TO MAKE A PASTE.

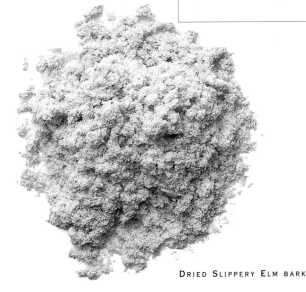

DRIED SLIPPERY ELM BARK

COMBINATIONS
For digestive problems it may be used with Marshmallow.

Umbilicus rupestris

PLANT FAMILY CRASSULACEAE

PENNYWORT

I have found Pennywort, or Navelwort, to be a specific in earache, but have come across no reference to this in the herbal literature. The fresh leaves are pressed to extract the juice, which can easily be done in a metal sieve. The juice, abundant in the succulent leaves, is introduced into the ear and kept in place by a plug of cotton wool. I have observed rapid and complete easing of the severe pain of earache in a very short time this way. This remedy may be safely used even with very young children. It is inadvisable if there is a suspicion of damage to the ear drum.

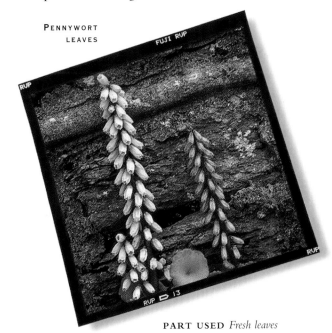

PENNYWORT LEAVES

PART USED *Fresh leaves*

ACTIONS *Demulcent, anodyne*

PREPARATION AND DOSAGE

EXTERNAL USE

PICK OFF INDIVIDUAL LEAVES AND PRESS THEM TO SQUEEZE OUT THE JUICE. USE EXTERNALLY.

Urginea maritima

PLANT FAMILY LILIACEAE

SQUILL

Squill is a powerful expectorant used in chronic bronchitis, especially where there is little sputum production, which causes a dry irritable cough. A more fluid mucus secretion is produced with Squill, which in turn facilitates an easier expectoration. The mucilage content eases and relaxes the bronchiole passages, thereby balancing the stimulation of the glycosides. It may be used in bronchial asthma and whooping cough. It has a stimulating action on the heart and has been used for aiding cases of heart failure and water retention when there is heart involvement.

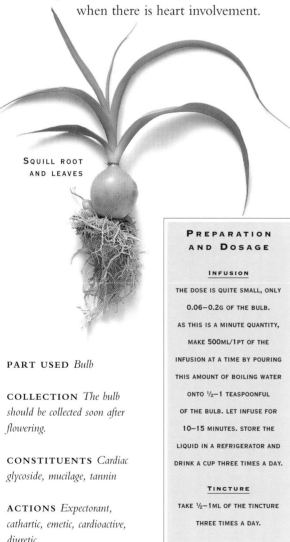

SQUILL ROOT
AND LEAVES

PART USED *Bulb*

COLLECTION *The bulb should be collected soon after flowering.*

CONSTITUENTS *Cardiac glycoside, mucilage, tannin*

ACTIONS *Expectorant, cathartic, emetic, cardioactive, diuretic*

PREPARATION AND DOSAGE

INFUSION

THE DOSE IS QUITE SMALL, ONLY 0.06–0.2G OF THE BULB. AS THIS IS A MINUTE QUANTITY, MAKE 500ML/1PT OF THE INFUSION AT A TIME BY POURING THIS AMOUNT OF BOILING WATER ONTO ½–1 TEASPOONFUL OF THE BULB. LET INFUSE FOR 10–15 MINUTES. STORE THE LIQUID IN A REFRIGERATOR AND DRINK A CUP THREE TIMES A DAY.

TINCTURE

TAKE ½–1ML OF THE TINCTURE THREE TIMES A DAY.

COMBINATIONS

For bronchitis it may be used with White Horehound and Coltsfoot, for whooping cough with Sundew.

Urtica dioica

PLANT FAMILY URTICACEA

NETTLE

Nettles are one of the most widely applicable plants we have. They strengthen and support the whole body. They are a specific in cases of childhood eczema and beneficial in all the varieties of this condition, especially in nervous eczema. As an astringent they may be used for nose bleeds or to relieve the symptoms wherever there is hemorrhage in the body; for example, in uterine hemorrhage.

PART USED *Aerial parts*

COLLECTION *The herb should be collected when the flowers are in bloom.*

CONSTITUENTS *Histamine, formic acid, chlorophyll, glucoquinine, iron, vitamin C*

ACTIONS *Astringent, diuretic, tonic, alterative, rubefacient*

PREPARATION AND DOSAGE

INFUSION

POUR A CUP OF BOILING WATER ONTO 1–3 TEASPOONFULS OF THE DRIED HERB AND LEAVE TO INFUSE FOR 10–15 MINUTES. THIS SHOULD BE DRUNK THREE TIMES A DAY.

TINCTURE

TAKE 1–4ML OF THE TINCTURE THREE TIMES A DAY.

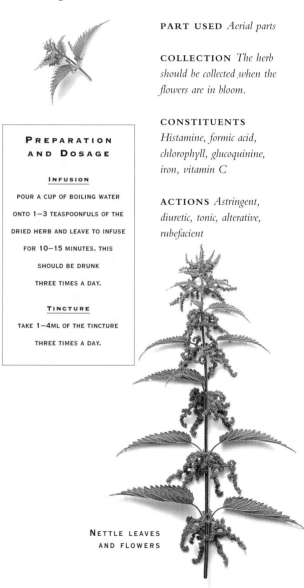

NETTLE LEAVES
AND FLOWERS

COMBINATIONS

Nettle will combine well with Figwort and Burdock in the treatment of eczema.

Valeriana officinalis

PLANT FAMILY VALERIANACEAE

VALERIAN

Valerian is one of the most useful relaxing nervines that is available to us. This fact is recognized by orthodox medicine, as is shown by its inclusion in many pharmacopeias as a sedative. It may safely be used to reduce tension and anxiety, over-excitability and hysterical states. It is an effective aid in insomnia. producing a natural healing sleep. As an anti-spasmodic herb it will aid in the relief of cramp and intestinal colic and will also be useful for the cramps and pain of periods. As a pain reliever it is most indicated where that pain is associated with tension. Valerian can help in migraine and rheumatic pain.

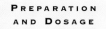

VALERIAN
LEAVES AND
FLOWERS

PREPARATION AND DOSAGE

INFUSION

POUR A CUP OF BOILING WATER ONTO 1–2 TEASPOONFULS OF THE ROOT AND LET INFUSE FOR 10–15 MINUTES. THIS SHOULD BE DRUNK WHEN NEEDED.

TINCTURE

TAKE 2–4ML OF THE TINCTURE THREE TIMES A DAY.

DRIED
VALERIAN ROOT

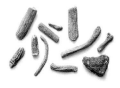

PART USED
Rhizome and roots

COLLECTION *The roots are unearthed in the late Fall. Clean thoroughly and dry in the shade.*

CONSTITUENTS
Volatile oil including valerianic acid, isovalerianic acid, borneol, pinene, camphene; volatile alkaloids

ACTIONS *Sedative, hypnotic, anti-spasmodic, hypotensive, carminative, aromatic, nervine*

COMBINATIONS

For the relief of tension it will combine most effectively with Skullcap. For insomnia it can be combined with Passion Flower and Hops. For the treatment of cramps it will work well with Cramp Bark.

Verbascum thapsus

PLANT FAMILY SCROPHULARIACEAE

MULLEIN

Mullein is a very beneficial respiratory remedy, useful in most conditions that affect this vital system. It is an ideal remedy for toning the mucous membranes of the respiratory system, reducing inflammation whilst stimulating fluid production and thus facilitating expectoration. It is considered a specific in bronchitis where there is a hard cough with soreness. Its anti-inflammatory and demulcent properties indicate its use in inflammation of the trachea and associated conditions. Externally an extract made in olive oil is excellent in soothing and healing any inflamed surface.

PART USED *Dried leaves and flowers*

MULLEIN
SHOOT, LEAVES
AND FLOWER

COLLECTION *The leaves should be collected in mid-summer before they turn brown. Dry them in the shade. The flowers should be gathered between mid-summer and early Fall during dry weather. They should be dried in the shade or with artificial heat not higher than 40°C/104°F. The flowers turn brown if damp, and become ineffective.*

PREPARATION AND DOSAGE

INFUSION

POUR A CUP OF BOILING WATER ONTO 1–2 TEASPOONFULS OF THE DRIED LEAVES OR FLOWERS AND LET INFUSE FOR 10–15 MINUTES. THIS SHOULD BE DRUNK THREE TIMES A DAY.

TINCTURE

TAKE 1–4ML OF THE TINCTURE THREE TIMES A DAY.

CONSTITUENTS *Mucilage and gum, saponins, volatile oil, flavonoids including hesperidin and verbascoside; glycosides including aucubin*

ACTIONS *Expectorant, demulcent, diuretic, sedative, vulnerary, anti-catarrhal, emollient, pectoral*

COMBINATIONS

In bronchitis it combines well with White Horehound, Coltsfoot and Lobelia.

Verbena officinalis

PLANT FAMILY LABIATAE

VERVAIN

Vervain is a herb that will strengthen the nervous system whilst relaxing any tension and stress. It can be used to ease depression and melancholia, especially when this follows illness such as influenza. Vervain may be used to help in seizure and hysteria. As a diaphoretic it can be used in the early stages of fevers. As a hepatic remedy it will be found of help in inflammation of the gall-bladder and jaundice. It may be used as a mouthwash against caries and gum disease.

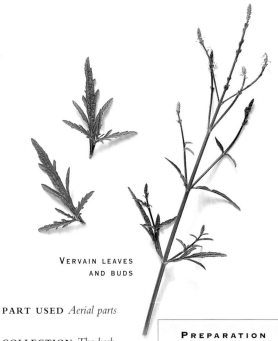

**VERVAIN LEAVES
AND BUDS**

PART USED *Aerial parts*

COLLECTION *The herb should be collected just before the flowers open, usually in mid-summer. Dry quickly.*

CONSTITUENTS
Bitter glycosides called verbenalin; essential oil, mucilage, tannin

ACTIONS *Nervine tonic, sedative, anti-spasmodic, diaphoretic, possible galactagogue, hepatic, analgesic, anti-bilious, emmenagogue, expectorant, pectoral*

PREPARATION AND DOSAGE
INFUSION
POUR A CUP OF BOILING WATER ONTO 1–3 TEASPOONFULS OF THE DRIED HERB AND LEAVE TO INFUSE FOR 10–15 MINUTES. THIS SHOULD BE DRUNK THREE TIMES A DAY.
TINCTURE
TAKE 2–4ML OF THE TINCTURE THREE TIMES A DAY.

COMBINATIONS
In the treatment of depression it may be used with Skullcap, Oats and Lady's Slipper.

Veronicastrum virginicum

PLANT FAMILY SCROPHULARIACEAE

BLACK ROOT

Black Root is used as a reliever of liver congestion and for an inflamed gall-bladder (cholecystitis). When jaundice is due to liver congestion, also use Black Root, as it will help whenever there is any sign of liver problems. Chronic constipation can often be due to a liver dysfunction, in which case this herb is also ideal.

PART USED
Rhizome and root

COLLECTION *This root, which was introduced to European herbalism via the Seneca Indians, should be dug up in the Fall and stored for a year before use.*

CONSTITUENTS
Leptandrin, a bitter principle, glycosides, phytosterols, saponins, tannins, resin

ACTIONS *Cholagogue, mild cathartic, diaphoretic, anti-spasmodic, hepatic, tonic*

PREPARATION AND DOSAGE
DECOCTION
PUT 1–2 TEASPOONFULS OF THE DRIED HERB IN A CUP OF COLD WATER AND BRING TO THE BOIL. SIMMER FOR 10 MINUTES. TAKE ONE CUP THREE TIMES A DAY.
TINCTURE
TAKE 2–4ML OF THE TINCTURE THREE TIMES A DAY.

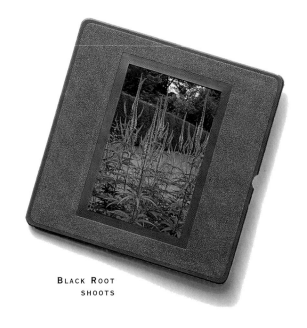

**BLACK ROOT
SHOOTS**

COMBINATIONS
Black Root will combine well with Barberry and Dandelion.

Viburnum opulus

PLANT FAMILY CAPRIFOLIACEAE

CRAMP BARK

Cramp Bark shows by its name the richly deserved reputation it has as a relaxer of muscular tension and spasm. It has two main areas of use. Firstly in muscular cramps and secondly in ovarian and uterine muscle problems. Cramp Bark will relax the uterus and so relieve painful dysmenorrhea. In a similar way it may be used as a protection against threatened miscarriage. Its astringent action gives it a role in the treatment of excessive blood loss in periods and especially bleeding associated with the menopause.

PART USED *Dried bark*

COLLECTION *Collect the bark in mid-spring and late spring, cut into pieces and dry.*

CONSTITUENTS *A bitter called viburnin, valerianic acid, salicosides, resin, tannin*

ACTIONS *Anti-spasmodic, sedative, astringent, emmenagogue, nervine*

PREPARATION AND DOSAGE

DECOCTION

PUT 2 TEASPOONFULS OF THE DRIED BARK INTO A CUP OF WATER AND BRING TO THE BOIL. SIMMER GENTLY FOR 10–15 MINUTES. THIS SHOULD BE DRUNK HOT THREE TIMES A DAY.

TINCTURE

TAKE 4–8ML OF THE TINCTURE THREE TIMES A DAY.

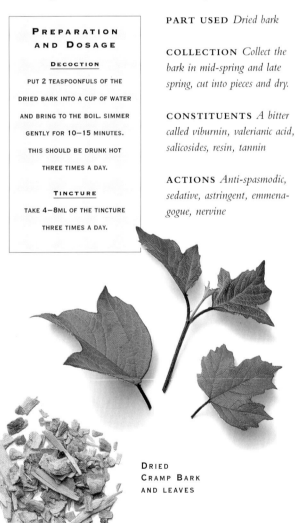

DRIED CRAMP BARK AND LEAVES

COMBINATIONS

For the relief of cramp it may be combined with Prickly Ash and Wild Yam. For uterine and ovarian pains or threatened miscarriage it may be used with Black Haw and Valerian.

Viburnum prunifolium

PLANT FAMILY CAPRIFOLIACEAE

BLACK HAW

Black Haw has a very similar use to Cramp Bark, to which it is closely related. It is a powerful relaxant of the uterus and is used for dysmenorrhea and false labour pains. It may be used in threatened miscarriage as well. Its relaxant and sedative actions explain its power in reducing blood pressure, which happens through a relaxation of the peripheral blood vessels. It may be used as an anti-spasmodic in the treatment of asthma.

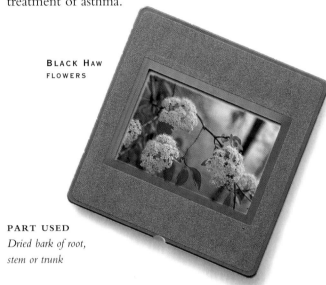

BLACK HAW FLOWERS

PART USED
Dried bark of root, stem or trunk

COLLECTION *The bark from the roots and the trunk is collected in the Fall. The shrubs should be dug out and the bark stripped from roots and trunk. The bark from branches should be collected in spring and summer. In both cases the bark should be dried in the shade.*

CONSTITUENTS
Triterpenoids, coumarins, bitter principle, valerianic acid, salicosides, tannin

ACTIONS *Anti-spasmodic, sedative, hypotensive, astringent, emmenagogue, nervine, tonic*

PREPARATION AND DOSAGE

DECOCTION

PUT 2 TEASPOONFULS OF THE DRIED BARK IN A CUP OF WATER, BRING TO THE BOIL AND SIMMER FOR 10 MINUTES. THIS SHOULD BE DRUNK THREE TIMES A DAY.

TINCTURE

TAKE 5–10ML OF THE TINCTURE THREE TIMES A DAY.

COMBINATIONS

For threatened miscarriage it will combine well with False Unicorn Root and Cramp Bark.

Vinca major

PLANT FAMILY APOCYNACEAE

PERIWINKLE

Periwinkle is an excellent all-round astringent that may be used internally or externally. Its main use is in the treatment of excessive menstrual flow, either during the period itself (menorrhagia) or with blood loss between periods (metrorrhagia). It can be used in digestive problems such as colitis or diarrhea where it will act to reduce the loss of fluid or blood whilst toning the membranes. It may also be used in cases of nose bleed, bleeding gums, mouth ulcers or sore throats. It has a reputation for aiding in the treatment of diabetes.

PERIWINKLE LEAVES
AND FLOWER

PREPARATION AND DOSAGE

INFUSION

POUR A CUP OF BOILING WATER ONTO 1−2 TEASPOONFULS OF THE DRIED HERB AND LET INFUSE FOR 10−15 MINUTES. THIS SHOULD BE DRUNK THREE TIMES A DAY.

TINCTURE

TAKE 1−2ML OF THE TINCTURE THREE TIMES A DAY.

PART USED *Aerial parts*

COLLECTION *This herb is collected in the spring.*

CONSTITUENTS *Alkaloids, tannins*

ACTIONS *Astringent, sedative*

COMBINATIONS

It will combine well with Cranesbill and Agrimony. For menstrual problems it may be used with Beth Root.

Viola odorata

PLANT FAMILY VIOLACEAE

SWEET VIOLET

Sweet Violet has a long history of use as a cough remedy and especially for the treatment of bronchitis. It may also be used to aid in the treatment of upper respiratory catarrh. With the combinations of actions present, it has a use in skin conditions such as eczema and in a long-term approach to rheumatism. It may be used for urinary infections. Sweet Violet has a reputation as an anti-cancer herb; it definitely has a role in a holistic approach to the treatment of cancer.

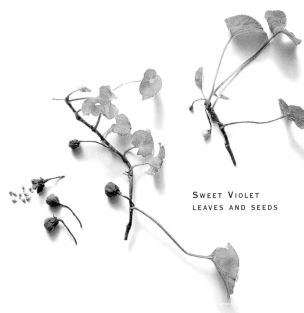

SWEET VIOLET
LEAVES AND SEEDS

PREPARATION AND DOSAGE

INFUSION

POUR A CUP OF BOILING WATER ONTO 1 TEASPOONFUL OF THE HERB AND LET INFUSE FOR 10−15 MINUTES. THIS SHOULD BE DRUNK THREE TIMES A DAY.

TINCTURE

TAKE 1−2ML OF THE TINCTURE THREE TIMES A DAY.

PART USED
Leaves and flowers

COLLECTION *The leaves and flowers are gathered mid-spring to late spring. Dry with care.*

CONSTITUENTS
Saponins, menthyl salicylate, alkaloids, flavonoids, essential oil

ACTIONS *Expectorant, alterative, anti-inflammatory, diuretic, anti-neoplastic*

Viola tricolor

PLANT FAMILY VIOLACEAE

PANSY

Pansy, or Heartsease, is used mostly in three areas, the skin, lungs and urinary system. It may be used in eczema and other skin problems where there is exudate (often called weeping) eczema. As an anti-inflammatory expectorant it is used for whooping cough and acute bronchitis where it will soothe and help the body heal itself. For urinary problems it will aid in the healing of cystitis and can be used to treat the symptoms of frequent and painful urination.

PART USED *Aerial parts*

COLLECTION *The herb can be collected throughout its growing season from early spring to late summer.*

CONSTITUENTS *Salicylates, saponins, alkaloid, flavonoids, tannin, mucilage*

ACTIONS *Expectorant, diuretic, anti-inflammatory, anti-rheumatic, laxative*

> ### PREPARATION AND DOSAGE
>
> #### INFUSION
> POUR A CUP OF BOILING WATER ONTO 1–2 TEASPOONFULS OF THE DRIED HERB AND LEAVE TO INFUSE FOR 10–15 MINUTES. THIS SHOULD BE DRUNK THREE TIMES A DAY.
>
> #### TINCTURE
> TAKE 2–4ML OF THE TINCTURE THREE TIMES A DAY.

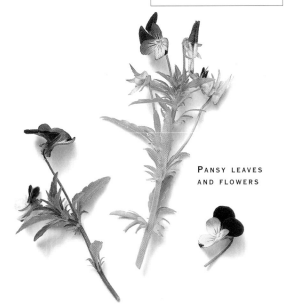

PANSY LEAVES AND FLOWERS

COMBINATIONS
For lung conditions Pansy may be used with Coltsfoot. For skin problems use it with Red Clover, Nettles and Cleavers. For cystitis combine it with Couchgrass and Buchu.

Viscum alba

PLANT FAMILY LORANTHACEAE

MISTLETOE

Mistletoe is an excellent relaxing nervine indicated in many cases. It will quiet, soothe and tone the nervous system. This remedy acts directly on the vagus nerve to reduce heart rate while strengthening the wall of the peripheral capillaries. It will thus act to reduce blood pressure and ease arteriosclerosis. Where there is nervous quickening of the heart (nervous tachycardia) it may be very helpful. Headache due to high blood pressure is relieved by it. It has been shown by current cancer research to have some anti-tumour activity.

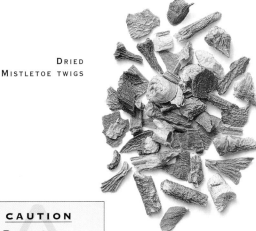

DRIED MISTLETOE TWIGS

> ### CAUTION
> DO NOT USE THE BERRIES.

PART USED
Dried leafy twigs

COLLECTION *Collect the young leafy twigs in the spring.*

CONSTITUENTS *Viscotoxin (a cardio-active polypeptide), triterpenoid saponins, choline, histamine, anti-tumour proteins*

ACTIONS *Nervine, hypotensive, cardiac depressant, possibly anti-tumour, antispasmodic, hypnotic, tonic*

> ### PREPARATION AND DOSAGE
>
> #### INFUSION
> POUR A CUP OF BOILING WATER ONTO 1–2 TEASPOONFULS OF THE DRIED HERB AND LEAVE TO INFUSE FOR 10–15 MINUTES. THIS SHOULD BE DRUNK THREE TIMES A DAY OR AS NEEDED.
>
> #### TINCTURE
> TAKE 1–4ML OF THE TINCTURE THREE TIMES A DAY.

COMBINATIONS
It combines well with Hawthorn Berries and Lime Blossom in the treatment of raised blood pressure.

163

Vitex agnus-castus

PLANT FAMILY VERBENACEAE

CHASTE TREE

Chaste Tree has the effect of stimulating and normalizing pituitary gland functions, especially its progesterone function. It may be called an amphoteric remedy as it can produce apparently opposite effects, though in truth it is simply normalizing. It has for instance a reputation as both an aphrodisiac and an anaphrodisiac! It will always enable what is appropriate to occur. The greatest use of Chaste Tree lies in normalizing the activity of female sex hormones and it is thus indicated for dysmenorrhea, pre-menstrual stress and other disorders related to hormone function. It is especially beneficial during menopausal changes. In a similar way it may be used to aid the body to regain a natural balance after the use of the birth control pill.

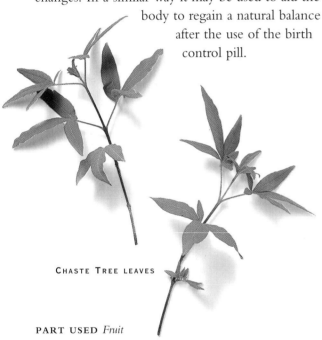

CHASTE TREE LEAVES

PART USED *Fruit*

COLLECTION *The very dark berries should be picked when ripe, which is between mid-Fall and late Fall. They may be dried in sun or shade.*

CONSTITUENTS *Iridoid glycosides, which include aucbin and agnoside; flavonoids including casticin, isovitexin and orientin; essential oil*

ACTIONS *Emmenagogue, tonic*

> ### PREPARATION AND DOSAGE
>
> #### INFUSION
>
> POUR A CUP OF BOILING WATER ONTO 1 TEASPOONFUL OF THE RIPE BERRIES AND LEAVE TO INFUSE FOR 10–15 MINUTES. THIS SHOULD BE DRUNK THREE TIMES A DAY.
>
> #### TINCTURE
>
> TAKE 1–2ML OF THE TINCTURE THREE TIMES A DAY.

Zanthoxylum americanum

PLANT FAMILY RUTACEAE

PRICKLY ASH

Prickly Ash may be used in a way that is similar to Cayenne, although it is slower in action. It is used in many chronic problems such as rheumatism and skin diseases. Any sign of poor circulation calls for the use of this herb, such as chilblains, cramp in the legs, varicose veins and varicose ulcers. Externally it may be used as a stimulation liniment for rheumatism and fibrositis. Due to its stimulating effect upon the lymphatic system, circulation and mucous membranes, it will have a role in the holistic treatment of many specific conditions.

> ### PREPARATION AND DOSAGE
>
> #### INFUSION
>
> POUR A CUP OF BOILING WATER ONTO 1–2 TEASPOONFULS OF THE BARK AND LET INFUSE FOR 10–15 MINUTES. THIS SHOULD BE DRUNK THREE TIMES A DAY.
>
> #### TINCTURE
>
> TAKE 2–4ML OF THE TINCTURE THREE TIMES A DAY.

PART USED
Bark and berries

COLLECTION *The berries are collected in late summer and the bark is stripped from the stems of the shrub in the spring.*

CONSTITUENTS *Alkaloids, volatile oil in the berries*

ACTIONS *Stimulant (especially circulatory), tonic, alterative, carminative, diaphoretic, hepatic, sialagogue*

PRICKLY ASH
LEAVES AND BERRIES

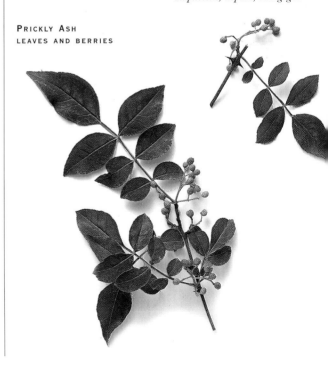

CORN SILK

Zea mays

PLANT FAMILY GRAMINACEAE

As a soothing diuretic, Corn Silk is helpful in any irritation of the urinary system. It is used for renal problems in children and as a urinary demulcent combined with other herbs in the treatment of cystitis, urethritis, prostatitis and the like.

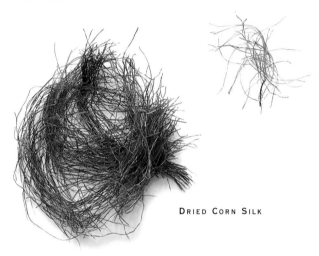

DRIED CORN SILK

PART USED *Stigmas from the female flowers of maize. Fine soft threads 10–20cm/ 4–8in long*

COLLECTION *The stigmas should be collected just before pollination occurs, the timing of which depends on the climate. It is best used fresh, as some of the activity is lost in time.*

CONSTITUENTS *Saponins, a volatile alkaloid, sterols, allantoin, tannin*

ACTIONS *Diuretic, demulcent, tonic, anti-lithic*

PREPARATION AND DOSAGE

INFUSION

POUR A CUP OF BOILING WATER ONTO 2 TEASPOONFULS OF THE FRESH OR DRIED HERB AND LEAVE TO INFUSE FOR 10–15 MINUTES. THIS SHOULD BE DRUNK THREE TIMES A DAY.

TINCTURE

TAKE 3–6ML OF THE TINCTURE THREE TIMES A DAY.

COMBINATIONS

With Couchgrass, Bearberry or Yarrow in the treatment of cystitis.

GINGER

Zingiber officinale

PLANT FAMILY ZINGIBERACEAE

Ginger may be used as a stimulant of the peripheral circulation in cases of bad circulation, chilblains and cramp. In feverish conditions, Ginger acts as a useful diaphoretic, promoting perspiration. As a carminative it promotes gastric secretion and is used in dyspepsia, flatulence and colic. As a gargle it may be effective in the relief of sore throats. Externally it is the base of many fibrositis and muscle sprain treatments.

GINGER ROOT

PREPARATION AND DOSAGE

INFUSION

POUR A CUP OF BOILING WATER ONTO 1 TEASPOONFUL OF THE FRESH ROOT AND LET IT INFUSE FOR 5 MINUTES. DRINK WHENEVER NEEDED.

DECOCTION

IF YOU ARE USING THE DRIED ROOT IN POWDERED OR FINELY CHOPPED FORM, MAKE A DECOCTION BY PUTTING 1½ TEASPOONFULS TO A CUP OF WATER. BRING IT TO THE BOIL AND SIMMER FOR 5–10 MINUTES. THIS CAN BE DRUNK WHENEVER NEEDED.

TINCTURE

THE TINCTURE IS AVAILABLE COMMERCIALLY IN TWO FORMS; WEAK TINCTURE, WHICH SHOULD BE TAKEN IN A DOSE OF 1.5–3ML THREE TIMES A DAY, AND STRONG TINCTURE WHICH SHOULD BE TAKEN IN A DOSE OF 0.25–0.5ML THREE TIMES A DAY.

PART USED *Rootstock*

COLLECTION *The rootstock is dug up when the leaves have dried. The remains of the stem and root fibres should be removed. Wash thoroughly and dry in the sun.*

CONSTITUENTS *Rich in volatile oil, which includes zingiberene, zingiberole, phellandrene, borneol, cineole, citral; starch, mucilage, resin*

ACTIONS *Stimulant, carminative, rubefacient, diaphoretic, aromatic, emmenagogue, sialagogue*

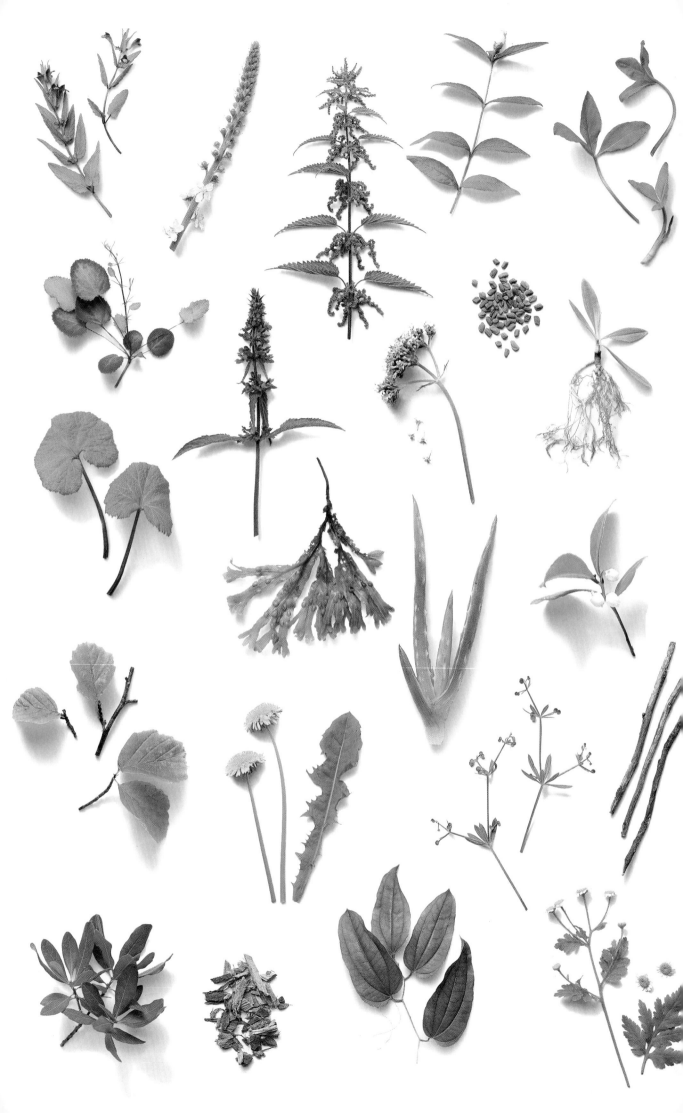

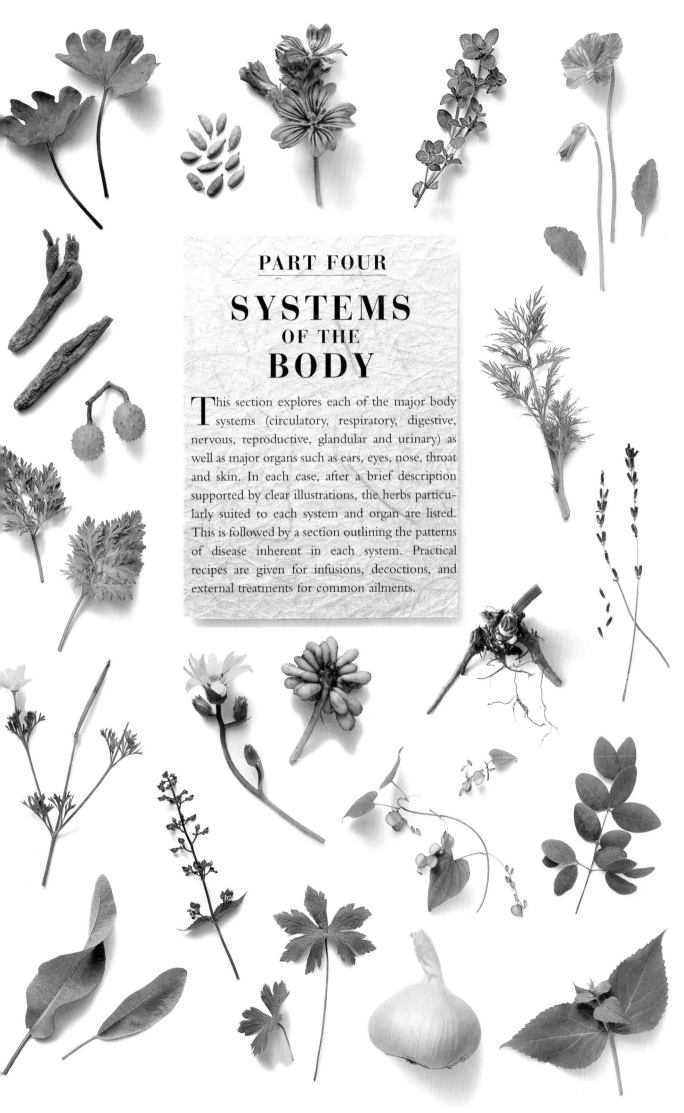

PART FOUR

SYSTEMS
OF THE
BODY

This section explores each of the major body systems (circulatory, respiratory, digestive, nervous, reproductive, glandular and urinary) as well as major organs such as ears, eyes, nose, throat and skin. In each case, after a brief description supported by clear illustrations, the herbs particularly suited to each system and organ are listed. This is followed by a section outlining the patterns of disease inherent in each system. Practical recipes are given for infusions, decoctions, and external treatments for common ailments.

THE CIRCULATORY SYSTEM

We begin our trip through the systems of the body by having a look at the circulatory system, as it connects all the others and affects all of them.

When we look at the body in a holistic way and treat any disease from this perspective, we recognize that all organs and systems are connected and influence each other. We have to look at what each one individually contributes to the whole picture. The heart vessels may be involved in any condition, and must be helped and aided in the healing process.

The vitality and tone of the whole circulatory system is fundamental to life and to the integration of all the parts of the body. If there is weakness or congestion present, it will have profound effects on the tissues and organs involved. If the blood supply to the organs is not adequate, there will be problems. Similarly, if waste materials produced in the metabolic process are not removed properly, damage to tissue will quickly result.

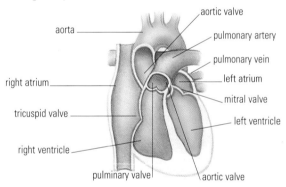

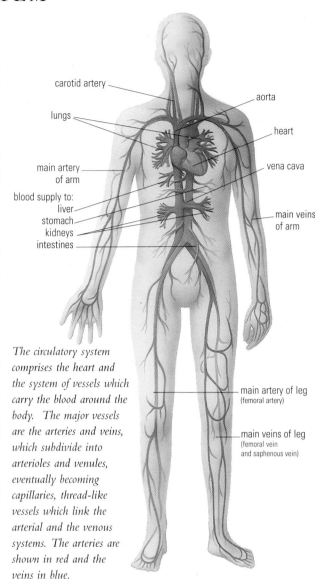

The circulatory system comprises the heart and the system of vessels which carry the blood around the body. The major vessels are the arteries and veins, which subdivide into arterioles and venules, eventually becoming capillaries, thread-like vessels which link the arterial and the venous systems. The arteries are shown in red and the veins in blue.

A cross-section of the heart, showing the four chambers and the aorta, the main artery of the body

Prevention of circulatory problems is easy, and a number of guidelines are set out below. However, when major heart problems are already apparent, care must be taken. Herbal medicine has a lot to offer in the healing of heart failure and cardiac conditions, but any treatment has to be under qualified supervision. Tell your doctor about all the herbal remedies you are taking.

Prevention of Circulatory Disease

Prevention is far better than having to resort to curing a disease that has developed, and prevention means finding ease for body, mind and spirit. There are specific guidelines relating to the cardio-vascular system that should be borne in mind. They apply not only to anyone who already has problems with this particular system, or whose way of life puts them into a 'high risk category' for developing cardio-vascular conditions. They also apply to anyone who does not want to develop problems in that area.

EXERCISE AND DIET

It is vital for the whole system that it is used and at least occasionally stretched and is properly fuelled.

As far as the circulatory system is concerned, the most important single factor that causes problems is the intake of fat. Most people in the West eat far too much of it. Over the last couple of years we have heard a lot about a relationship between the consumption of saturated fats and the level of choles-terol (one of these fats) in the blood, leading to various cardiovascular problems. One recommended way out was to eat unsaturated fats instead of the dangerous saturated ones, mainly by changing from animal fats to vegetable fats. According to new research, however, it is not all that simple. The evidence is pointing to dangers in the consumption of unsaturated fats too; it seems sensible, for the present, to reduce your total fat intake. It is better to eat a small amount of additive-free, organic fat such as butter, than larger amounts of over-processed 'low-fat' spread. This means a decrease in the consumption of visible fat (in meat, butter, oils) and also invisible fat (in cakes, pastries, thick soups, mayonnaise, dairy products, eggs), which often make up the bulk of our fat intake. Instead, most of our food should consist of plenty of fresh fruit and vegetables, whole grains, beans and peas, the latter two being considered capable of reducing the cholesterol level in the blood. The minimum of salt should be added.

SMOKING AND DRINKING

Anyone with concerns about their health, and especially about the heart and blood vessels, should stop smoking and keep their intake of alcohol to a reasonable amount.

DEALING WITH STRESS

There is a close correlation between the level of stress in your life and the occurrence of health problems, particularly with problems in the cardio-vascular system. 'Stress' is a relative concept. It would be more appropriate to consider the individual's ability to deal with the stress in his or her life than to look at the stress itself.

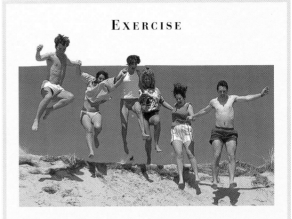

EXERCISE

The only way to ensure that heart and blood vessels are truly used is to exercise so the heart beat is speeded up and we become short of breath. This does not mean that people should jog themselves into exhaustion every day! Regular exercises that feel right and are enjoyable are the key. Moderation in all things, exercise included.

There are a number of tools available to us today to help us take responsibility in our lives and to deal with stress and emotional tensions. It is possible to help with tension by using herbal remedies, but it is far better and more realistic to go to the underlying cause within us and change it. This involves consciousness and sometimes courage. Relaxation therapy, meditation and a clear-eyed re-evaluation of your life patterns all have much to offer in identifying the stress points surrounding your daily life.

Disease can be prevented by bringing ease into our lives. Psychological and spiritual harmony will create the inner environment for bodily harmony.

A BALANCED DIET

Healthy eating plays a major role in preventative medicine. A good diet should deliver useful nutrients to support the body and its systems rather than clog it up with unnecessary sugars and fats, which could eventually cause disease, especially in the circulatory system. Good eating need not mean dull eating, however.

If you are worried that your diet contains too much processed, convenience or non-nourishing food, make the change gradually by introducing more fresh fruit and vegetables, pasta, whole grain food, oily and white fish, while cutting down on red meat, fats and sugar, and substituting goat's milk and cheese for cow's milk products.

Herbs for the
Heart and Circulation

As with all systems of the body, an identification of herbs for that system is a necessary simplification. The body is an integrated whole and the herbal approach to healing recognizes this. Any problems arising in a particular system may be caused by the state of health and vitality in any other part of the body, and therefore any herb can have a role to play in the treatment of any system. However, to enable our limited human comprehension to grasp the basics of herbalism, it is valid to identify herbs that have a specific role to play in this system.

To keep things simple and to avoid complex groupings, the herbs will be differentiated into those that have a direct action on the heart, and those that affect the peripheral vessels.

HEART TONICS

The most important herbal agents for the heart include *Broom, Bugleweed, Figwort, Hawthorn Berries, Lily of the Valley, Motherwort* and *Night Blooming Cereus.*

Herbs such as *Foxglove* (Digitalis) and *Mediterranean Squill* have been left out of the list, even though these plant remedies are used extensively by orthodox medicine as effective treatments for heart failure. However, as there are marked dangers with the use of *Foxglove,* this poisonous plant has been left out. This does not mean that effective heart remedies are not available to us. By far the most important one on the list is *Lily of the Valley.*

Crataegus laevigata
Hawthorn Berries
normalize heart activity.

• Lily of the Valley: A Case Study

The remedies often used to treat the heart are rich in a group of chemicals called cardiac glycosides *(see page 35)*. These complex chemicals stimulate the muscles of the heart, strengthen their contraction and ensure that more blood is pumped through the body. The efficiency of the heart is thereby increased, but with the help of these chemicals the oxygen required by the heart muscle for this work is not increased and thus we do not have to worry about any oxygen deficiency.

With Foxglove, however, there is an added danger as some of its constituents can accumulate in the body and lead to poisoning, which does not happen with *Lily of the Valley.* As pharmacological analysis shows, there are a number of different cardiac glycosides present in *Lily of the Valley,* but only two act directly on the heart, and of these the most important one is Convallatoxin. To a pharmacist this would imply that the rest are useless, which could not be further from the truth, as the other glycosides have been found to increase the solubility of the active ones by up to 500 times. This means that a smaller dose can be given, as an increase in solubility will also increase the 'bio-availability'. Furthermore it was found that though Convallatoxin has a fast effect and is oxidized and excreted rapidly, the whole plant has a longer effective time in the body. Others of the apparently inactive glycosides are converted by the body into the directly active ones as and when needed. A danger of poisoning does not exist with *Lily of the Valley,* as its glycosides have a unique chemical structure which ensures that they are easily excreted and do not build up in the body. Even so, make sure that you always consult a practitioner when using this herb.

In *Lily of the Valley* we have a good example of the synergistic way in which herbs can work. From all this analytical and biochemical study we can see that the whole is indeed more than the sum of its parts. The action of the whole plant cannot be predicted by knowing the separate chemical constituents, as the effects are brought about through complex, integrated interactions.

Let us now have a closer look at the specific heart tonics mentioned previously. They all act in a way that tones and strengthens heart functions, and will be given here with some brief indications of their use in the circulatory system. Please consult The Herbal for more details.

• Lily of the Valley
This can be used where the strength of the heart is insufficient, as in angina or in the treatment of the ageing heart, especially when there are deposits in the blood vessels.

• Night Blooming Cereus
This can be used similarly to *Lily of the Valley* and is especially useful where there is any change in the rhythm of the heart beat.

• Hawthorn Berries
These constitute one of the

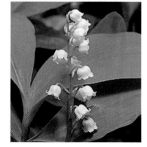

Convallaria majalis
Lily of the Valley, *a powerful herb for the heart*

most valuable remedies for the cardiovascular system, strengthening the force of the contraction of the heart muscle while also acting to dilate the vessels of the coronary circulation. They can be used in most circulatory problems as they are amphoteric (ie they will relax or stimulate the heart according to its need) and normalize the heart function.

- **Motherwort** This herb is a relaxing nervine and a valuable emmenagogue. Its value for the circulatory system is noted in its Latin name, *Leonurus cardiaca*. It will greatly strengthen and normalize the function of the heart.

Leonurus cardiaca
Motherwort *strengthens the normal function of the heart.*

- **Broom** It can be considered as the primary heart diuretic. Whilst it strengthens and normalizes the heart beat, broom also rids the body of any build-up of water that is caused by insufficient heart strength. Care has to be taken though, as it may also increase blood pressure.
- **Figwort** Although this is primarily a herb known for skin problems, it also increases the strength of the heart contractions.
- **Bugleweed** Whilst this herb increases the strength of the heart beat it also reduces its rate. It is a valuable relaxant as well.

HERBS FOR THE CIRCULATION

As with herbs for the heart, there is a vast range of remedies available to help and heal the vessels of the circulatory system, but here we limit ourselves to specific ones.

The most important herbal agents for the circulation include *Broom, Buckwheat, Cayenne, Dandelion, Ginger, Hawthorn, Horsechestnut, Lime Blossom, Mistletoe* and *Yarrow*.

As you can see, some of these are also heart tonics, while some are diaphoretics and stimulate the peripheral circulation (*Cayenne, Ginger*), and yet others are diuretics (*Yarrow*). This again goes back to the fact that the body will manifest problems in an area because of a whole range of causes and contributing factors stemming from the interdependence of all the systems.

DIURETICS

When circulatory problems arise there is often a need to aid the body in the removal of water from the system. When the heart is weak and fails to circulate the blood efficiently through the kidneys a build-up of water in parts of the body can occur and in such conditions diuretics such as *Broom, Dandelion, Lily of the Valley* and *Yarrow* can help. Perhaps the most important diuretic for circulatory problems is *Dandelion*. When any other remedy is used to increase the power of the heart, there is always the danger of causing a potassium deficiency in the body, which in turn would aggravate the heart problem. However, as *Dandelion* already contains a high level of potassium, there is an overall gain of it whenever *Dandelion* is used as a diuretic, which makes its value apparent.

The cardio-active herbs *Broom* and *Lily of the Valley* are included here as *Broom* is a strong diuretic and because *Lily of the Valley* also acts as a strong diuretic if the root of the problem lies in the heart.

NERVINES

Anxiety and stress can lead to cardiovascular problems, and it is often impossible to pinpoint any particular cause. Any specific problem is a manifestation of the whole interacting web of lifestyle, inner reality and physical tendencies. Whenever there is a cardiovascular problem, the use of relaxing nervines has to be considered, as in many cases anxiety and stress are involved, and sometimes are even caused by the problem.

The most useful nervines for cardiovascular problems are *Balm, Hops, Lime Blossom, Motherwort, Pasque Flower, Skullcap* and *Valerian*. Each case needs to be individually assessed. The appropriate nervines to be used by any individual should be selected by comparing their associated actions in The Herbal section of this book (*see pages 52–165*).

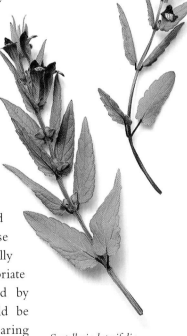

Scutellaria laterifolia
Skullcap *is a useful nervine for stress-based heart and circulation problems.*

Patterns of Circulatory Disease

Conventional medicine divides heart problems into many categories, but when using herbs it is not usually necessary to do this, as we are working with herbs that have an overall strengthening effect.

HEART WEAKNESS

To strengthen the heart, the following mixture should be taken over an extended period of time.

Hawthorn Berries	2 parts	🗡
Motherwort	2 parts	▣
Lily of the Valley	1 part	◉

Drink a cup of this three times a day. If there is any water retention, one part of *Dandelion* should be added to the mixture. If tension or anxiety is present, use the following combination.

Balm	1 part	🗡	
Lime Blossom	1 part	▣	◉

This tea should also be drunk three times a day or as often as needed.

If this does not prove strong enough, use *Skullcap* and *Valerian* instead, as described in the section on The Nervous System *(see pages 202–11).*

PALPITATIONS

Quite separate from any organic heart disease, racing of the heart beat can occur and can be caused by a whole range of factors, from menopause and allergies to fear and sexual excitement.

There are a number of effective remedies that will reduce erratic and fast heart beats without affecting the heart in an adverse way. In addition to the remedies described for normalizing heart activity, *Broom, Bugleweed, Mistletoe, Motherwort, Passion Flower* and *Valerian* are indicated.

A common occurrence is the speeding up of the heart rate due to anxiety and stress. An excellent basic mixture for this problem is the following.

Motherwort	2 parts	🗡
Mistletoe	1 part	▣
Valerian.	1 part	◉

This should be drunk three times a day or as needed.

If there is any suggestion of heightened blood pressure or heart problems, *Hawthorn Berries* should be added.

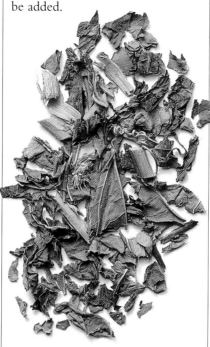

Passiflora incarnata
Passion Flower *helps to reduce palpitations.*

ANGINA PECTORIS

This painful and distressing condition is brought about when the blood supply to the heart itself is deficient and leads to a lack of usable oxygen in the heart tissue, often brought about by physical exertion or emotional stress.

A twofold process has to bring this about. Initially the vessels can be dilated to allow more blood to flow through, but as a long-term treatment, any blockage that is present in the vessels has also to be cleared. The key to this is the use of

Hawthorn Berries, which will do both, if given enough time and taken regularly.

An addition of *Lime Blossom* leads to excellent results, as it has the unique ability to clear any cholesterol deposits in vessels and guard against any further build-up. A basic mixture comprises:

Hawthorn Berries	3 parts	🗡
Motherwort	2 parts	▣
Lime Blossom	2 parts	◉
Lily of the Valley	1 part	

This tea should be drunk three times a day over a long period; it will not immediately relieve the pain of an attack.

If there is an additional problem with high blood pressure, *Mistletoe* should be added to the mixture.

Angina has to be treated within the context of the complete state of health; the individual must be treated as a whole being and any other problem should also be taken into account.

HIGH BLOOD PRESSURE

High blood pressure (hypertension) is a very common problem in our society. It can be caused by a range of primarily physical problems, in which case these must be seen to as appropriate, but it may also occur without any clear cause.

There is often a genetic disposition, but this tendency need not actually manifest physically if steps for its prevention are taken.

Stress and anxiety play a large part in this condition. Emotional problems, work pressure, and the state of the world can all contribute to a state of mind that is reflected in the body by a pattern of tension, inflexibility and constriction, a tightening of the whole being, so raising the blood pressure. The direct relationship between mind and body, mediated through the nerves, leads to a constriction of the peripheral blood vessels and influences the heart beat.

Relaxation therapy and body-work techniques such as massage are very valuable in such cases, as they ease up the body.

There are a number of herbs that will dilate the peripheral blood vessels, thereby increasing the total volume of the system. Similarly, there are herbs that will help the kidneys to pass more water, thus reducing the amount of fluid in the system. There are others to normalize the activity of the heart, safely decreasing the force with which the blood is pumped through the body. The most important remedies in this group are *Buckwheat, Cramp Bark, Garlic, Hawthorn Berries, Lime Blossom, Mistletoe* and *Yarrow.*

As always, the actual approach to each individual will vary. As a basic guide, the following mixture is effective:

Hawthorn Berries	2 parts
Lime Blossom	2 parts
Yarrow	2 parts
Mistletoe	1 part

This tea should be drunk three times a day.

In addition to this, *Garlic* may be eaten, preferably raw. If there is a lot of tension in the body, one part of *Cramp Bark* should be included in the mix. If there is much anxiety and stress, include *Skullcap* and *Valerian.* When headaches accompany high blood pressure, include one part of *Wood Betony* in the mixture.

CAUTION: *Do not use* Broom *as a diuretic in cases of raised blood pressure.*

By using this mixture over a period of time, blood pressure will return to a normal level. The mixture is safe and does not artificially depress the blood pressure.

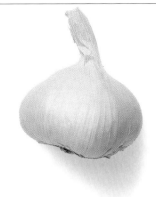

Allium sativum
Garlic *is well-established in folk medicine as a blood cleanser which can keep cholesterol levels down.*

ARTERIOSCLEROSIS

Arteriosclerosis is characterized by a thickening and hardening of the artery walls, restricting the flow of blood to the cells of the body. Cholesterol and fatty deposits in the artery walls lead to a speedy degeneration of the vessels and cause profound problems. These fatty deposits are called atheroma. They can build up in the aorta, in the arteries of the heart and in the brain. Arteriosclerosis is one of the most common causes of death in the Western world.

Arteriosclerosis is a primary product of inappropriate lifestyle and a lot can be done to heal the body by making necessary changes to diet, exercise, stress levels, as well as smoking and alcohol intake.

There are also a number of herbs that can help in this condition, above all *Lime Blossom*, as it has a specific anti-atheroma action. In long-term use it will guard against the deposition of cholesterol, also helping the body in the removal of any that has already built up. The long-term use of *Garlic,* in pill form or as part of the diet, has a similar effect.

Specific herbs for this condition include *Garlic, Hawthorn Berries, Lime Blossom, Mistletoe* and *Yarrow.* These are also herbs found to be most effective in the treatment of raised blood pressure, which often accompanies arteriosclerosis. The same mixture as for high blood pressure can be used, if the proportion of *Lime Blossom* is increased to three parts.

THROMBOSIS AND PHLEBITIS

When there is a build-up of atheroma, there is an added danger that a piece of it or clotted blood may enter the bloodstream. Both can cause a vessel to be blocked, which leads to a deficiency of oxygen downstream from the blocked blood vessel.

The seriousness of this thrombosis depends on where in the body the block occurs. It can be a minor problem, but it also is a possible cause of death. It must be treated to make sure that no new focus for thrombus formation develops. The treatment should be based on herbs that ensure a healthy circulatory system, together with the advice given for arteriosclerosis.

Symphytum officinale
Comfrey *makes a useful compress for pain caused by phlebitis.*

When a clot occurs in the veins of the legs, the condition is labelled phlebitis. In cases of local inflammations and pains, lotions, compresses or poultices are most effective. *Arnica, Comfrey, Hawthorn Berries* and *Marigold* can all be used in the external treatment of these conditions.

173

VARICOSE VEINS

Lack of exercise, obesity, pregnancy, and anything that reduces the circulation in the legs, such as tight clothing or sitting with crossed legs, can contribute to the development of varicose veins, a name for veins that have become enlarged, twisted and swollen.

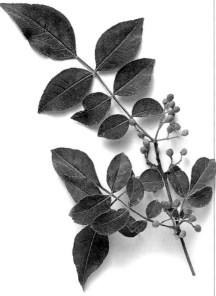

Zanthoxylum americanum
Prickly Ash *can help relieve varicose veins by stimulating blood flow.*

They can appear anywhere in the body, but are most commonly found in the legs. It is essential that adequate exercise be taken and that the feet are elevated when sitting for a long time, to counteract the effects of gravity.

Herbal medicine has a lot to offer in this condition, as long as its action is supported by exercise. The diet should be rich in fruit and green vegetables.

Constipation has to be avoided. Vitamins B-complex, C and E should be added to the diet. The herbs to be used in this condition should stimulate the peripheral circulation and thereby aid the flow of blood in the legs.

Appropriate herbs are *Cayenne, Ginger* and *Prickly Ash Bark* (or *Berries*). Furthermore, herbs that strengthen the blood vessels have

to be included, for example *Buckwheat, Hawthorn Berries* or *Horsechestnut*. If there is any water retention that leads to swelling, a diuretic such as *Dandelion* or *Yarrow* has to be included.

This mixture approaches the problem from all angles.

Hawthorn Berries	3 parts	
Horsechestnut	3 parts	
Prickly Ash Bark★	2 parts	
Yarrow	2 parts	
Ginger	1 part	
★or berries		

This should be drunk three times a day.

When there is a local inflammation with pain, a lotion or compress of *Witch Hazel* will often ease the discomfort, otherwise *Marigold, Comfrey* or *Hawthorn Berries* can be used externally.

VARICOSE ULCERS

If varicose veins become chronic, the altered pressures in the capillaries cause protein to leak from them and fibrin to be deposited in extracellular tissue. This makes the skin more vulnerable to injury and slower to heal, leading to the formation of varicose ulcers. They are notoriously difficult to heal. Here it is even more important that adequate exercise be taken and that the feet are elevated, to counteract the effect of gravity on the legs.

The herbs to be used here are the same as for varicose veins, but a higher proportion of diuretics and alteratives have to be used.

External treatment is vital here. If there is any secondary infection, it can be treated by a compress made from *Marigold, Marshmallow* and *Echinacea*, which has to be changed often. When the infection has subsided, change the compress for a poultice of powdered *Comfrey*,

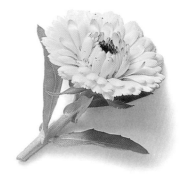

Calendula officinalis
Marigold *in a poultice can help soothe varicose ulcers.*

Marigold and *Marshmallow* made into a thick paste and applied to the surrounding tissue of the ulcer and kept in place with the aid of an elastic bandage.

BAD CIRCULATION AND CHILBLAINS

When the circulation of the extremities is not adequate, leading to cold hands and feet, the following mixture can be very helpful.

Prickly Ash Bark★	3 parts	
Hawthorn Berries	3 parts	
Ginger	1 part	
★or berries		

This should be drunk three times a day.

When there are any unbroken chilblains, they can be treated successfully by the application of a thin layer of *Cayenne* ointment, applied very sparingly.

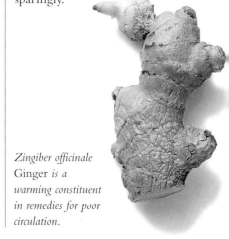

Zingiber officinale
Ginger *is a warming constituent in remedies for poor circulation.*

THE LYMPHATIC SYSTEM

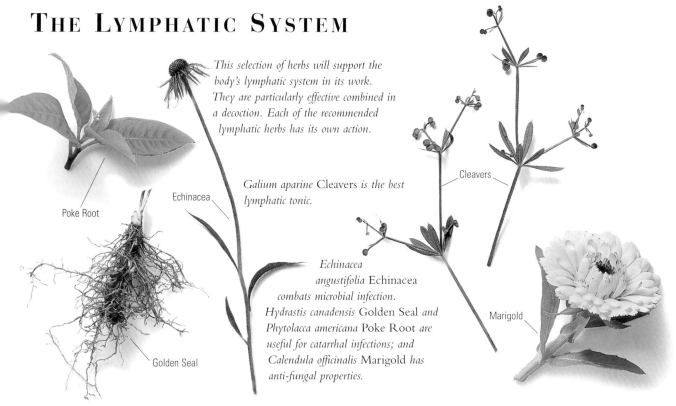

This selection of herbs will support the body's lymphatic system in its work. They are particularly effective combined in a decoction. Each of the recommended lymphatic herbs has its own action.

Galium aparine Cleavers *is the best lymphatic tonic.*

Echinacea angustifolia Echinacea *combats microbial infection.* Hydrastis canadensis *Golden Seal and* Phytolacca americana *Poke Root are useful for catarrhal infections; and* Calendula officinalis *Marigold has anti-fungal properties.*

Poke Root

Echinacea

Golden Seal

Cleavers

Marigold

The lymphatic system is a series of vessels running parallel to the circulatory system whose job is to return inter- and intra-cellular fluid back to the blood stream.

However, in the process of this apparently passive job of transport, much vital work goes on. It is through the lymphatic drainage of the cells, tissues and organs that cleansing largely occurs. The proper flow and coherence of the lymphatic system is thus vital to the body function and must be considered when approaching the body from a holistic point of view.

A second major function of this system occurs in the lymphatic glands, as the anti-microbial activity of the body is partially located there. This function is considered in various parts of the book, but especially in the section on ears, nose, throat and eyes *(see pages 184–7)*. Swollen glands may occur wherever there are lymph glands, common sites being the throat, under the arm, the breasts and the tops of the legs in the groin. Herbs such as *Cleavers,*

Echinacea, Golden Seal, Marigold and *Poke Root* may be considered to be lymphatic cleansers and may be used as such wherever they are needed.

A cleansing diet is called for wherever there is any suspicion of lymphatic trouble. A fruit-based cleansing diet would be best. In such a diet, the following sources of food should be avoided or kept to a minimum. This will give the lymphatic system a rest from overload with inappropriate foods:

- *Red meats*
- *Greasy, fatty foods and fried foods*
- *Cheese, butter, cream, milk*
- *Vinegar and pickles*
- *Alcohol*
- *Sugar and sugar-based products*
- *Artificial additives, preservatives, colourings, flavourings*

Avoidance of these foods will help the body, but with the use of the right foods, an active cleansing through the diet can take place. Fresh fruit and vegetables provide

the basis here. For a thorough cleansing, it is best to go on a fruit diet for three or four days at the most and then reintroduce other foods. The following is a short list of appropriate foods:

- *Fresh fruits, especially oranges, grapes and apples*
- *Fresh green vegetables*
- *White meat and white fish if desired*

Whenever you undertake a cleansing diet or a fruit only regime, always consult a practitioner first. Never use extreme diets during pregnancy.

A herbal mixture that will aid the lymphatic system wherever the problem arises is the following.

Echinacea	2 parts	
Cleavers	1 part	
Golden Seal	1 part	
Poke Root	1 part	

This should be drunk three times a day.

This sort of mixture could be used in other conditions wherever it is thought that the lymphatic drainage needs support.

THE RESPIRATORY SYSTEM

The air we breathe is spiritual ecology in action. When we draw in the breath of life, we share that air with all other human beings, all life on our planet. It is through respiration that our oneness with the trees becomes a manifest fact, and our communication with the oceans has immediate impact.

Every minute, usually unconsciously, we breathe in and out between ten and fifteen times. We move enough air to and fro every day to blow up several thousand balloons. In this way the body extracts the oxygen it needs from the air and discharges waste carbon dioxide from the blood.

Whilst only one-fifth of the air is oxygen, this is needed by every cell in the body to release the energy that is locked in food reserves. Many cells can survive for a period of time without oxygen, others need a constant supply. Brain cells die – and cannot be replaced – if they lack oxygen for more than a few minutes. Supplying the cells of the body with oxygen is the responsibility of the respiratory and circulatory systems. This process is controlled by the brain via the medulla oblongata in the brain stem, where messages concerning blood composition are integrated with other information, thus regulating the appropriate breathing rhythm.

If there are respiratory disturbances that inhibit gas exchange in the lungs, they can lead to a lowering of the body's vitality, an increase in metabolic disorders, and degeneration of tissue.

The anatomy and physiology of the respiratory system are complex and beautiful embodiments of integration and wholeness.

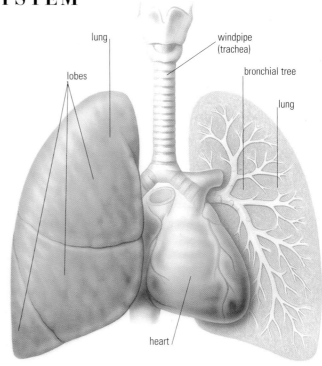

Air enters the lungs via the windpipe when we breathe. The bronchial tree of blood vessels in each lung is responsible for the exchange of gases, which takes place in the grape-like clusters of the alveoli. Oxygen is taken in and carbon dioxide is breathed out.

lung
windpipe (trachea)
lobes
bronchial tree
lung
heart

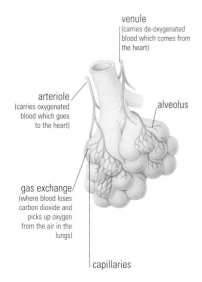

venule
(carries de-oxygenated blood which comes from the heart)

arteriole
(carries oxygenated blood which goes to the heart)

alveolus

gas exchange
(where blood loses carbon dioxide and picks up oxygen from the air in the lungs)

capillaries

In the alveoli of the lungs oxygen diffuses into the blood and carbon dioxide escapes.

Prevention of Respiratory Disease

We are not only what we eat, but also what we breathe. Any problems with breathing will not only affect other organs and systems, but may well cause disease in these systems. However, as the body is a whole, the reverse is also true. When the lungs need to be treated, we also have to look at the circulatory system; much of what has been said about the heart and the circulation is relevant to the lungs. We should also look at the condition of the digestive system, and especially of the organs of elimination, as the lungs share the role of removing waste with the bowels, the kidneys and the skin. If a problem develops in any of these systems, the body compensates by increasing the load on the others. There are limits to the amount of waste the lungs can put up with if, for instance, the bowels become clogged up.

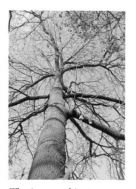

The inner architecture of the lungs is very like the structure of a tree, with a central trunk and branches that subdivide into smaller elements.

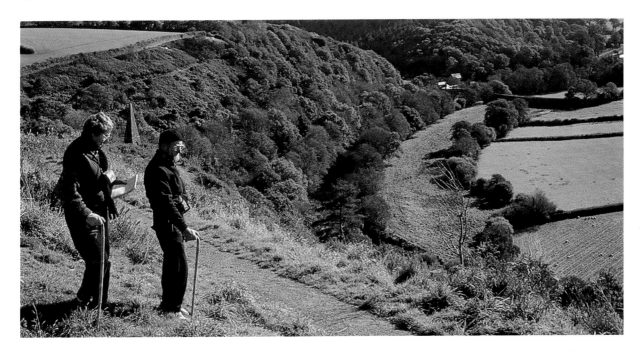

Most pathological changes in tissue can be prevented if the environmental milieu of the cells is constantly rich in oxygen. The amount of oxygen which the circulation supplies to the tissue is largely controlled by respiration.

From all this it is apparent that the best preventative measures for this system are regular exercise and good breathing. While we take breathing for granted, conscious and proper breathing is regarded, even in orthodox medical circles, as invaluable. The central role of the breath in many spiritual paths should perhaps give us a clue here.

As with all disease, the best prophylactic is the right lifestyle. Diet, exercise and quality of life all have a profound influence on the health of the lungs.

To ensure healthy lungs, the inner environment must be in harmony, and so also must be the outer environment. If the air we breathe is polluted it will disrupt the ecology of the lungs just as it disrupts the ecology of any forest. Air contaminated with chemicals and particles, gases and smoke, should be avoided. Which brings us to tobacco. Smoking puts a wall of tar and ash between the individual and the world so that a free ecological flow cannot take place in the lungs. This can lead to an impressive host of problems, from bronchitis to cancer, without taking into account all the effects of a diminished oxygen supply to the rest of the body. If we are to heal ourselves and our world, here is a good place to start.

Help your respiratory system by taking time out from city life to take in some good clean air. Walking is an excellent all-round exercise for stamina and if you can walk in the countryside you will be inspiring your whole system.

Eating a whole-food diet and living in the country pales a bit when faced with twenty cigarettes a day!

There are other specific dangers which can be recognized and avoided. In the case of infections, the simplest answer is to just avoid contact with them.

However, as this is often socially impossible, we need to maintain our natural defences at their peak. A word is in place here about the questionable or too frequent use of antibiotics.

The body, if given the chance, is capable of great feats of self-defence, as long as we provide a balanced, vitamin-rich diet in combination with a lifestyle that is healthy in thought and feeling as much as in action. In this context it is vital to curb the misuse of antibiotics. While these drugs, used at the right time in the right way, can save lives, they can also reduce the innate defence systems of the body to impotence. In addition to the reduction of our defence, they also in the long run create – in an evolutionary sense – highly resistant bacteria, so that problems become more and more difficult to treat.

Over the last thirty years doctors have had to watch alarming developments in this direction. With correct lifestyle and the use of herbal remedies when needed, antibiotics can often be avoided.

If you make exercise fun, it will be easier to build it into your everyday life.

177

Herbs for the Respiratory System

All aspects of the respiratory system can benefit from appropriate herbal remedies. Herbs can aid the activity of the mucous membranes and ensure that gas exchange through these membranes can occur; they can activate the secretion of lung tissue so that the air is sufficiently moistened and the membranes protected; they can augment neurological responses regulating the breath; they can tone up the circulation and ensure that blood bathes the tissues properly, and help by stimulating the whole of the glandular and excretory process to ensure a clean and harmonious inner environment.

Although it is inadvisable to classify herbs strictly by their actions, it may be of value to lay some broad guidelines. We will look at respiratory stimulants, respiratory relaxants, amphoteric remedies and respiratory demulcents.

RESPIRATORY STIMULANTS

Herbs in this category act as stimulants to the nerves and muscles of the respiratory system by triggering a neurological reflex via the sensory endings in the digestive system. This causes 'expectoration'.

Expectorants encourage the loosening and subsequent expulsion of mucus from the respiratory system. Plants that fit into this category include *Bittersweet, Cowslip, Daisy, Senega, Soapwort, Squill* and *Thuja*.

RESPIRATORY RELAXANTS

The primary actions of these plants is to relax the tissue of the lungs, which will be most useful in any problems concerned with tension and over-activity. The easing of tension promotes the flow of mucus and thus allows expect-oration to occur. Many plants can be

Primula veris
Cowslip *flowers, which are becoming increasingly rare, ease reactions to stress and tension, facilitating restful sleep.*

Asclepias tuberosa
Pleurisy Root *(above left)* and *Verbascum thapsus*
Mullein *(above right)* both help to maintain the acid/alkali balance in the respiratory system.

included in this group, but *Angelica, Aniseed, Coltsfoot, Elecampane, Ephedra, Flax Seed, Grindelia, Hyssop, Plantain, Pill-bearing Spurge, Sundew, Thyme, Wild Cherry Bark* and *Wild Lettuce* are representatives.

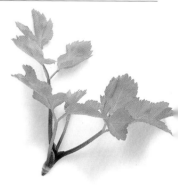
Angelica archangelica Angelica *is o the herbs that helps to relax the tiss of the lungs.*

AMPHOTERIC REMEDIES

The concept of amphotericity is of great value when we deal with the apparently contradictory actions of many plants. The term is borrowed from chemistry where it is used to describe a substance that is capable of acting as either an acid or an alkali. Amphoteric herbs, which are normalizers, change and adapt their actions, depending on the conditions. Amphoteric herbs work in a way that suits the system at a particular time, using the body's wisdom to do that which is appropriate. The best respiratory amphoterics are *Blood Root, Lobelia, Mullein, Pleurisy Root* and *White Horehound*.

DEMULCENTS

Demulcents soothe, relieve and soften irritated or in-flamed mucous membranes, as their mucilagi-nous, slippery characteristics enable them to coat, protect and lubricate the membranes and other tissue surfaces. Under their protective help, healing can take place.

Many of the herbs already mentioned are demulcents, the most valuable ones for the lungs being *Comfrey Root, Coltsfoot, Flax Seed, Licorice, Lungwort Moss, Marshmallow Leaf* and *Mullein*.

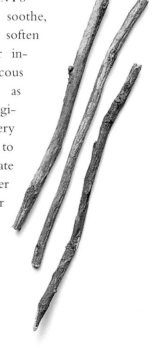
Glycyrrhiza glabra
Licorice, *here shown as a root, relieves and soothes inflamma-tion in the mucous membranes.*

Patterns of Respiratory Disease

In practice, the various respiratory diseases and syndromes that have been labelled with a name can be viewed as the manifestation of two sorts of respiratory defect: congestion or spasm. Congestion is brought about by an overburdening of the lungs with mucus, either excessive production or inadequate excretion of it, which in time leads to degenerative effects. Spasms of the bronchial muscles constitute the other group of respiratory problems and can be caused by a number of factors.

CONGESTION

Organisms can only thrive within the body if the 'soil' is right. In the case of the lungs, congestion provides the right soil for infection, but this is not a healthy and normal state of affairs. Removing only the infection does nothing for the underlying problem; instead the congestion also has to be treated to prevent a recurrence of the symptoms.

One factor that is most often related to congestion is the mucus content of the diet. If the body's need for mucus-forming foods is exceeded, it will get rid of it by increasing secretion, for instance into the lungs. If this natural cleansing process is inhibited by antibiotics the seeds are sown for chronic and perhaps degenerative diseases as the result of congestion.

Therefore, in any respiratory condition where there is excessive mucus, it is essential that a diet low in mucus-forming foods be embarked upon. Whenever there is a build-up of catarrh such as sinus congestion, a diet that limits the intake of food that feeds the catarrh-forming metabolic paths would help. Even in normal conditions, some people think that accumulations of catarrh, or mucus, are sites in which metabolic waste and toxic material build up, which may eventually overload the body and lead to degenerative disease.

Marrubium vulgare White Horehound, like many medicines, tastes nasty but is effective. It is used as a cough remedy, but has to be combined with a sweetener such as Licorice.

There is nothing inherently wrong with mucus; it is a natural body carbohydrate acting as a lubricant and a waste disposal medium. It is only the excess that we need to watch, and the dietary promoters of mucus formation which are:

- *Dairy products, including goat's milk and yoghurt*
- *Eggs*
- *Grains, especially gluten-rich ones such as wheat, oats, rye and barley*
- *Sugar*
- *Potatoes and other starchy root vegetables like swedes and turnips*

Replace these foods with fresh fruit and juices when following a mucus-free diet.

COUGHS

Coughs can be treated herbally in many ways and every herbalist will have a favourite herb or mixture. *Coltsfoot* is by far the best standard remedy to have available. Sometimes a combination can be more effective. A basic one with a quite pleasant taste can be made with the following ingredients.

Coltsfoot	1 part	↗
Mullein	1 part	■
Licorice	1 part	⏲

This can be taken up to every three hours, although three times a day would be best.

Another highly effective remedy is *White Horehound*, but because of its unpleasant taste it needs to be well masked by combining it with *Licorice* or *Aniseed*. This herb was the original constituent of old-fashioned cough candy – an infusion of *White Horehound* plus sugar, lots of it.

If the cough is causing any pressure on a weak heart, it might be useful to add *Motherwort* to the tea. This will help cardiac activity without forcing the heart.

A dry, irritable cough would benefit from respiratory relaxants and demulcents. *Wild Lettuce* and *Coltsfoot* are useful here. Sometimes such coughs can be nervous in origin, in which case it is more advisable to use nervine relaxants.

BRONCHITIS

Bronchitis is an infection of the bronchi, the tubes that take air to the lungs.

Tussilago farfara Coltsfoot is the favourite herbal specific for coughs and is particularly effective for dry, irritating hacking.

179

Thymus vulgaris
Thyme *helps to clear mucus and soothe sore tissue; it is very useful in bronchitis.*

The best herbs to use are pectorals that combine expectorant actions to clear the sputum with demulcent properties to soothe the inflamed tissue. They include *Aniseed, Angelica Root, Blood Root, Coltsfoot, Comfrey Root, Elecampane Root, Flax Seed, Hyssop, Lobelia, Lungwort, Mouse Ear, Mullein, Senega, Thyme* and *White Horehound*. Consult the Herbal section for more details on each of these, in order to choose the most appropriate herb or combination for your own case.

Anti-microbial herbs are also indicated to fight against any infection. Perhaps the most important one amongst the many available is *Garlic*, which may be taken in any form, either raw or as *Garlic* oil in capsules.

The antiseptic oil in *Garlic* is excreted through the lungs and so directly affects any bacteria there. Other good anti-microbials for bronchitis are *Echinacea, Eucalyptus*

and *Thyme*. The antiseptic volatile oils contained in *Eucalyptus* and *Thyme* can also be of value in the form of inhalations or baths.

In addition to the above it might be helpful to aid the lymphatic system, especially if there are swollen glands. As it would be beneficial to stimulate elimination as well, *Cleavers* and *Poke Root* can be recommended.

PLEURISY

When an infection has given rise to pleurisy or developed into pneumonia, the most important thing is to treat the person for fever, thus helping the whole body and specifically the chest. To this end diaphoretics are invaluable, usually combined with respiratory demulcents. *Boneset, Cayenne, Comfrey Root, Hyssop, Garlic, Pleurisy Root* and *Mullein* will be found especially useful. Choose the appropriate ones, depending on the

condition of the whole body, and combine them into an infusion.

In addition to this internal help, pleurisy is a condition where a poultice or a compress is called for.

Alternatively, a compress using an infusion of *Cayenne* may be of value (*see the Preparation of Herbs section, pages 22–31*).

WHOOPING COUGH

As this condition can lead to unfortunate complications and to a constitutional weakness in later life, it should be treated thoroughly.

The herbs *Sundew* (which may make the urine darker than usual) and *Mouse Ear* can be regarded as specific remedies and should be included in a mixture.

Mouse Ear	2 parts	
Sundew	1 part	↗
Coltsfoot	1 part	◼
Thyme	1 part	◷
White Horehound	1 part	

TO MAKE A FLAX SEED POULTICE

A poultice made from *Flax Seed* is excellent for chest complaints.

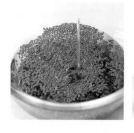

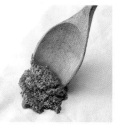

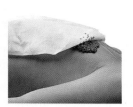

1 *Take a handful of Flax Seed and stir thoroughly with boiling water, until it reaches the consistency of thick paste.*

2 *Spread the paste about 1cm/¹/2in thick on linen, leaving the sides of the linen free and avoiding lumps forming.*

3 *Apply it as hot as possible, covering the whole chest, and leave for two hours. Renew it some hours later or the next day.*

After removing the *Flax Seed* poultice, sponge the area with warm water, then dry it well. To increase its power, you can sprinkle some *Mustard* powder on the poultice, but do not use *Mustard* for young children or people with sensitive skin.

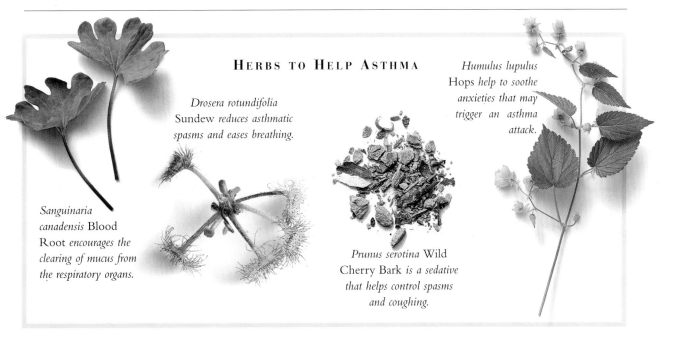

HERBS TO HELP ASTHMA

Drosera rotundifolia
Sundew *reduces asthmatic spasms and eases breathing.*

Humulus lupulus
Hops *help to soothe anxieties that may trigger an asthma attack.*

Sanguinaria canadensis Blood Root *encourages the clearing of mucus from the respiratory organs.*

Prunus serotina Wild Cherry Bark *is a sedative that helps control spasms and coughing.*

This should be drunk three times a day.

The mixture may be flavoured with *Aniseed* or *Licorice*. If vomiting is accompanying the cough attacks, it is best to give the drink after a spasm to ensure that it stays down. A *Flax Seed* poultice may be helpful.

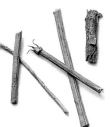

Ephedra sinica
Ephedra, *also known to Chinese herbalists as Ma Huang, is very useful for asthmatic attacks prompted by allergy.*

In more serious or chronic respiratory conditions – such as emphysema or bronchiectasis – herbal therapy can play a major part in the treatment.

Particularly remedies that clear sputum – such as *Elecampane* or *Comfrey Root* – should be considered. The herbs recommended for asthma will be useful to regain tissue tone, but above all there is the need for breathing exercises.

ASTHMA
Asthma can stem from a combination of causes. There is often an allergic component

that triggers asthmatic attacks. In some cases the cause is purely genetic whilst in others it may be an acquired reaction due to exposure to an irritant. The state of the nervous tone of the body can also lead to bronchial spasms. In predisposed people, tension, anxiety, hyperactivity or exhaustion can cause so much stress that an asthma attack is triggered off. Similarly, spasms or difficulty in breathing could be caused by osteopathic problems that happen to affect the spot where the thoracic nerve comes out of the spine.

Asthma will respond well to herbal treatment, but it is impossible to give a prescription that is appropriate in all cases. Herbs that help reduce spasm and ease breathing include *Grindelia, Lobelia, Mouse Ear, Pill-bearing Spurge, Sundew* and *Wild Cherry Bark*.

If there is production of sputum – which of course must be got rid of – expectorants such as *Aniseed, Blood Root, Coltsfoot, Comfrey Root, Licorice* and *Senega* will help.

Where there is an allergic component, it is good to remember the use of the Chinese herb *Ephedra*.

If the attacks tax the strength of the heart – which they often do – *Motherwort* will be invaluable with its gentle strengthening action.

If any hypertension is involved, *Hawthorn Berries* and *Lime Blossom* will be useful. Anxiety and tension are best treated with *Hops, Skullcap* or *Valerian*.

Occasionally asthma responds well to the use of nervines alone, as fear is one of the most potent triggers for an asthma attack. It can even be fear of the attack itself. As such, anything that will augment the person's inner strength and self-image is called for. The nervines will help this process, but a psycho-therapeutic approach can also be invaluable in addition. Relaxation techniques can help, some of which are described on pages 204–5 in the section on The Nervous System.

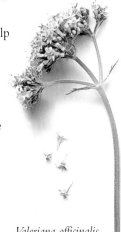

Valeriana officinalis
Valerian *can be used where asthmatic attacks are triggered by nervousness, anxiety or tension.*

181

EARS, NOSE, THROAT AND EYES

All the organs considered in this section share an anatomical closeness and a functional relationship, and are a major interface between the inner and outer environments. This interface is physical in that there is an exchange of gas in respiration and an input of food in eating for instance, but there is also the interface of awareness and communication.

With our ears we hear the sounds of our world, a sense that reflects the spiritual quality of comprehension. With our nose we smell, an outer reflection of spiritual discernment and idealism. Through the mouth the world of taste opens to us, itself a doorway to discrimination. The voice, generated in the throat, facilitates communication. Through the eyes, light is revealed to us, and also the doorway to divinity.

This interaction with our outer environment, and the close connection between these organs through the continuous layer of mucous membranes they share, explains many of the conditions which may occur. It is possible to simply say that a bacterial infection has occurred, or that an allergy reaction is due to a particular grass pollen, but this is a very limited way of looking at symptoms. The systemic root for a reduction of innate resistance must be sought, as must the cause of an immunological sensitivity.

There is a strong connection between the respiratory system and the ears, nose and throat. A beautiful example of the body's synergy and self-healing is given by the way that mucus is dealt with by the mucous membranes. Part of the function of the mucus is to trap particles and protect the underlying membranes from invasion. The mucus is disposed of by the 'mucociliary escalator'. The cells lining the nose and throat have little hairs on them called cilia. These beat in one direction, moving material inexorably downwards towards the esophagus and thus into the sterilizing stomach. The lining of the bronchial tubes has cilia that move material upwards to the same fate. Under healthy conditions this works perfectly. However, if there is a change in the consistency of the mucus the mechanism cannot operate efficiently. Much of the herbal treatment of mucous conditions is therefore based on changing the consistency of the mucus; the cilia will do the rest.

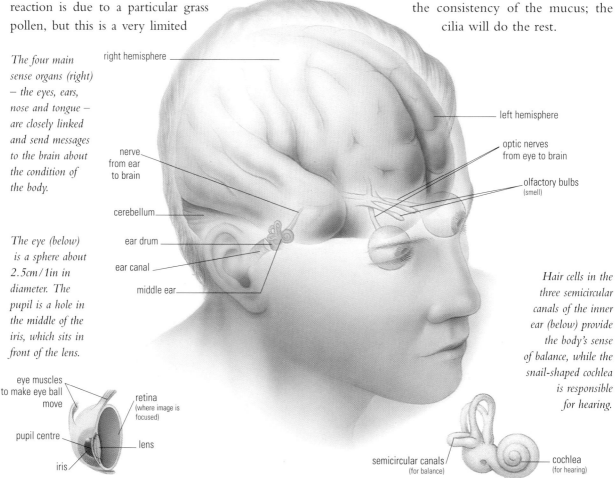

The four main sense organs (right) – the eyes, ears, nose and tongue – are closely linked and send messages to the brain about the condition of the body.

right hemisphere

left hemisphere

optic nerves
from eye to brain

nerve
from ear
to brain

olfactory bulbs
(smell)

cerebellum

The eye (below) is a sphere about 2.5cm/1in in diameter. The pupil is a hole in the middle of the iris, which sits in front of the lens.

ear drum

ear canal

middle ear

Hair cells in the three semicircular canals of the inner ear (below) provide the body's sense of balance, while the snail-shaped cochlea is responsible for hearing.

eye muscles
to make eye ball
move

retina
(where image is
focused)

pupil centre

lens

iris

semicircular canals
(for balance)

cochlea
(for hearing)

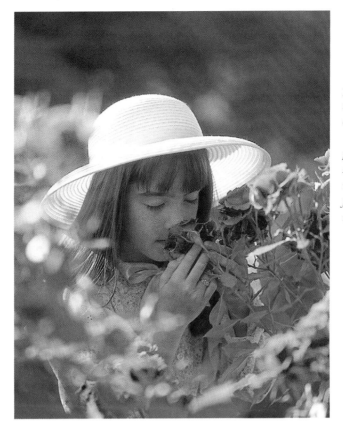

When you smell a flower, your nose is detecting molecules of the volatile essential oil in the plant. These oils can have a physical effect — soothing, stimulating or relaxing — which is why the scent of flowers can change your mood so effectively.

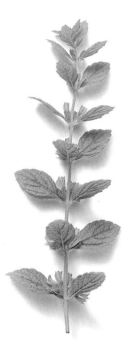

Melissa officinalis Balm is an aromatic herb rich in essential oil, which can be easily detected by smell.

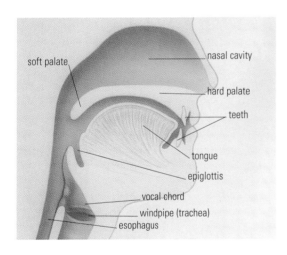

soft palate
nasal cavity
hard palate
teeth
tongue
epiglottis
vocal chord
windpipe (trachea)
esophagus

White light is composed of a spectrum of seven colours (below), as demonstrated when a beam of light is refracted through a prism. Human eyes are designed to see best in daylight and in colour.

The retina is equipped with a layer of special cells, rods which detect brightness levels and cones which detect colour.

The senses of smell and taste (above), are closely allied. Airborne scent molecules enter the nasal cavity where they are caught on a patch of mucous membrane packed with sensitive receptors called olfactory hairs. The scents are analysed in the olfactory centre of the brain. Taste is detected on the tongue, where taste buds are clustered in

groups. Bitterness is detected at the back of the tongue, sourness at the sides, saltiness at the front and sweetness at the tip.

Light reflected from an object (below), enters the eye through the cornea and is turned upside-down on the retina at the back of the eye.

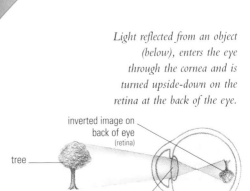

inverted image on
back of eye
(retina)

tree

lens

Herbs for Ears, Nose, Throat and Eyes

As most of the diseases that manifest in this system stem from problems with the mucous membranes, we usually have to deal with catarrh and infections. Whilst we have to remember that these conditions can only be treated in the context of the whole body, certain groups of remedies are especially indicated. For any catarrhal problem, astringents and anti-catarrhal plants should be used, but herbs rich in volatile oils can also be very useful. As there is often a microbial involvement, anti-microbials should be considered, as should alteratives to aid the lymphatic system in its defensive and cleansing work *(see page 175)*.

Especially suited for use in this system are *Balm of Gilead, Boneset, Echinacea, Elder Flower, Eyebright, Golden Seal, Golden Rod, Hyssop, Marshmallow Leaf, Peppermint, Poke Root, Sage, Silverweed* and *Wild Indigo*.

Patterns of Disease

THE EARS

We are most familiar with the ears' responsibility for hearing, but besides this perception of sound-waves they send impulses to the brain that tell which way up we are and also information about the movement of the body in the three dimensions of space. To fulfil all these functions, the body has evolved an architecturally beautiful structure that facilitates these complex activities in a miraculously efficient way.

It is beyond the scope of this book to explore problems in the inner ear. We shall concern ourselves only with conditions due to infections and catarrh that are within the field of home treatment.

• **Infections** of the middle ear often originate in the throat and spread via the eustachian tube. The most important herbs to use are anti-microbial remedies like *Blue Flag, Echinacea, Garlic* and *Wild Indigo*, which are also anti-catarrhal and alterative, with *Echinacea* being the most useful one in all infections of ears, nose and throat. The herbs rich in antiseptic oils may be useful but are more indicated in throat or

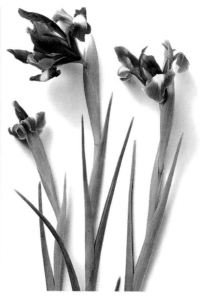

Iris versicolor Blue Flag *is a very useful anti-microbial herb for middle-ear infections.*

nose complaints. The lymphatic tonics such as *Cleavers* and *Poke Root* have to be considered, as should the anti-catarrhal and mucous membrane tonics *Elder Flower, Golden Rod* and *Golden Seal*.

The appropriate herbs should be combined into a tea (except maybe for *Golden Seal*, which because of its bitter taste often has to be given as a powder in capsules, particularly for children). Whilst this internal treatment will be effective, in cases of earache there may in addition be the need for an external treatment.

• **Earache** can be very painful, particularly in children, and can cause much distress, but there are a number of ways to ease such pain. The quickest way I know to relieve earache is to use *Pennywort* juice. Crush a couple of leaves in a sieve and collect the expressed juice. Put a couple of drops (which have to be at body temperature) of this green juice into the painful ear and plug it with some cotton wool.

Mullein oil can be used in the same way, as can warm *Almond* oil or the tincture of *Lobelia*. If none of these is available, make a strong infusion of *Chamomile, Yarrow* or *Hyssop* and use a couple of drops in the same way.

While any of these remedies will relieve the earache, we have to remember that the infection itself which is causing the pain also needs to be treated.

• **Mastoiditis,** not an uncommon condition, is an infection of the mastoid process, just behind the ear, which may produce an abscess or a boil that affects the outer or middle ear. This condition should be treated in the same way as boils, as a systemic infection *(see the section on The Skin, pages 212–14)*.

• **Deafness and Hearing Problems** may be due to neurological causes or a catarrhal blockage of the middle ear. Such blockages can be successfully treated with the approach described for nasal catarrh. A build-up of wax

Hyssopus officinalis Hyssop *in an infusion is a very effective earache remedy.*

Solidago virgauria Golden Rod *effectively combines astringent and anti-catarrhal properties.*

in the outer ear canal can also contribute to deafness and should be removed by a competent practitioner.

• **Tinnitus** is a condition in which a noise is heard within the ear. It can be caused by catarrhal congestion, but regardless of the cause it may be treated effectively, with *Golden Seal* or *Black Cohosh*, taken as a tea or in capsules over a period of time.

THE NOSE

The nasal passages are lined with mucous membranes. They constantly produce mucus, to protect the underlying membranes from drying out and to remove and sterilize any irritant that enters the nose when we breathe. This natural production of mucus can be stimulated by various factors and lead to problems of excess mucus, such as catarrh and colds. The reason can lie in external irritants, such as tobacco or petrol fumes, dust particles or bacteria, but most commonly stems from internal problems, from a state of internal build-up of toxins due to an in-appropriate lifestyle, particularly an inappropriate diet *(page 195)*.

If this is the cause, the body will use the mucus of the upper respiratory tract as one of its vehicles for waste removal. The first step in a treatment of such conditions is to examine your diet. In all the following suggestions for herbal

treatment it is assumed that a diet that is low in mucus-producing foods is followed.

• **Catarrh** Nasal catarrh may be the result of systemic factors and can also involve infections and allergies. To treat this sometimes intransi-gent problem effectively, we can use herbs that work on the mucous membranes in the nose, while we also treat the body in a wider context.

Herbs such as *Golden Rod, Elder Flower* and *Eyebright* bring specific relief, as they are anti-catarrhal and astringent, with *Golden Rod* normally being the most useful. *Golden Seal* is another specific remedy for nasal catarrh, but should be used with discretion as some people find that it has too much of a drying action on the mucous membranes.

Catarrh is often accompanied by an infection, so anti-microbial remedies like *Echinacea, Garlic* or *Wild Indigo* should be used. As the lymphatic system will be under

stress, *Poke Root* should be included, which is a good tonic for the system and at the same time is anti-catarrhal.

Besides using a mixture of these herbs as a tea, we can also make an excellent balm of antiseptic, volatile oils to relieve nasal congestion. It may be applied in a very small amount to the nostril and so be inhaled, or it can be rubbed on the chest at night so that the vapours will be inhaled.

Peppermint Oil	15ml/1tbsp
Eucalyptus Oil	15ml/1tbsp
Pine Oil	15ml/1tbsp
Petroleum Jelly	500g/1lb

Melt the petroleum jelly without over-heating it. When it just turns liquid, add the oils and stir them in. Pour the mixture into pots and seal them when the balm has reached room temperature.

Another way to inhale volatile oils is to use the method of steam inhalation. We can either use some of the balm, or an aromatic herb such as *Eucalyptus, Pine Needles* or even *Chamomile.*

TO MAKE A EUCALYPTUS STEAM INHALATION

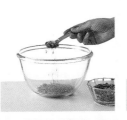 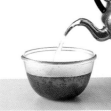 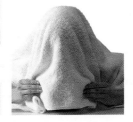

1 *For a steam inhalation of* Eucalyptus, *put three teaspoons of leaves in a basin.*

2 *Pour 2l/4pt of boiling water onto the* Eucalyptus *leaves.*

3 *Put your head over the basin and cover with a towel, to prevent a loss of the volatile oils. For about ten minutes, inhale through the nose.*

Do not go out immediately afterwards, as the mucous membranes will be very sensitive for a while. Repeat the process two or three times a day.

• **Colds** The common cold is usually seen as an inconvenience that should be suppressed as soon as possible. It is a typical example of the way we perceive an 'illness'; we tend to see it as something that has to be combated, rather than taking it as an indicator that points to something being out of balance in the body.

The aim should not be to suppress the indicator and to stay out of balance, but rather to find our way back to inner harmony, and thus make the indicator unnecessary. We 'catch' a cold when the conditions in our body are right for a virus to thrive. If our inner environment were sound and in harmony, we would not 'catch' a cold, no matter how many viruses were 'thrown' at us.

The first step in the treatment of a cold is to work on the causes of mucus build-up *(see under catarrh)*. In most cases it will mean cutting out all mucus-forming foods from the diet.

The next step is to treat the cold herbally. My favourite is a combination of *Elder Flower, Peppermint* and *Yarrow* in equal parts, a tea that combines the anti-catarrhal and mucous membrane-toning properties of *Elder Flower* with the stimulating, decongestant action of *Peppermint* and the diaphoretic and diuretic powers of *Yarrow*. The tea should be drunk at least three times daily as hot as possible. If the cold is accompanied by feverishness, use an additional diaphoretic such as *Boneset*.

Sambucus nigra
Elder Flower *is a demulcent and anti-catarrhal that can help in colds and flu. It combines well with* Achillea millefolium Yarrow *and* Mentha x piperita Peppermint.

Vitamin C should also be considered. Its value cannot be overstressed, both in the treatment and in a long-term prophylaxis of a cold. I recommend taking 2g of the vitamin – divided over the day – at the first sign of a cold until a few days after it clears, then to lower the dosage to 500mg. It should be taken in the form of *Rosehips* or *Acerola Berries* or as extracts from these, since both are also rich in bioflavonoids, necessary for the absorption and action of vitamin C.

• **Influenza** A herb that should be in every home in case of flu is *Boneset*, as it will relieve the aches and pains while also easing some of the malaise of this unpleasant infection. A useful mix is:

Boneset	2 parts	
Elder Flower	1 part	
Peppermint	1 part	

Drink a cup as hot as can be taken every two hours. If the tea is too bitter, especially for children, it may be sweetened with *Licorice*.

The depression that sometimes accompanies the flu or follows it may be eased by using *Skullcap* or *Vervain*. If antibiotics have been taken, it is good to take vitamin C and eat live yoghurt afterwards. Vitamin C eases the stress caused to the body by the antibiotics and by the fever. A live yoghurt helps the new growth of beneficial bacteria in the intestines, as antibiotics tend to kill them all.

• **Sinusitis** is an infection of the sinus cavities, which often turns from an acute state into a chronic one, and can develop into a very persistent and almost constant state. For a short-term treatment, an effective method is:

Echinacea	1 part	
Golden Rod	1 part	
Golden Seal	1 part	
Marshmallow Leaf	1 part	

Drink a cup of this tea every two hours.

This mixture combines the anti-microbial properties of *Echinacea*, the anti-catarrhal actions of *Golden Rod*, the tonic and anti-catarrhal actions of *Golden Seal*, and the invaluable demulcent contribution of *Marshmallow Leaf*. Besides using the tea, the balm and the steam inhalation mentioned for catarrh *(see page 185)* can also prove to be very beneficial.

• **Hayfever** and other conditions such as allergic rhinitis are caused by an immunological reaction to an external allergenic substance. To treat and alleviate the symptoms of hayfever, the following combination of herbs can be most effective.

Elder Flower	2 parts	
Ephedra	1 part	
Eyebright	1 part	
Golden Seal	1 part	

A cup of this tea should be drunk two or three times a day.

To prevent hayfever occurring and to be really effective, the treatment should start at least a month before the person's particular hayfever season begins, as the tonic and anti-allergenic properties need time to take effect. The low-mucus diet may be beneficial here as will a regular daily intake of vitamin C and a diet that includes plenty of *Garlic* (or *Garlic* capsules if you do not care to eat the vegetable itself).

• **Polyps** Nasal polyps can be a recurring problem and have to be examined and treated in the context of the condition of the whole body. Locally they can best be treated with a snuff made from equal parts of *Blood Root* and an astringent such as *Rhatany,* which should be made into a fine powder. The snuff should be used twice a day over a long period. Additionally, the nasal polyps may also be painted twice daily with the fluid extract of *Thuja* using a fine brush.

• **Nosebleed** is purely a symptom of something else that is wrong in the body. It may be a minor sign or can indicate a serious problem, for example, high blood pressure, but if it is a recurring event, get professional advice.

The symptom itself can easily be treated by the use of an astringent. Soak some cotton wool in distilled *Witch Hazel* and put a small plug into the nostril.

THE THROAT

The throat may be affected by the problems originating in the lungs, the nose, the sinuses, the stomach and the mouth, and also by systemically-based problems. They may take the form of tonsillitis, pharyngitis, or laryngitis, but these conditions must always be seen in the wider context. A good example of this wider view is the holistic approach to tonsillitis.

• **Tonsillitis** The glandular tissue that is called the tonsils is a variety of the lymphatic tissue, and shares with other lymphatic glands a role in the defence of the body from infection. The inflammation of the tonsils – tonsillitis – demonstrates that the glands fulfil their purpose

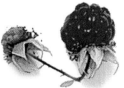

Rubus idaeus Raspberry *can help in tonsillitis, either drunk as an infusion or used as a gargle.*

of protecting the body. The appropriate treatment aims at supporting the body herbally, to aid the glands in the work they are doing. To this end, anti-microbial remedies such as *Echinacea, Myrrh* or *Red Sage* are called for, together with lymphatic alterative tonics such as *Cleavers, Poke Root, Marigold* or *Golden Seal.* Astringents and demulcents may also be used. A good mixture for internal use is:

Echinacea	2 parts	
Poke Root	2 parts	
Red Sage	2 parts	
Balm of Gilead	1 part	

Take a cup every two hours, which may be sweetened with *Licorice.*

Agrimony and *Raspberry* have a good reputation in tonsillitis. An infusion of equal parts drunk three times a day may help. Use the infusion as a gargle as well.

A gargle of *Red Sage* or *Golden Seal* can be used, which can also be sprayed onto the tonsils using a hand spray that is obtainable from chemists.

• **Laryngitis** The advice given for tonsillitis is also applicable for laryngitis. *Red Sage* – if not available, *Garden Sage* – makes an especially invaluable mouthwash and gargle. Put two tablespoons of *Sage Leaves* into 500ml/1pt of cold water and bring it to the boil. Cover it and let it infuse for a further ten minutes. Reheat the mixture whenever needed and gargle often.

THE EYES

The treatment of the eye is beyond the scope of this book. However,

conditions that affect the eyelids and tear glands may be treated herbally.

The herbs *par excellence* for the treatment of the eyes is *Eyebright.* It can be used internally and externally in all eye problems, and will help the eyeball and the surrounding tissue, but it can also be combined with other herbs. When treating styes, inflammation of the eyelids or other infections such as conjunctivitis, it is best to treat the problem both internally and externally. Internally, the herbs should be anti-microbial, detoxifying and toning for the whole body, to strengthen it to the point where it can 'throw off' the infection itself. A good example of such a combination would be:

Blue Flag	1 part	
Cleavers	1 part	
Echinacea	1 part	
Eyebright	1 part	
Poke Root	1 part	

A cup of this should be drunk three times a day.

Externally, an eyewash or a compress may be made with *Eyebright.* Put one tablespoon of the dried herb in 500ml/1pt of water, boil it for ten minutes and let it cool. Use it as an eyewash or apply it as a compress by moistening cotton wool, gauze or muslin in the warm liquid and placing it over the eyes for about 15 minutes. This should be repeated several times a day.

Other remedies that may be used in a similar way externally are *Marigold* and *Golden Seal.*

Euphrasia officinalis Eyebright *is the most important herb in the treatment of eye complaints. It can be used internally or externally.*

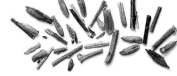

THE DIGESTIVE SYSTEM

The digestive system has been described as a tube passing through the body, as a sort of factory where food is processed and made available for the body to use. This description indicates how narrow our awareness of our bodies often is today. In fact, the digestive system is one of the major interfaces between our inner world and the outer, with a total surface that is some hundred times larger than our skin, with a complexity of reactions that are still beyond our understanding. For instance, the number of living microbes that inhabit the digestive system equals the total number of cells in the body, but how exactly the mixture of these microbes influences our well-being, and how our state of health influences their condition, is still largely unresearched.

The digestive system is richly supplied with nerves, a whole network of integrated con-trol that works in conjunction with a

wide array of hormones, both local and systemic. This has been described as a web of enteric brains. Enteric means to do with the gut and in this context means the local nervous system of the digestive system. This gut level intelligence can usually run the digestive system quite adequately. The degree of interactions and synergy between the various parts of the digestive tract is quite astounding and the more research done by the physiologists, the more is revealed.

As we are what we eat, our health and vitality depends to a large degree on how well our digestive system functions in providing the building blocks for our physical body. It is not just a matter of what substance we put into our mouth, but also essentially one of how it is processed so that it can be assimilated and used by the body.

If there is a functional problem in the digestion, then no matter what is being

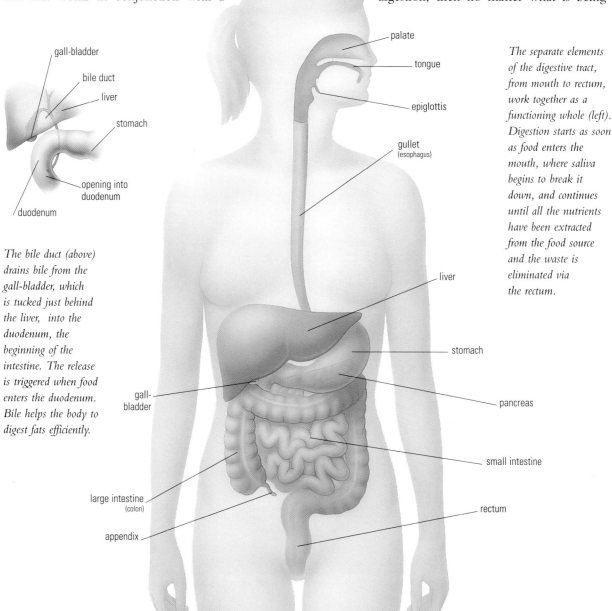

The bile duct (above) drains bile from the gall-bladder, which is tucked just behind the liver, into the duodenum, the beginning of the intestine. The release is triggered when food enters the duodenum. Bile helps the body to digest fats efficiently.

The separate elements of the digestive tract, from mouth to rectum, work together as a functioning whole (left). Digestion starts as soon as food enters the mouth, where saliva begins to break it down, and continues until all the nutrients have been extracted from the food source and the waste is eliminated via the rectum.

gall-bladder
bile duct
liver
stomach
opening into duodenum
duodenum

palate
tongue
epiglottis
gullet (esophagus)
liver
stomach
pancreas
small intestine
rectum
gall-bladder
large intestine (colon)
appendix

eaten it will not be properly absorbed, and deficiency will be experienced. It must be stressed that this refers to functional problems, where the system does not work as well as it could, not to organic conditions caused by injury or a structural abnormality of the organs and tissue involved. An example of a functional, as opposed to an organic, problem in this system would be tension during irregular and rushed meals, leading to indigestion. Food enters an unprepared gut too fast, and fails to be properly absorbed; malabsorption leads to discomfort. The fault can lie either in the eating habits, the content or amount of digestive juices, or in a dysfunction of the intestinal walls. These problems can give rise to a whole range of diseases.

An equally important activity of the digestive system is elimination. Not all the food that is eaten is absorbed. Some is not digestible and needs to be disposed of. The body also produces a lot of metabolic waste products that it has to eliminate, partly through the digestive system. The condition of the bowels and the state of their content will fundamentally affect the rest of the body. In addition to the physiological influences that affect the functioning and health of the digestive system, there is a constant interplay between the state of mind and digestion. Emotions profoundly influence both the functioning and structure of tissue in the stomach and intestines. To approach the healing of digestive problems in a holistic way, an appreciation of these psychological influences must be included.

Prevention of Digestive Disease

Most of the digestive problems that commonly occur are easily avoided by changes of lifestyle and habits. Some clear guidelines to follow in preventing problems include our attitudes towards alcohol, tobacco, stress and diet.

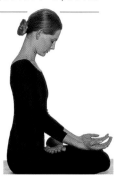

Yoga is a gentle, effective body therapy that can help to reduce stress and so minimize the digestive problems caused by it.

Excess alcohol acts as a major irritant on the walls of the intestine and is a specific threat to the liver. It should ideally be kept to a minimum. Tobacco presents a similar problem. It has been proven that nicotine slows the healing of gastric ulcers and may promote the development of duodenal ulcers. The tar that gets swallowed acts as an irritant.

Stress and anxiety are major contributors to illness and impede the healing process. Their effect is particularly strong on the digestive system via the influence of the autonomic nervous system. Such states of stress and anxiety should be actively reduced. The diet should be as mixed, natural and as high in roughage as possible. Artificial chemical additives should be avoided. The specific details of diet should be determined individually according to personal needs and philosophical approach.

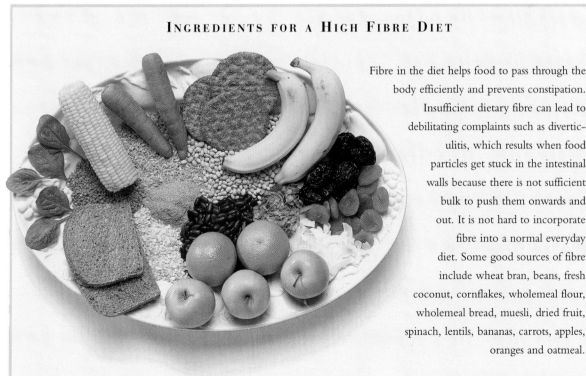

INGREDIENTS FOR A HIGH FIBRE DIET

Fibre in the diet helps food to pass through the body efficiently and prevents constipation. Insufficient dietary fibre can lead to debilitating complaints such as diverticulitis, which results when food particles get stuck in the intestinal walls because there is not sufficient bulk to push them onwards and out. It is not hard to incorporate fibre into a normal everyday diet. Some good sources of fibre include wheat bran, beans, fresh coconut, cornflakes, wholemeal flour, wholemeal bread, muesli, dried fruit, spinach, lentils, bananas, carrots, apples, oranges and oatmeal.

Herbs for the Digestive System

There are a multitude of plant remedies that have a use in the treatment of digestive disorders. This is not surprising if herbs are viewed as food – as vegetables. Most herbs are taken by mouth and therefore absorbed through the digestive system where their healing powers will start to be effective immediately.

Rather than give an endless list of digestive herbs, they will be reviewed by their actions, with a few outstanding examples given. A more exhaustive list of herbs is given in the section on The Action of Herbs (see pages 36–9).

Actions can be broadly grouped into those that stimulate various parts of the system to increase or better activity – the digestive stimulants – and those that relax the tissue or reduce any overactivity in the system – the digestive relaxants.

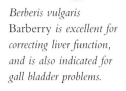

Berberis vulgaris
Barberry *is excellent for correcting liver function, and is also indicated for gall bladder problems.*

DIGESTIVE STIMULANTS

• **Bitters** While having a large range of other properties and chemical constituents, the bitter herbs all have in common an intensely bitter taste. This bitterness promotes appetite and in a complex way aids digestion. If these herbs are given in capsule form and cannot be tasted, their digestive properties do not come into play. Out of the many bitters, the most valuable ones are *Barberry, Centaury, Gentian Root, Golden Seal, White Horehound* and *Wormwood*.

Of course a large range of other actions are also represented here. For example, *White Horehound* can be used in a bronchitic condition where the appetite is weak and the digestion sluggish, or as a digestive remedy in cases where there is a lung weakness.

• **Sialagogues** The importance of the saliva in the digestive process cannot be overstressed. Digestion starts in the mouth and initiates a process that is continued in the gut. The saliva breaks down large carbohydrates into smaller units which can then be processed in other parts of the system. If time is not taken to chew food properly the saliva is not able to mix with it thoroughly enough and the whole digestive process is affected. Besides the bitters, which all stimulate the flow of saliva, other types of sialagogue are *Cayenne, Ginger, Licorice* and *Rhubarb Root*.

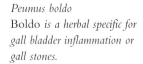

Peumus boldo
Boldo *is a herbal specific for gall bladder inflammation or gall stones.*

• **Hepatics** are herbs that strengthen, tone and stimulate the secretionary function of the liver. This causes an increase in the flow of bile. Remedies that also promote the discharge of this bile into the duodenum are called cholagogues.

In treating the whole body, it is often beneficial to aid the liver and its function as this most important organ is intimately involved in all body functions and the health of all tissues.

There are many hepatic herbs available to us, and the most useful are *Balmony, Barberry, Black Root, Blue Flag, Boldo, Dandelion Root, Fringetree Bark, Golden Seal, Vervain, Wahoo, Wild Yam* and *Yellow Dock*.

Gentiana lutea
Gentian Root *is a bitter which stimulates digestion, combats flatulence and counteracts poor appetites.*

• **Laxatives and Evacuants** Many herbs can promote the evacuation of the bowels, ranging from very mild laxatives to more violent and drastic purgatives. Such strong purgatives should only be used in extreme cases and under qualified supervision. The best laxatives are those that stimulate the natural secretion of the digestive juices such as bile (the cholagogues), thus promoting evacuation. Some of these are *Balmony, Barberry, Dandelion Root, Licorice, Wahoo* and *Yellow Dock.*

For a more powerful evacuant, consider *Rhubarb Root,* which in small dosage is also a mild astringent. Other valuable ones to consider are *Aloe, Buckthorn, Cascara Sagrada* and *Senna.* These stronger evacuants work mainly by chemical or neurological stimulation, irritating the lining of the intestines and causing an active expulsion of material.

● **Emetics** There are situations where rapid expulsion of the contents of the stomach is highly desirable, as in poisoning where vomiting is often the appropriate treatment. Many plants can cause this reflex by either acting on the controlling nerves or by irritating the gastric lining. Good ones to use would be *Balm, Ipecacuanha, Lobelia* and *Senega.*

● **Anthelmintics** The anthelmintics are a group of stimulating herbs that do not really act on the digestive system itself but rather against parasitic worms that might be present. Refer to the section on Infections and Infestations *(pages 40–5)* for more information.

Geranium maculatum American Cranesbill *is an astringent useful in diarrhea, dysentery and hemorrhoids.*

DIGESTIVE RELAXANTS

● **Demulcents** When the membranes of the digestive tract are irritated or inflamed, demulcent herbs can soothe and protect them. Out of the many demulcents that are active in different parts of the body, *Comfrey Root, Hops, Iceland Moss, Irish Moss, Marshmallow Root, Oats, Quince Seed* and *Slippery Elm* are the ones which are most effective for the digestive system.

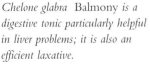

Chelone glabra Balmony *is a digestive tonic particularly helpful in liver problems; it is also an efficient laxative.*

● **Carminatives** Many aromatic herbs contain volatile oils that affect the digestive system by relaxing the stomach muscles, increasing the peristalsis of the intestine and reducing the production of gas in the system. They thus support the movement of material through the system and relieve distension caused by gas. Of the many carminatives, *Angelica, Aniseed, Calamus, Caraway, Cardamon, Cayenne, Chamomile, Coriander, Fennel, Ginger, Peppermint* and *Thyme* are among the best ones for the digestive system.

● **Astringents** The action of astringents lies mainly in their ability to contract cell walls, thus condensing the tissue and making it firmer and arresting any unwanted discharge. *Agrimony, American Cranesbill, Bayberry, Meadowsweet, Nettles, Oak Bark, Pilewort* and *Tormentil* are suitable for the digestive system.

● **Anti-spasmodics** are remedies that rapidly relax nervous tension that may be causing digestive spasms or colic. The tension of our current lifestyle can manifest in many digestive conditions that necessitate the use of relaxing nervines or muscular anti-spasmodics.

The best ones to use in cases of digestive problems are *Chamomile, Hops, Lobelia, Mistletoe, Pasque Flower, Skullcap* and *Valerian.* Consult The Herbal section for more details on each of these, in order to choose the best herb or combination for your individual case.

● **Anti-microbials** Infections can be the cause of digestive problems; they can also arise easily if the digestive system has been weakened by a disease. In either case, the use of anti-microbials will be helpful. Many of the herbs already mentioned are anti-microbials, such as *Pulsatilla, Thyme* and *Wormwood,* but the two outstanding ones are *Echinacea* and *Myrrh.*

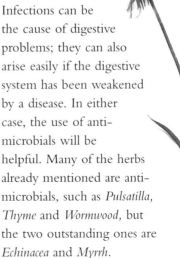

Echinacea angustifola Echinacea *is a powerful anti-microbial which is very useful as a mouthwash to combat infections of the mouth or gums.*

Patterns of Digestive Disease

In this section we shall review the digestive system, starting with the mouth and ending with the rectum, referring to the common conditions but explaining their treatment in terms of the whole. It is valuable first to recognize a number of general symptoms that are common to many diseases affecting the whole system but which have a particular relevance to digestion. These are constipation, diarrhea, vomiting, stomach pain and loss of appetite.

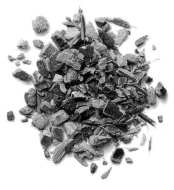

Rhamnus pushiana
Cascara Sagrada *is a well-established member of the herbal medicine chest which has been used for many years as a folk remedy; it is extremely useful for chronic constipation.*

GENERAL SYMPTOMS

• **Constipation** Contrary to common belief, constipation is not a disease but a symptom of some underlying problem. This could be inappropriate diet, a liver problem or even a physical blockage in the system. Constipation, especially in those over 50 years of age, can signify a more serious illness. If it persists for more than a week, medical advice should be sought.

In any case, the cause must be identified and treated, as the long-term use of laxatives in chronic constipation can eventually lead to other symptoms such as headaches, colic or even jaundice. In cases of chronic constipation, the muscles of the intestines have to be retrained to move the bowel content. The movement of the intestinal wall is a complex and highly integrated example of muscle control, designed to push

the content onwards at the right time and with the right force. This natural peristaltic movement can be blocked by the long use of laxatives. Two things should be done to retrain the intestines: meals should be eaten regularly (at the same time each day) and small amounts of appropriate herbs should be used to re-stimulate the peristalsis, for instance *Cascara Sagrada*.

A further factor that should not be underestimated is the attitude and state of mind of the person who is constipated. Somebody who is tense and tight, who wants to hold on to everything and everyone, who cannot relax and let go, will often also be constipated. In such cases, relaxation exercises or meditation can be the best laxatives.

When constipation is the result of a disease process, it is important to relieve the symptom whilst treating the cause, otherwise the body might well absorb some of

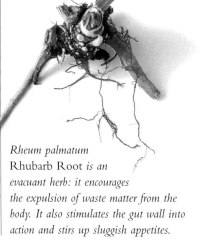

Rheum palmatum
Rhubarb Root *is an evacuant herb: it encourages the expulsion of waste matter from the body. It also stimulates the gut wall into action and stirs up sluggish appetites.*

the stagnant material from the intestine.

Of all the evacuant herbs available, perhaps the most widely applicable is *Rhubarb Root,* as it is a prime example of a normalizing herb. While in a large dose it is a purgative, taken in small doses it tones the intestine wall, promotes appetite and can disperse any gas that develops.

Any of the evacuant herbs will work well on their own, but the following mixture combines a number of valuable actions. *Barberry* aids the liver and the gall-bladder, *Boldo* stimulates the digestive process, *Cascara Sagrada* acts on the peristaltic movement, *Licorice* is mainly included to mask the bitter taste of some of the herbs, *Rhubarb Root* is included in a small dose for the above mentioned reasons, and *Ginger* will guard against any colic.

Barberry	2 parts	
Boldo	2 parts	
Cascara Sagrada	1 part	
Licorice	1 part	
Rhubarb Root	1 part	
Ginger	1 part	

Take a cup of this tea before going to bed.

As an alternative to *Boldo, Dandelion* can be used and *Fennel* can be substituted for *Ginger,* both in the same quantities.

• **Diarrhea** A diarrhea that does not last more than a day or two is a very common symptom and can be caused by an acute infection or inflammation of the intestine wall or by psychological stress, for instance by over-excitement or by a long journey. Persistent diarrhea, especially in children or the elderly, calls for medical advice.

In most cases diarrhea sets in when the body has to remove

Filipendula ulmaria Meadowsweet *is one of the best all-round herbs for all digestive problems. Both the leaves and flowers are used. It reduces the excess acidity that causes heartburn and gastritis, but is very gentle in its action and therefore suitable for children.*

digestive poisons from its system, and as such it should not be suppressed.

However, it can be useful to control the process and help the system with herbs that tone the lining of the intestine wall and which are mildly astringent. For persistent, long-standing diarrhea, seek the advice of a skilled practitioner.

By far the best mild digestive astringent is *Meadowsweet,* which can safely be used in all cases of diarrhea. In cases of childhood diarrhea, a good remedy is a tea made of equal parts of *Lady's Mantle* and *Meadowsweet,* which can be sweetened with some honey and should be taken often. For an acute attack in adults, a very good mixture would be:

American Cranesbill	1 part	
Bayberry	1 part	☑
Meadowsweet	1 part	◪
Oak Bark	1 part	⏱

This tea should be drunk every hour until the symptoms subside and then before every meal until the digestion is normal.

• **Pain** in the digestive system is an indicator of the type of illness present. Any extreme, acute abdominal pain necessitates immediate medical supervision.

Less acute pain will often accompany digestive disorders. Colic and griping pains are due to intense muscle spasms in the gut,

and usually indicate the body's attempt to remove a blockage that could be caused by wind or fecal matter, or perhaps a muscle spasm.

Flatulent colic will be relieved by the carminative herbs but all causes must be treated to clear the pain. Useful anti-spasmodics in this case are *Caraway, Ginger, Valerian* and *Wild Yam.*

Pain from stomach ulcers and similar problems can be eased by using demulcents such as *Marshmallow* or *Comfrey.* Of course, the roots of the problem must be treated in all cases where pain is a symptom.

• **Loss of Appetite** The appetite can be a good indicator for the state of the digestive system. If there is a gastric problem, the appetite will often diminish for a period of time. This way the stomach will have a better chance to recover, as it has to process less food. A similar pattern can evolve with liver problems when the liver is over-burdened.

If there is a loss of appetite in the recovery phase of an illness such as influenza, digestive stimulants such as *Gentian* or *Wormwood* should be used to restore healthy function. Persistent appetite loss is a serious symptom for which medical advice should be sought.

• **Anorexia Nervosa** is characterized by an extreme loss of appetite, practically an aversion to food, and often the inability to eat anything, which consequently leads to a drastic loss of weight. Anorexia nervosa is caused by psychological problems and has thus to be approached

psychotherapeutically under medical supervision. Herbally, the process can be aided with the use of digestives and nervines, for instance with the following tea.

Chamomile	1 part	
Condurango	1 part	☑
Gentian	1 part	◪
Skullcap	1 part	⏱

This should be drunk three times a day.

THE MOUTH

The health of the mouth, the gateway to the digestive system, will affect the whole of the system.

If there is a chronic tooth problem that is making proper chewing painful, or if there is an infection such as an abscess, the system downstream will be affected and polluted.

Similarly, if there is not enough saliva or if the composition of saliva is not adequate, the digestive process will then be slowed down. Oral hygiene therefore cannot be stressed too much. Problems in the gut can also give mouth problems such as bad breath or recurrent mouth ulcers.

• **Teeth** When problems arise, teeth must be treated by a dentist, but herbs can help to prevent tooth decay.

Althaea officinalis Marshmallow Root *is a powerful demulcent and is strongly recommended for all inflammations in any part of the digestive tract.*

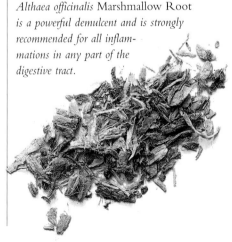

Glycyrrhiza glabra
Licorice Root *is used to help gastritis, colic and stomach ulcers. It also has a history as a herbal toothbrush.*

Long before tooth-brushes made of bristle or plastic were developed, roots like *Marshmallow, Licorice, Alfalfa* or *Horseradish* were used to clean teeth. *Licorice Root* for instance can be prepared very easily, simply by peeling the bark off one end and flaying the fibres.

If you want to use toothpaste, many herbal ones are now available, the best ones being those that contain the anti-microbial herbs *Myrrh* and *Echinacea.*

For the first-aid treatment of toothache, chew some *Cloves,* as they are rich in the analgesic oil eugenol. Alternatively, you can soak a pad of cotton wool in *Clove* oil and place it by the tooth. *Peppermint* oil also acts as an analgesic, but it is not as effective.

• **Gingivitis** is a common infection of the surface tissue of the gums, caused by a lack of oral hygiene and inappropriate diet.

The herbal anti-microbials such as *Echinacea, Eucalyptus* and *Myrrh* can be used very effectively in the form of tinctures. Depending on the severity of the infection, you can either wash the gums daily with a tincture of *Myrrh* or, if a stronger remedy is needed, you can use a mixture of equal parts of tincture of *Myrrh* and tincture of *Echinacea.* Alternatively, massage the gums before going to bed with oil of *Eucalyptus* and wash out the mouth in the morning with distilled *Witch Hazel.*

• **Pyorrhea** This chronic deg-enerative disease of the gums must be treated systemically with the use of alteratives that are anti-microbials and lymphatic cleansers as well.

For a treatment use the approach described under gingivitis to treat the gums themselves, and combine this with a high dosage of vitamin C. Most important is the use of a mixture of:

Echinacea	2 parts	
Blue Flag	1 part	✍
Cleavers	1 part	📓
Poke Root	1 part	⏲

This tea should be drunk three times daily for a number of weeks until the condition clears.

• **Abcess** This very painful condition can best be helped by the use of the tea described under pyorrhea. This treatment will also protect the whole system from a spreading of the infection which could occur, as the existence of the abscess indicates that the defence capacity of the body is reduced. Any treatment that aims at encouraging the body to absorb the abscess should be avoided.

• **Mouth Ulcers** are very often indicators of a run-down general condition and are best treated by increasing general health.

They commonly occur after the use of antibiotics, or during recovery from influenza. In both cases the body has been exposed to considerable physiological stress, resulting in a general weakening. This in turn affects the normal ecology of the mouth and of other areas and, as one symptom, the ulcer appears. They can also arise during psychological stress.

To treat the ulcer, *Red Sage* (in the form of a mouthwash, made preferably from the infusion of fresh leaves) is very simple and effective. The fresh leaves can also be chewed. Alternatively a mouth-

HOW TO MAKE A HERBAL TOOTHBRUSH

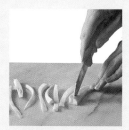 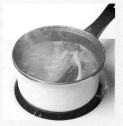 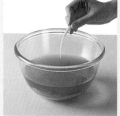

1 *Choose a straight Marshmallow root and cut it into 12cm/ 5in pieces.*

2 *Peel the ends and boil in water, together with Cinnamon sticks and Cloves until the sticks are tender.*

3 *Put the pieces carefully – as they break easily – into brandy and let them soak for a day.*

Take them out and let them dry. Before you use them, soak the ends for a short time in hot water. You will not even need to use toothpaste, since all the necessary ingredients are in the root.

wash of tincture of *Myrrh* in an equal amount of water will usually be effective.

At the same time, vitamin B-complex and vitamin C should be taken to help deal with the stress involved, whatever the cause is. If ulcers persist, seek medical advice.

THE STOMACH

The stomach is the organ that takes the brunt of the liberties we sometimes take with the food and drink we consume. Too much alcohol, too much refined food, too many cigarettes, too many aspirins, all will affect the stomach.

The main task of the stomach is to prepare the food for further processing in the small intestine, which it accomplishes by mixing it with hydrochloric acid and powerful enzymes.

Before we look at the stomach, two problems with the esophagus (the tube down which swallowed food travels) will be examined. If there is a burning sensation in the esophagus or acid rising to the mouth, the symptom is due to a problem in the stomach. It can be treated with the help of demulcents, but the condition of the stomach has also to be examined. If there is a problem with swallowing (dysphagia), it should be examined professionally. It is often due to nervous tension and anxiety and may be relieved by the use of nervines such as *Hops, Valerian* or *Wild Lettuce.*

• **Indigestion** The label 'indigestion' is used for a wide range of symptoms, all of which are due to a functional problem in the stomach that is caused by inappropriate eating habits.

Indigestion can be accompanied by pain, flatulence, heartburn and other symptoms. The causes of these symptoms can be grouped into four categories.

• **Irregular Eating** The functioning of the body is characterized by rhythms, and the stomach – and in fact the whole digestive system – is no exception to this. If meals are taken irregularly, these rhythms are disturbed and functional problems may result.

• **Overeating and Eating too Quickly** If too much food goes into the stomach, either at any one time or in total over the day, the stomach will be overloaded and thus work with reduced efficiency. Overloading causes problems which may affect the whole system. Obesity is the most common result. Also when food is swallowed too quickly and not chewed thoroughly it causes problems; food will not be digested properly and may pass through the system in an undigested state.

• **Eating the Wrong Food** Many people are allergic to certain foods, even though the symptoms might not be very obvious. Any food that causes a problem should be eliminated from the diet altogether.

• **Nervous Tension** The stomach, like the whole digestive system, is easily affected by stress and anxiety.

By taking all these factors into account and by changing your diet and lifestyle accordingly, indigestion can be treated. There are a number of herbs that will speed up the healing process, but they will have to be chosen according to the cause.

The most important remedy is *Meadowsweet,* which will settle the stomach and reduce any excess acidity. The demulcents can be very useful, a good one being *Irish Moss.*

If the digestion is sluggish, bitters such as *Gentian, Golden Seal* and *Wormwood* will help.

If there is flatulence, the carminatives should be used as well. Good ones for the stomach are *Aniseed, Balm, Cardamon, Fennel* and *Peppermint.*

If there is nervous tension involved, the nervine relaxants are indicated, especially those that also aid digestion, such as *Chamomile, Hops, Lavender, Rosemary* and *Valerian.* In all cases consult The Herbal section to choose the most appropriate herb or combination of them to use in the individual case.

Artemisia absinthum Wormwood *is a bitter herb which stimulates the digestion. It is probably best-known as the major ingredient in vermouth, the aperitif drink.*

• **Gastritis** When a disturbance in the stomach changes from a functional one such as indigestion to a structural one, the first stage is an inflammation of the lining of the stomach wall. It may last only for a short time and can be due to an infection or a reaction to food, or it might be more chronic. If it lasts for a while, the causes that should be looked at are: eating the wrong foods, alcohol, cigarettes (swallowed tar) and stress. Usually a combination of these factors will be involved.

The treatment of gastritis is based on diet and herbs. As far as diet is concerned, the primary short-term need is to avoid irritants that may cause or aggravate the inflammation. These may involve temperature, or irritants of a chemical or mechanical nature.

• **Very Hot Foods or Drinks** should be abstained from, as these will directly aggravate the inflammation. Cold things will usually have a similar painful effect. Spicy food, curries, rich and greasy foods will all have an unpleasant effect.

• **Chemical Irritants** will have an immediate impact. Commonly used foodstuffs which contain vinegar, which is diluted acetic acid, must be avoided. Vinegar should not be added to food; pickles must similarly be avoided.

• **Alcohol** in any form is out, as this acts on the stomach lining in a similar way to vinegar. Tobacco will also aggravate the problem as much of the tar is swallowed.

• **Mechanical Irritants** will cause discomfort as well. When there is acute

Hydrastis canadensis
Golden Seal *has many roles in the herbal repertoire, but is particularly useful in gastritis, colitis and ulcers.*

inflammation it is best to have a diet that is very low in fibre, as fibre may have a similar effect to sandpaper on a cut.

A bland diet is called for: no coarse bread, nuts, tomatoes etc.

As soon as an improvement is established, then reintroduce roughage, as it is an essential component of a healthy diet.

Herbally, the following mixture will effectively soothe and heal the stomach lining.

Comfrey Root	2 parts
Marshmallow Root	2 parts
Meadowsweet	2 parts
Golden Seal	1 part

Take this tea after each meal, until the condition clears.

If a lot of flatulence accompanies the inflammation, add one part of *Calamus* to the mixture. Similarly, if stress is part of the problem, *Valerian* may be added as a suitable nervine.

• **Gastric Ulcer** When abuse of the stomach has continued, perhaps unconsciously, for too long, an inevitable breakdown occurs in the lining of the stomach. As the mucous membranes of the wall no longer deal with the unhealthy condition, the acid and the digestive enzymes can reach the wall and take their toll. A gastric ulcer develops.

The herbal treatment of these ulcers is quite straightforward and apparently fast. However, a relief of the pain must not be confused with the healing of the underlying problem. The herbal remedies will ease the symptoms and start the healing process, but a complete healing will take time and has to include a close

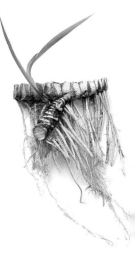

Acorus calamus
Calamus *stimulates the appetite and is a very good tonic for the whole digestive system. It is particularly useful in colic caused by wind.*

look at your lifestyle, including diet, work and sleep patterns.

By developing a gastric or a duodenal ulcer, the body is telling you that something in the whole web of your lifestyle is inappropriate. It may just be the diet, but it may also often be the work pattern or a relationship.

Herbs can heal the ulcer, but it may return very quickly unless the lessons that are being offered are recognized consciously and are acted upon.

The treatment is based on a careful diet and on the use of herbs. A useful herbal tea to be drunk cold consists of:

Comfrey Root	1 part
Golden Seal	1 part
Marshmallow Root	1 part
Meadowsweet	1 part

A cold infusion of the demulcents is more mucilaginous and soothing than tea or tincture. For details see the section on preparing herbs *(pages 22–31)*.

The *Comfrey* and *Marshmallow* provide excellent soothing demulcent action combined with a healing effect upon the mucous membranes.

Slippery Elm may be added to the diet or taken as tablets. The *Meadowsweet* will settle the stomach content and reduce the impact of over-acidity.

The *Golden Seal* will prove beneficial for the membranes and act to tone the tissue whilst providing a general tonic action upon the body. If bleeding occurs within the stomach, *American Cranesbill* may be added to the mixture. If there is a stress component – and there usually is – *Valerian* or *Hops* may be considered.

The diet should be very low in fibre during the acute phase of the illness. In addition there should be little protein, thereby giving the stomach less work to do. When the symptoms recede, fibre and a variety of proteins may slowly be reintroduced. Of great importance is the avoidance of alcohol and tobacco. With tobacco, withdrawal may produce nervous tension and therefore make things worse. If this is the case, then try to keep going – you were hooked!

THE SMALL INTESTINE

The small intestine makes up the longest part of the digestive system with a total length of about 6m/20ft, which is divided into three sections, the duodenum, the jejenum and the ileum.

The long stretch of the small intestine is the site where most nutrition is absorbed into the body.

Thus any problems in the small intestine will affect the nutritional state, causing apparent deficiencies which are really malabsorption problems. Stress has a marked impact on this part of the body, as is demonstrated by duodenal ulcers.

• **Duodenal Ulcers** The duodenum, the first stretch of the small intestine, starts at the pyloric sphincter, a valve at the end of the stomach. This valve controls the release of parts of the stomach contents into the duodenum, and if it does not function properly, too much stomach acid can get into the duodenum and cause problems.

When too much of the highly acidic stomach juices seep into the alkaline duodenum, the walls of the duodenum will become inflamed and ultimately develop ulcers.

A number of factors can cause the seepage, but by far the most common ones are stress and tension.

The approach to healing a duodenal ulcer is threefold, consisting of a herbal treatment, dietary changes and a consideration of the factors that are causing stress and tension.

The herbal treatment is based on a number of actions. Demulcents are called for to soothe the

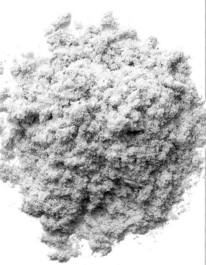

Ulmus rubra
Slippery Elm Bark *is another well-known digestive remedy, soothing and particularly suitable for sensitive or convalescent digestions.*

ulcer and the surrounding tissue. If a vulnerary action can be added to speed up the healing process then all the better. This may be done with both *Marshmallow* and *Comfrey Root*. The specific mucous membrane-healing properties of *Golden Seal* will aid the healing of the lining of the intestine. An appropriate astringent such as *American Cranesbill* should be used in order to strengthen the tissue. As a duodenal ulcer is often accompanied by a general debility and a reduction in vitality due to toxins from the ulcer entering into the blood and lymph system, appropriate alteratives and lymphatic tonics such as *Echinacea* should be used. A good basic mixture would therefore consist of:

Comfrey Root	2 parts	
Marshmallow Root	2 parts	⬈
American Cranesbill	1 part	⬛
Echinacea	1 part	⏱
Golden Seal	1 part	

This tea should be drunk three times a day before meals. If you are fasting, drink it at the times you would usually eat.

The diet should be low in fibre and low in proteins as long as the symptoms persist and must be followed by a gradual return to a normal wholefood diet. An excellent soothing food to take during the peak of the problem is *Slippery Elm.* It can be made into a thick gruel and as such will provide nutrition as well as a demulcent action on the ulcerated tissue.

To deal with stress and tension, nervines are indicated for a short-term treatment. But the body is sending a signal and giving a clue by developing a symptom like an ulcer, and it is best to take the hint. Take a look at your lifestyle and purpose in life. Is your life fulfilling and meaningful? Many valuable techniques are available to help you re-evaluate your life and clear these problems, ranging from simple relaxation techniques to psychotherapy. Stress management and relaxation are discussed in the next section.

Herbally, a good nervine mixture to treat tension can be made of equal parts of *Skullcap* and

Valerian, which should be made into a tea and drunk whenever needed. Other appropriate relaxing herbs, though not as strong, are *Balm, Chamomile, Lavender* and *Lime Blossom,* which can also be made into a tea and drunk whenever needed.

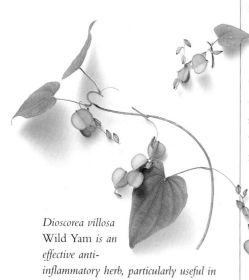

Dioscorea villosa
Wild Yam *is an effective anti-inflammatory herb, particularly useful in cases of diverticulitis.*

• **Enteritis** This name is given to an inflammation that can occur in any section of the small intestine and sometimes can even occur along its whole length.

When it appears in one of the sections, it can be called accordingly, duodenitis, jejuvenitis or ileitis, but the treatment will always be the same. In most cases, the guidelines and treatment suggested for duodenal ulcers will be found sufficient. However, it would be good to add one part of *Wild Yam* to the tea indicated for duodenal ulcers to further ease the inflammation and pain.

• **Malabsorption** A very common – though frequently unrecognized – condition is a diminished ability of the small intestine to absorb food in general or specific components, like minerals. This can lead to symptoms of malnutrition, apparent mineral or vitamin deficiencies, anemia and weight loss, abdominal pain or a more insidious state of vague ill-health.

Most commonly the malabsorption stems from an allergic reaction to particular foods, which leads to problems in the lining of the intestine wall. The allergic reaction might be extreme and obvious, as in the case of celiac disease due to a strong allergy to gluten, or it can take a mild form and not produce obvious symptoms. In any case of suspected malabsorption, it is always worth removing potential allergens from the diet.

A complete list of potential allergens would include all food, as everything can trigger an allergic reaction, but the majority of cases are found to be caused by just four types of food: gluten-containing foods, primarily all products made from wheat; milk and milk products, like cheese and butter; sugar, and foods rich in sugar and eggs. Eliminate these foods from your diet for a number of weeks and see if anything changes. If so, leave the food that is causing the allergy out of your diet; if not, see if your diet contains other food that you might suspect, such as coffee or tea, or tomatoes.

Herbal remedies can help to soothe, heal and renew the lining of the intestine. Demulcents such as *Comfrey Root, Marshmallow Root* and *Slippery Elm* will soothe the mucous mem-branes. Anti-inflammatory herbs, such as *Wild Yam* and *Meadow-sweet,* should be considered as well as astringents such as *Bay-berry, Agrimony* and

Myrica cerifera
Bayberry *is an astringent which is very useful in diarrhea and dysentery.*

Meadowsweet. Carminatives such as *Cardamon, Chamomile* and *Hops* will be invaluable, with the last two also acting as relaxing nervines. It may be necessary to guard against infection, thus *Echinacea* would be used.

For more serious problems in this category, such as celiac syndrome or Crohn's disease, seek the help of a qualified practitioner.

THE LARGE INTESTINE

The main function of the large intestine – or colon – is to absorb water and minerals. Little or no other food is extracted, as this has occurred in the small intestine. The bacteria in the gut, or gut flora as they are known, make some of our vitamins here and protect against some toxic bacteria.

• **Colitis** is an inflammation of part of the colon, and is the most common complaint affecting the large intestine. The intensity and the particular symptoms depend on the extent of the inflammation. Whilst the symptoms vary to some extent from person to person, colitis is characterized by alternating bouts of diarrhea and constipation, by a general lowering of vitality and often depression. This distressing condition will usually respond well to herbal medication and the use of an appropriate diet. A useful mixture is:

Wild Yam	3 parts	
Bayberry	2 parts	
Agrimony	1 part	
Comfrey Root	1 part	
Golden Seal	1 part	
Marshmallow Root	1 part	

This tea should be drunk three times a day.

This combination of herbs soothes and heals the lining of the large intestine with demulcents (*Comfrey, Marshmallow*), astringents (*Bayberry, Agrimony, Comfrey*) and an anti-inflammatory herb (*Wild Yam*). Other astringents such as *American Cranesbill, Periwinkle, Oak Bark* and *Shepherd's Purse* may also be considered. It may also be necessary to include alteratives and anti-microbials, such as *Echinacea* or *Garlic,* depending on the condition.

When stress and anxiety accompany the colitis, then relaxing nervines such as *Lime Blossom, Skullcap* and *Valerian* should also be considered.

The key to diet in the treatment of colitis is the avoidance of anything that will irritate the colon wall: by physical irritation, by its temperature, because of a chemical action or because it causes an allergic reaction.

• **Physical Irritation** can be avoided by excluding any fibrous food from the diet. Bran and wholemeal flour, raw vegetables, fruit skins, fruits with pips (such as raspberry), nuts and cooked fibrous vegetables (such as cabbage) should all be avoided. The temperature of food should be medium; hot or cold foods or drinks should be avoided.

• **Chemical Irritants** should be avoided, namely alcohol, vinegar and vinegar products (such as pickles), spicy condiments, strong cheese and fried foods.

• **Food that Causes Allergic Reactions,** such as cow's milk products, should be avoided, as should coffee and pork products. Instead, goat's

milk or soya milk can be substituted. Other permissible foods include eggs, tender and light meats, fish, liver, poultry, bland soups, lightly cooked vegetables and fruit (bananas and avocados may be eaten raw), products of unbleached white flour, fine cereals and *Slippery Elm* food *(see under Duodenal Ulcers, page 197)*, which also has a very healing action.

Meals should be small and eaten often, rather than large and eaten three times daily. The diet should be followed whilst the inflammation is acute, but once the symptoms are eased, high fibre foods should be slowly reintroduced. The chemical irritants and foods causing allergies should be avoided permanently.

• **Diverticulitis** Due to the unnatural and unhealthy food that is the usual diet of so many in the 'civilized' world today, there is a high occurrence of weakness of the colon wall. This weakness can lead to the development of a pouch in the wall, called a 'diverticulum'. Sometimes a few small ones develop, sometimes a lot, and in many cases they can also grow into large ones. Often these diverticula cause little or no apparent trouble, but they can also be the site for inflammations and for the build-up of waste

Agrimonia eupatoria
Agrimony *is a tonic and an astringent, particularly useful in mucous colitis.*

Senna alexandrina
Senna Pods *are probably the best known herbal remedy among non-herbalists. Senna is a very powerful cathartic and should be used with caution.*

material. Once an inflamed state is reached, any fibrous or indigestible material such as tomato skins can cause intense pain and discomfort.

Diverticulitis – the inflamed state – can be treated by a combined herbal and dietary approach. An efficient basic herbal mixture can be made from:

Wild Yam	3 parts	
German Chamomile	2 parts	
Marshmallow	1 part	
Calamus	1 part	

This tea should be drunk three times a day.

If the diverticulitis is accompanied by flatulence, then more carminatives, such as *Ginger* and *Calumba,* should be added, and if there is also constipation, laxatives such as *Rhubarb Root* or *Senna* may be included.

The dietary approach seems paradoxical. Even though the problem arises from a lack of roughage in the diet over a period of time, when the inflammation is acute, roughage would aggravate the problem and has to be avoided. Instead, the diet should be bland and low in fibre and rich in demulcent food such as *Slippery Elm*. Only when the inflammation has been brought under control should whole foods and roughage gradually be reintroduced. A natural and healthy diet is the best way to control diverticulitis in the long term.

199

• **Appendicitis** An infection of the appendix can manifest in two ways, either in an acute and severe attack or in a more chronic form. A sudden and acute attack calls for immediate medical attention as it can develop into peritonitis, a condition where the appendix bursts, which is very dangerous.

The symptoms of a chronic infection can take the form of recurring attacks of abdominal pain on the lower right side, accompanied by a rise in temperature, by nausea and perhaps vomiting. This can be treated with a mixture of:

Echinacea	2 parts
Wild Yam	2 parts
Agrimony	1 part
Chamomile	1 part

This tea should be drunk three times a day over a period of time.

While this mixture may also ease the symptoms of an acute appendicitis, proper medical attention is called for in the case of a sudden attack. Even though constipation often accompanies appendicitis, laxatives should not be used as they may aggravate the condition.

• **Hemorrhoids,** or piles, is a distressing condition of the rectum and anus. They may be internal or external. In most cases they respond well and quickly to the use of herbal remedies, taken internally and used as external applications.

It is of paramount importance to trace the cause of this problem and treat it as a priority. If this is not done, the piles will recur. The most common cause is chronic constipation. The treatment of this has already been reviewed. Another common cause is a congested liver.

The following herbal approach will usually help in the most intransigent cases. The most important herbs needed here are astringents, especially ones that also tone the vessel involved. The herb to choose is *Pilewort* (of course!). In addition *Witch Hazel, Periwinkle* and *Tormentil* may be considered, if a simple infusion of *Pilewort* should not suffice. If constipation is caused by a congested liver, hepatics may help through their gentle laxative and tonic actions. Consider *Barberry, Dandelion Root, Golden Seal* or *Yellow Dock.*

A very soothing ointment for piles can be made from *Pilewort,* which should be applied after each motion.

THE LIVER AND GALL-BLADDER

The liver is the largest organ of the human body and it is involved, directly or indirectly, in all physiological processes. Here is not the place to investigate in depth the workings of this incredible organ, but it is appropriate to mention briefly its main functions, to show how vital its health is to the body.
• The liver is involved in the metabolism of carbohydrates and is the most important organ for the maintenance of blood sugar levels.
• The liver is involved in the metabolism of proteins and is the main site for the breakdown of amino acids and for the synthesis of blood plasma proteins such as globulins and clotting factors.
• The liver is involved with the metabolism of fats, for instance with the synthesis of cholesterol and its subsequent breakdown into the bile salts.
• The liver is involved in the storage and metabolism of vitamins. The fat soluble vita-

Chionanthus virginicus Fringetree Bark *is particularly useful for liver complaints and any jaundice that accompanies them.*

mins depend on bile for their absorption; the vitamins A, D, K and B^{12} are stored in the liver and many of the vitamins are metabolized in the liver.
• The liver is involved in inactivating hormones like the estrogens, the corticosteroids and the other steroids.
• The liver is involved in the detoxification of drugs to protect our inner ecology from disruption by drugs, pollutants, artificial food additives and other potentially poisonous substances. This function will put the liver under stress from constant work.
• The liver produces and excretes bile, a digestive juice essential for the digestive process.

These few examples demonstrate that the liver plays an integral part in maintaining the health of the blood, in the proper function of the endocrine system and of the digestive process and in metabolism in general. As the liver is connected with many other functions of the body, any dysfunction or disease will affect the liver and reflect in its activity. Similarly, a state of minor liver dysfunction may manifest itself as a symptom elsewhere in the body far from the actual liver itself. Skin disorders are a good example of this.

The liver can be helped by the use of hepatics, the most important of which include *Balmony, Barberry, Black Root, Blue Flag, Boldo, Dandelion, Fringetree Bark, Golden Seal, Vervain, Wahoo, Wild Yam* and *Yellow Dock.*

• **Supporting the Liver** There is often the need to aid the liver even when no specific 'disease' is present. A wide spectrum of functional problems can occur, which may be described as 'liverishness'.

Folk remedies that were used as 'spring tonics' were often based upon liver stimulants, to ensure that after a winter of bad food the liver would be strengthened and could thus help in cleansing and toning the whole body.

While the modern diet in developed countries can be well balanced and nutritious throughout the year, it is nevertheless contaminated with a range of chemicals with which the body has great difficulties in dealing. Thus we can need a 'spring tonic' at any time of the year.

The simplest way of helping the liver and the whole digestive process is to use bitters, such as *Gentian, Golden Seal* or *Wormwood.* A more specific decongestant action on the liver is supplied by all the hepatics mentioned above. *Dandelion* is the simplest and most widely applicable one. The root or leaves of *Dandelion* are excellent hepatics that also work on the kidney and so help the cleansing of the body through that organ. Whilst treating the liver in this way it is helpful to aid the stomach as well by using *Meadowsweet.* Similarly any other aspect of the whole system that needs aid should be taken into account. A useful liver tonic is:

Dandelion	2 parts
Meadowsweet	2 parts
Fringetree Bark	1 part
Golden Seal	1 part

This infusion should be drunk after each meal.

• Diet for Liver and Gall-Bladder

In any problem related to the function of the liver or the gall-bladder, it is vital that strict dietary guidelines are followed, to ease the digestive burden on the liver and to ensure that there is no unnecessary pain caused. The dietary guidelines are simple: avoid all fatty and roasted foods and reduce all fats to an absolute minimum; drink alcohol only in moderation.

• Jaundice

is a symptom, not a disease. It indicates congestion within the liver which leads to a build-up of bile in the blood. This causes the yellowish colour of the skin in jaundice. The cause for the congestion has to be identified to guarantee real healing. It can be caused by an overburden of chemicals, it can be due to an infection or it can be due to physical damage, and thus has to be treated accordingly. However, the treatment can be supported by a decoction that will aid the recovery in most forms of jaundice.

Balmony	1 part
Black Root	1 part
Dandelion	1 part
Fringetree Bark	1 part
Golden Seal	1 part

A small cup of this should be drunk every two hours during the day while symptoms last.

• Gall-Bladder Inflammation

This extremely painful condition usually responds well to herbal remedies. The diet must be carefully examined and the recommendations that are given above must be strictly followed. A mixture that will ease the pain and reduce the inflammation can be made from:

Marshmallow Root	2 parts
Dandelion	1 part
Fringetree Bark	1 part
Wahoo	1 part
Mountain Grape	1 part

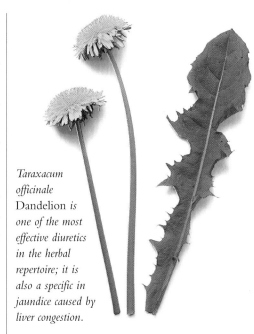

Taraxacum officinale Dandelion *is one of the most effective diuretics in the herbal repertoire; it is also a specific in jaundice caused by liver congestion.*

This tea should be drunk three times a day.

With the extreme pain that often accompanies this condition, relaxing nervines such as *Valerian* might be useful.

• Gallstones

The cause of the development of gallstones is not entirely clear. Herbs can in some cases help the body to eliminate the stones with a minimum of pain. However, this may take some time. A mixture that can do this is:

Marshmallow Root	2 parts
Balmony	1 part
Boldo	1 part
Fringetree Bark	1 part
Golden Seal	1 part

This tea should be drunk three times daily.

The *Golden Seal* in this mixture may be substituted with *Barberry* or *Mountain Grape,* as all contain very similar alkaloids.

The whole of the digestive system must be helped in a case of gallstones, so it has to be treated with the appropriate digestive herbs. If the nervous system is under stress, then it should be treated accordingly.

THE NERVOUS SYSTEM

The body's nervous system is controlled by the brain and its functions are carried out by the sets of nerves that run out from the spinal column. Nerves monitor the state of the body, relay the information to the brain which gives instructions or modifications to keep the system in balance.

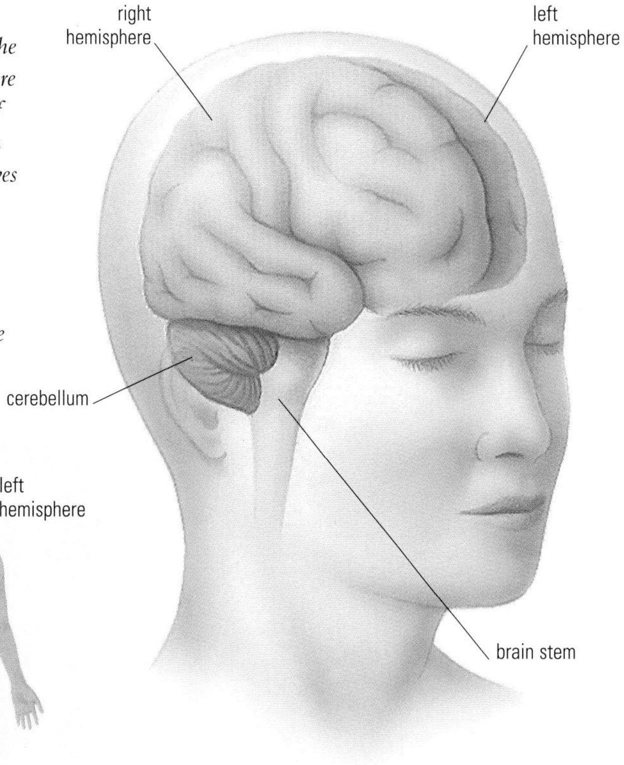

right hemisphere

left hemisphere

cerebellum

brain

cerebellum

spinal column

spinal nerves

right hemisphere   left hemisphere

The cerebellum of the brain comprises the left and right hemispheres (above), which are linked to the brain stem.

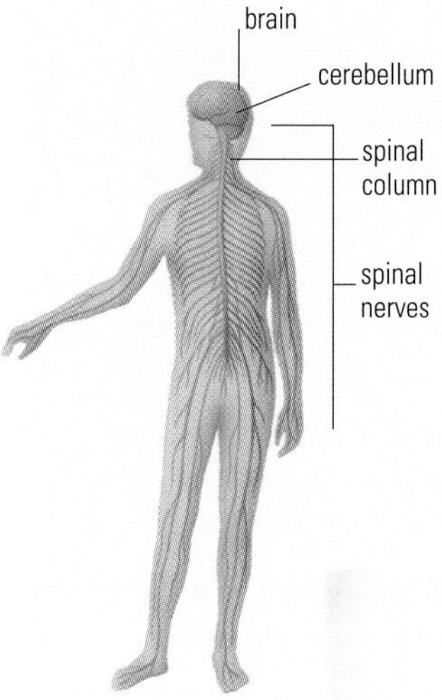

brain stem

The nerves of the body are organized into two main systems (above): the central nervous system (brain and spinal cord) and the peripheral nervous system, with its 31 pairs of spinal nerves.

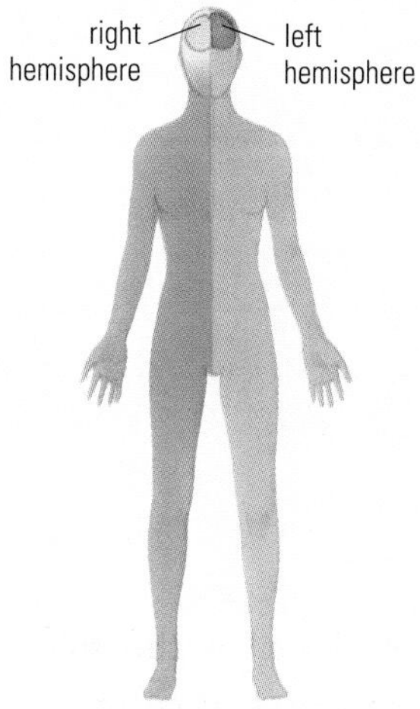

The left hemisphere of the brain controls the right side of the body and vice-versa.

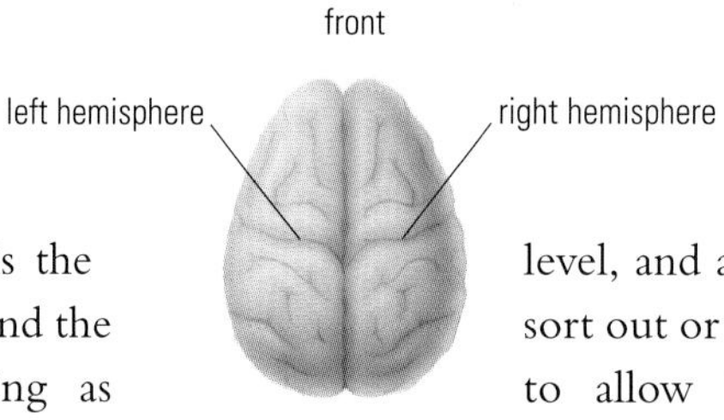

front

left hemisphere   right hemisphere

The brain's two cerebral hemispheres seen from above, with the fissure that separates them in between

In no other system of the body is the connection between the physical and the psychological aspects of our being as apparent as in the nervous system. Clearly, the nervous system is part of the physical make-up of the body and, just as clearly, all psychological processes take place in the nervous system. Therefore, if there is disease on the psychological level, it will reflect in the physical; and when there is disease on the physical level, this will inevitably reflect in the psychological.

A holistic approach to herbal healing acknowledges this interconnectedness, and regards nervous tissue and its functions as a vital element in the treatment of the whole being.

Traditional allopathic medicine tends to reduce psychological problems to the mere biochemical level, and assumes that 'appropriate' drugs will sort out or at least hide the problem sufficiently to allow 'normal' life to continue. Many techniques in the field of alternative medicine assume or imply the other extreme, namely that psychological factors are the cause of any disease and that treatment of the psyche is the only appropriate way of healing, and will take care of any physical problem.

By bringing these two reductionist views together, we come closer to a holistic approach; with herbal medicine we can treat the nervous system and part of the whole body and can feed and strengthen it and help the psyche. For our being to be wholly healthy, we have to take care of our physical health through right diet and right lifestyle, but we are also responsible for a healthy emotional, mental and spiritual life.

Herbs for the Nervous System

There are a number of ways in which herbs can benefit the nervous system in addition to the rather simplistic ones of stimulation and relaxation.

NERVINE TONICS

Perhaps the most important contribution herbal medicine can make in this area is in strengthening and feeding the nervous system. In cases of shock, stress or nervous debility, the nervine tonics strengthen and feed the tissues directly.

One of the best and certainly the most widely applicable remedy to feed nervous tissue is *Oats,* which can either be taken in the form of tinctures, or combined as needed with relaxants, stimulants, or any other indicated remedy, or can simply be eaten, in the form of old-fashioned porridge, not instant oatmeal.

Other nervine tonics that have, in addition, a relaxing effect include *Damiana, Skullcap, Vervain* and *Wood Betony.* Of these, *Skullcap* is often the most effective, particularly for problems related to stress.

Scutellaria laterifolia Skullcap *is an effective nervine tonic, particularly useful for stress-related nervous problems.*

NERVINE RELAXANTS

In cases of stress and tension, the nervine relaxants can do much to alleviate the condition. A representative list of the nervine relaxants include *Black Cohosh, Black Haw, California Poppy, Chamomile, Cramp Bark, Hops, Hyssop, Jamaican Dogwood, Lady's Slipper, Lavender, Lime Blossom, Mistletoe, Motherwort, Pasque Flower, Passion Flower, Rosemary, St John's Wort, Skullcap* and *Valerian.* As can be seen from this list, many of the relaxants also have other properties and can be selected to aid in related problems.

In addition to the herbs that work directly on the nervous system, the anti-spasmodic herbs – which affect the peripheral nerves and the muscle tissue – can have an indirect relaxing effect on the whole system. When the physical body is at ease, ease in the psyche is promoted.

The demulcents can also help in conjunction with nervines, as they soothe irritated tissue and promote healing by protecting the area from further damage.

NERVINE STIMULANTS

Direct stimulation of the nervous tissue is not very often indicated. In most cases it is more appropriate to stimulate the body's innate vitality with the help of nervine or even digestive tonics, which work by augmenting bodily harmony and thus have a much deeper and longer-lasting effect than nervine stimulants.

When direct nervine stimulation is indicated, the best herb to use is the *Kola.* Drinking *coffee, maté tea* and *black tea* should also be remembered. A problem with these commonly used stimulants is the fact that they have a number of side-effects and can be involved in causing many minor psychological problems such as anxiety and tension.

Some of the herbs rich in volatile oils are also valuable stimulants, the best being *Peppermint.*

BACH FLOWER REMEDIES

The Bach Flower Remedies, developed by Dr Edward Bach (1887-1936), represent an approach to herbalism that is an alchemical amalgam of the spiritual essence of the flower in co-operation with the emotional/mental need of the person.

They are not used directly for physical illness, but for the individual's worry, apprehension, hopelessness, fear, irritability, and so on. The state of someone's psychic being has a major bearing on the causation, development and cure of any physical illness. The remedies appear to work with the life-force, allowing it to flow freely through or around the block and so speed healing and a return to wholeness.

These flower remedies are ideal for self-use. They are inherently benign in action with no unpleasant reactions and can be used by anyone. There are 38 remedies, all of which are easy to obtain at health stores or pharmacies.

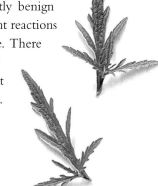

Verbena officinalis Vervain *is a sedative herb, useful for depression, especially that suffered after a viral illness.*

Patterns of Nervous Disease

The connection between physical and psychological factors in illness is recognized by orthodox medicine in the concept of psychosomatic and somatopsychic illness. Psychological factors can predispose or aggravate physical problems (psychosomatic concept) or physical factors can affect the psychological state (somatopsychic concept). It is perhaps far more appropriate to view all illness as part of a profound relationship between body, mind and soul.

A number of conditions have an especially strong relationship with the nervous system, whilst not producing neurological symptoms. These conditions can often be helped greatly by strengthening the nerves and toning the whole system. A representative list includes:

Panax ginseng Ginseng *is an excellent rejuvenator and is useful for depression and exhaustion, either mental or physical.*

- The circulatory system: high blood pressure and coronary disease
- The respiratory system: asthma, hayfever and irritable coughs
- The digestive system: peptic ulcer, colon disorder, flatulence and dyspepsia
- The skin: eczema, psoriasis
- The glandular system: thyroid problems and other endocrine disorders
- The reproductive system: many problems associated with menstruation

This list suggests conditions in which nervines are often appropriate, which does not imply that the conditions are 'all in the mind'. It means that to promote healing in the whole being, the nervous system may need more help here than usual.

The nervous system is perhaps the easiest system in the body in which to see the relevance of discussing dis-ease rather than disease. It may seem like a quibble, but this usage demonstrates the holistic view that the proper functioning of the whole body can be seen in terms of harmony and energy flow. By viewing disease from this standpoint it is possible to differentiate between psychological and neurological problems without resorting to a dualistic separation of mind and body.

There is a plethora of relaxation and meditation techniques which can help attain a relaxed state. We each have to find those most suitable for us. For some of us complex relaxation programmes work best, whilst for others it might be a walk in the woods. Meditation can range from a gentle inner stilling to a profound process of inner transcendence. Whilst in a herbal of this kind it is not possible to explore these in depth, here are a couple of simple but effective methods.

RELAXATION EXERCISES

Breathing is of great value in relaxation, particularly during the initial stages. People who are at ease with themselves and their world breathe slowly, deeply and rhythmically. Breathing is the only autonomic function we are capable of controlling consciously and by doing so it is possible to influence all autonomic and, to a degree, emotional responses.

Here is a basic and safe breathing relaxation technique.

A BASIC AND SAFE RELAXATION TECHNIQUE

Ideally this should be done twice a day for 5-15 minutes in a quiet room free of disturbance.

1 Rest on your back with head and neck comfortably supported.

2 Rest hands on upper abdomen, close your eyes and settle into a comfortable position.

3 Breathe slowly, deeply and rhythmically. Inhalation should be slow, unforced and unhurried. Silently count to 4, 5 or 6, whatever feels right for you.

4 When inhalation is complete, slowly exhale through the nose. Count this breathing out, as when breathing in. The exhalation should take as long as the inhalation. There should be no sense of strain. If initially you feel you have breathed your fullest at a count of 3, that is all right. Try gradually to slow down the rhythm until a slow count of 5 or 6 is possible, with a pause of 2 or 3 between in and out breath.

5 This pattern of breathing should be repeated 15 or 20 times and, since each cycle should take about 15 seconds, this exercise should occupy a total of about 5 minutes.

6 Once the mechanics of this exercise have been mastered, introduce thoughts at different parts of the cycle. On inhalation try to sense a feeling of warmth and energy entering the body with the air. On exhalation sense a feeling of sinking and settling deeper into the surface you are lying on.

7 On completion do not get up immediately but rest for a minute or two, allowing the mind to become aware of any sensations of stillness, warmth, heaviness etc.

Once mastered, this exercise can be used in any tense situation with the certainty that it will defuse the normal agitated response and should result in a far greater ability to cope.

Often tension is focused in the muscles of the body itself, and the following exercise can release such tightness and so allow the mind to be at ease. It is best to precede this exercise with a few cycles of deep breathing.

1 Lie down or sit in a reclining chair.

2 Avoid distractions and wear clothes that do not constrict.

3 Starting with the feet, try to sense or feel that the muscles of the area are not actively tense.

4 Then deliberately tighten the muscles, curling the toes under and holding the tension for 5 or 10 seconds.

5 Then tense them even more strongly for a further few seconds before letting all the tension go and sensing the wonderful feeling of release.

6 Try consciously to register what this feels like, especially in comparison with the tense state in which they were held.

7 Progress to the calf muscles and exercise in the same way. First sense the state the muscles are in, then tense them, hold the position, and then tense them even more before letting go. Positively register the sense of relief. If cramp occurs, stop tensing that area immediately and go on to the next.

8 After the calf go on to exercise the knees, then the upper leg, thighs, buttocks, back, abdomen, chest, shoulders, arms, hands, neck, head and face. The precise sequence is irrelevant, as long as all these areas are 'treated' to the same process.

9 Some areas may need extra attention. For example, in the abdomen the tensing of muscles can be achieved either by contracting (pulling in the tummy) or by stretching (pushing outwards). This variation in tensing is applicable to many muscles in the body.

10 There are between 20 and 25 of these 'areas' depending upon how you go about it. Give each at least 5–10 seconds of tensing and a further 5–10 seconds of letting go and passively sensing the feeling. Thus 8–10 minutes should cover the whole technique. This should be followed by several minutes of an unhurried feeling of warm relaxed tranquillity.

11 Focus the mind on the whole body. Sense it as heavy and content, free of tension or effort. This can be enhanced by a few cycles of deep breathing.

12 Have a good stretch and then carry on with your daily life.

Passiflora incarnata Passion Flower *is a powerful yet gentle sedative and hypnotic, the first choice for cases of chronic insomnia.*

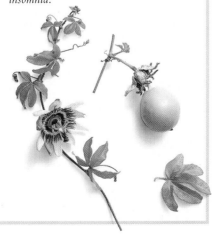

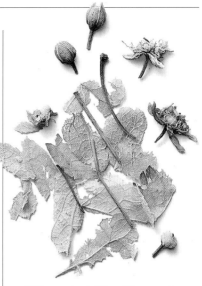

Tilia x *vulgaris* Lime Blossom *is a relaxing herb used to lower high blood pressure and relieve nervous tension. It is very pleasant drunk as an infusion.*

PSYCHOLOGICAL DISEASE

Our society is plagued by self-doubt, by fear and alienation, by de-humanization and violence. It is perhaps understandable that an epidemic of stress-related conditions characterizes the case-books of most doctors.

● **Stress** can be seen as any stimulus or change in the internal or external environment which disturbs homeostasis or inner harmony. This can be many things, from work conditions, relationships and bodily health to the state of the weather. The body responds in a similar way to any stress which involves hormonal and behavioural reactions.

A certain degree ·of stress-reaction is essential to survive in a modern city; the problems arise when an individual stress-response moves beyond that which aids, to a state that detracts.

By definition, stress itself cannot be treated, as it is a natural response to prevailing conditions. What can be done, however, is to aid the body as it responds. This is possible with the use of herbs and with the help of vitamins, but perhaps more important are relaxation exercises to give the body some chance for recovery. In addition, the situation causing the stress should be re-evaluated. Rather than alter the response to a situation, change the situation.

When stress does lead to a problem, the treatment can be based on a number of approaches. It is vital that the body's nutrition is adequate. It is often appropriate to supply the body with additional vitamin C and the vitamin B-complex, as it needs more of both when stressed. The nervine tonics will feed and tone the nervous system. The best ones in this case are *Skullcap* and *Oats,* but others may also be indicated, if there are related physical symptoms. *Ginseng* is an excellent herb to increase one's ability to cope with stress, when it is taken over a period of time. Of equal relevance and potency as an adaptogen is *Siberian Ginseng.*

• **Anxiety** We have all at some point in our lives experienced anxiety. Normally the feeling lasts only for a short time and is caused by some relevant external problem.

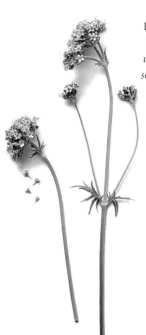

Valeriana officinalis Valerian *is a very useful relaxant and sedative, much used for insomnia. Its qualities are recognized by orthodox medicine as well as herbalism and homeopathy.*

ADAPTOGENS

It is worth exploring the concept of adaptogens here.

This is a relatively new concept to Western medicine and herbalism. However, in China and other countries in the East such ideas are the very basis of their preventative approach to health and wellbeing. Adaptogens act in such a way as to improve the body's adaptability. In other words, by helping it to adapt 'around' the problem, they enable it to avoid reaching a point of collapse or over-stress.

There is now much research into these potentially astounding remedies. The core of their action appears to lie in helping the body deal with stress. As we know, an inability to cope with external pressures leads to many internal repercussions. Thus many diverse forms of illness can develop. Adaptogens seem to increase the threshold of damage via support of adrenal gland and possibly pituitary gland function.

Some useful adaptogens are *Siberian Ginseng, Ginseng, Wild Yam, Borage, Licorice, Chamomile* and *Nettles.* They work via the adrenal or other endocrine glands to modify hormone production and flow. More information about the behaviour of the adrenal glands and the kinds of herbs that can support and encourage their function can be found in the section on The Glandular System *(see pages 226–9).*

By stretching the meaning of the word it can come to mean what in the past we called a tonic. This is especially relevant where a herb can have a normalizing effect, that is, produce contradictory actions depending on the body's needs. This restorative quality is a common and unique feature of herbal medicines.

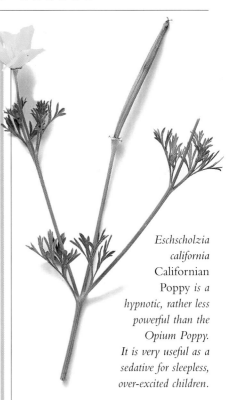

Eschscholzia california Californian Poppy *is a hypnotic, rather less powerful than the* Opium Poppy. *It is very useful as a sedative for sleepless, over-excited children.*

Sometimes, though, it becomes a habitual pattern, influencing our thoughts and behaviour. We then perceive the world filtered through our attitude of anxiety and we act accordingly. We enter a vicious circle where anxiety produces more anxiety.

Therapeutic counselling techniques and herbal medicine can ease the process.

All the nervine relaxants will ease anxiety and tension, the specific ones varying with each individual, as some are more effective with a particular mind than others. The most effective ones in the herbal repertoire are *Lady's Slipper, Lime Blossom, Mistletoe, Skullcap* and *Valerian.*

In addition to the nervine relaxants, the anti-spasmodic herbs are useful, as often in cases of anxiety there is also muscle tension, the relief of which helps the whole being to move to a state of ease and wellbeing, the perfect inner state within which to bring about healing.

A mixture of equal parts of *Skullcap* and *Valerian* is usually best;

the one drawback of this effective mixture is that its taste is not very pleasant.

Skullcap	1 part	
Valerian	1 part	

This tea can be drunk three times a day or when needed. Since it is safe at higher dosage for most people, take it in the amount which is effective for you.

• **Pre-menstrual Tension** This distressing problem, connected with the menstrual cycle, can create emotional and psychological disruption. To ease PMT in the short term, *Skullcap* and *Valerian* can be very effective. However, to really solve the problem, the state of hormonal balance in general has to be examined and treated. This is discussed in depth in the section on The Reproductive System *(pages 230–9)*.

• **Hyperactivity** A growing phenomenon is that of hyper-activity, particularly in children. Hyperactivity is not easy to define or diagnose, and many normal, healthy children have been classed as hyperactive just because they are more lively than their peers or parents. If a child has been correctly diagnosed as hyperactive, a number of steps should be taken. One of the central factors leading to hyperactivity is an accumulation of heavy metals in the body. Due to increased industrialization, our atmosphere and diet have become rather polluted by these substances.

The first step to combat hyperactivity is to provide a diet that is as pure and natural as possible, without any synthetic chemicals. Artificial food additives should also be avoided. It appears that young, developing nervous systems are particularly prone to

the damage or irritation that many food additives can cause. The effect is one of excessive activity with only a few hours' sleep each night, and because of the overactivity such children are more prone to accidents. There is some associ-ation with eczema and asthma, both of which will be aggravated by the overactivity. There may be difficulties in speech, balance and learning, even if the child has a high IQ.

Those parents with a child suspected of having this problem will be under extreme stress themselves. So there are two things to look at: ways to help the child and ways for the parents to cope.

A treatment that can be quite effective is based on a diet which cuts out all food and drink containing synthetic additives of any kind and certain natural chemicals.

A combination of the diet and good herbal treatment for any bodily symptoms the child has developed should be able to clear the problem.

To rid the body of the chemicals that have already been accumulated, alteratives should be used over a long period of time. The best one in this case is *Red Clover*, as it is also a nervine relaxant. For a short-term allevi-ation of the problem, other strong relaxants might be added and the person should also be treated for stress (as the body will be in a constant state of alert) with the aid of *Oats* and *Vervain* and the

vitamins C and B-complex. Gentle bitter tonics such as *Dandelion* or *Centaury* will quicken a return to stability.

• **Depression** can be a reaction to external factors or it can be an internally created state of mind, and often it is a combination of the two. Herbs can help to lift the depression, but at the same time the basic cause has to be treated.

An honest look at the factors involved and a courageous re-appraisal of your life is called for, as herbs by themselves will not solve the underlying problem.

Chamaemelum nobile Garden Chamomile *is a gentle sedative, particularly safe for children.*

They may, however, create the space and ease of mind to do so. The best anti-depressive herbs include *Damiana, Ginseng, Kola, Lady's Slipper, Lavender, Lime Blossom, Oats, Rosemary, Skullcap, Valerian* and *Vervain*.

When the depression is connected with a general debility of the whole body, affecting the nervous system, the following mixture is indicated:

Kola	2 parts	
Damiana	1 part	
Lavender	1 part	
Oats	1 part	
Rosemary	1 part	

This should be drunk three times a day.

Where there is not so much debility involved, use the following mixture:

Kola	1 part	
Lime Blossom	1 part	
Skullcap	1 part	

Lavandula angustifolia Lavender *is an effective anti-depressant, excellent for stress-induced headaches, and is a gentle remedy for sleeplessness.*

This tea should be drunk three times a day as well. If a more powerful approach is needed, *Valerian* may be added to the mixture.

As with all the mixtures recommended, remember that they may not be the ones you need. As all the herbs in this book are safe to use (within normal dosage), try out different mixtures. Read in The Herbal section about the herbs that can be used and choose accordingly. Use the teas over two or three days to give them time to work. If you are in doubt, consult a herbalist in your area. You may want to talk to someone confidentially about your problems, and a worthy herbalist will be a good listener.

• **Insomnia** At one time or another everyone has a sleepless night; stress during the day or anxiety about the next day can keep us awake and restless all through the night, or keep us from finding deep peaceful sleep. When this occurs only once in a while, there is nothing much wrong. However, it can become a repeated situation in which the whole body will suffer, as it is during sleep that most healing and revivifying takes place. There are many useful and powerful herb hypnotics that aid a

restful night's sleep, but often a gentle relaxation with the help of nervine relaxants is enough to allow the natural sleep process to take over.

The most effective sleep inducers are *Californian Poppy, Hops, Jamaican Dogwood, Passion Flower* and *Valerian*, with *Jamaican Dogwood* being particularly useful when sleeplessness is due to pain. A useful mixture is:

Passion Flower	1 part	
Valerian	1 part	

This tea should be drunk just before going to bed. The strength needed will vary from person to person, so experiment. The mixture is safe and it is impossible to overdose with these herbs. Most of the nervine relaxants will promote a restful, natural sleep. *Chamomile, Lime Blossom* and *Red Clover* are especially good and make delicious teas. They should be drunk last thing at night to relax any tension left over from the day and ease you into sleep.

Another very pleasant and excellent way to imbibe these herbs is through the skin when having a bath. This is a particularly good way to help children to sleep better. Thus, a *Lime Blossom* bath last thing at night will promote sleep, whilst a *Chamomile* one will in addition help with teething problems.

Trifolium pratense Red Clover *has relaxing properties and makes a soothing infusion to be drunk last thing at night.*

NEUROLOGICAL DISEASES

So far we have discussed problems manifesting mainly through psychological causes. We now turn to the herbal treatment of problems that manifest themselves within the nerve tissue itself. These can be overt organic ones such as multiple sclerosis or minor functional ones such as headaches.

• **Headaches** can be caused by a variety of psychological and physical dysfunctions, from stress and tension to digestive disorders and postural problems.

The list of herbs potentially useful for headaches is therefore extensive and includes *Balm, Cayenne, Chamomile, Elder Flower, Ground Ivy, Jamaican Dogwood, Lady's Slipper, Lavender, Marjoram, Peppermint, Rosemary, Rue, Skullcap, Tansy, Thyme, Valerian, Wood Betony* and *Wormwood*.

From this list it is apparent that actions other than that of pain relief (anodyne) will aid in the treatment of headaches. This, of course, reflects the diversity of possible causes, which range from pollution, bad lighting or domestic gas leaks (no matter how minute), to neck tension, eye strain, postural problems, bad diet, allergies or other factors.

Firstly, some general advice. You can take a relaxing bath with any of the herbs suggested above, if possible including *Lavender* as one of the ingredients. Or use one of the herbs that are rich in volatile oils (the best ones for headaches being *Lavender, Rosemary, Marjoram* and *Peppermint*), which can be used in the form of oils or as strong infusions. They can either be rubbed on the forehead and temples or their vapour can be inhaled, both methods often easing pain surprisingly fast. Besides using herbs, relaxing techniques can also be helpful: a walk in the woods or a meditation or whatever helps you feel at ease.

The most common physical causes of headaches are digestive disorders such as indigestion and constipation, muscular and nervous tension, and menstrual problems.

For stomach-related headaches, the use of carminatives and bitters

Hypericum perforatum St John's Wort *is an extremely versatile herb and can be used dried or as a volatile oil to soothe neuralgia and many other pains.*

is indicated, with the following mixture often being helpful:

| Skullcap | *1 part* | ▱ |
| Valerian | *1 part* | ▣ ◔ |

This tea can be drunk whenever it is needed.

If this is needed often, the digestion and diet will need attention. Where chronic constipation is the problem the advice given in the section on the digestive system should be followed.

Tension in the neck and shoulders, caused either by psychological stress or by postural problems (usually both together), will often bring on a headache. The use of nervine relaxants will ease this sort of headache, with *Valerian* often being the most effective herb.

Menstrual problems can also cause headaches and are best treated by correcting the hormonal balance, which is described in the later section on the reproductive system. However, for a short-term treatment the following tea is very helpful.

Balm	*1 part*	▱
Lavender	*1 part*	▣
Meadowsweet	*1 part*	◔

A cup of this tea can be drunk whenever needed.

● **Migraine** This distressing and intense headache is often accompanied by digestive disruptions like nausea and vomiting and by visual disturbances and photophobia. It can last for hours or days.

Like headaches, migraines can be triggered by a whole range of factors. Their treatment often involves both long-term attention to the cause and specific medications for an individual attack. To discover the underlying cause,

it is sometimes necessary to seek expert advice, as self-diagnosis can be difficult.

The invaluable herb *Feverfew* must be mentioned here. Whilst not quite the wonder remedy the media have led us to believe, the regular use of it, either fresh or as a tablet or a tea, will often clear the migraines after a month or so of treatment. A number of herbs will ease the pain of an attack, if they are taken at the first sign. These include *Black Willow, Jamaican Dogwood, Passion Flower, Valerian* and *Wood Betony.*

If there are also digestive symptoms such as nausea, vomiting or acid indigestion, herbs like *Black Horehound, Chamomile, Golden Seal* or *Meadowsweet* can be useful. Consult The Herbal section in order to decide which is the most appropriate herb or combination for the individual case concerned.

Tanacetum parthenium Feverfew *has long had a reputation as the herbal headache cure. The fresh leaves can be chewed when a headache comes on. It is also useful for migraines.*

The underlying cause can be one single factor, but often a number of contributing elements play a part in bringing about a migraine. The elements are most often found in one of the following categories of causes.

• **Diet** An allergic reaction to certain foods is the most common factor causing migraines. A comprehensive list of allergenic foods includes everything that can be eaten. However, the commonest triggers are red meat (especially pork), chocolate, dairy products, coffee, strong tea, white sugar, yeast products, vitamin B supplements, pickles, acid foods, animal fat, alcohol (especially red wine, sherry and port).

Passiflora incarnata Passion Flower *has pain-relieving properties that make it very helpful in cases of neuralgia and shingles. It can also calm fits and seizures.*

Often the reaction is not triggered by a single allergenic food but by a number of reactions to different foods accumulating and reaching a critical threshold. If you suspect a single allergy or such an accumulation as the cause, fast for two days and gradually reintroduce different foods. If a migraine is set off by a specific item, you have identified a trigger and can avoid it in the future. To support your digestive system, a regular treatment with *Balmony, Golden Seal, Meadowsweet* or *Wormwood* should be used for a number of months. After a while, fast again for two days, gradually reintroduce foods, and see if the reaction is still the same.

• **Stress** leading to tension is another common and potent trigger for migraines. It is best approached through relaxation therapy and sometimes even necessitates some form of psychotherapy. Typical examples of people susceptible to stress-induced migraines are those unable to cope with responsibilities, leading to a constant state of frustration, or at the other extreme, those who are over-conscientious perfectionists.

In both, the neurotic tension can lead to migraine. The appropriate herbs in such cases are nervine relaxants and tonics, such as *Hops, Mistletoe, Oats, Skullcap* or *Vervain*.

If instead the migraine is related to a debilitated state, nervine stimulants such as *Damiana* or *Kola* are appropriate.

One herb application in all cases of migraine caused by stress is *Ginseng*. It has to be taken for a number of weeks, though, before showing any clear effect.

• **Hormonal Problems** A common cause of migraine in women is hormonal problems associated with

Vitex agnus-castus Chaste Tree *is a very efficient normalizer and is particularly useful in stabilizing hormonal problems in women.*

the onset of periods or possibly menopause. A long-term treatment aiming at the balancing of the hormonal system, with the aid of herbs such as *Black Cohosh, Chaste Tree, Life Root, False Unicorn Root* or *Wild Yam,* may help. For more specific information, refer to the section on The Reproductive System *(pages 230–9).*

• **Structural Problems** A migraine can be brought about by structural problems in the neck or the spinal column, leading to muscular or nerve problems. A visit to a competent osteopath or chiropractor would be appropriate if any such problem is suspected.

• **Neuralgia** – or nerve pain – can range from excruciating pain that follows the length of a nerve, to a local pain where the nerve reaches the skin. The pain can be caused by an infection or by an osteopathic problem, but most commonly it is due to a general debilitated condition, brought about by wrong diet, stress and lack of rest.

To heal neuralgia, the underlying cause must be taken care of. If it is due to debility, the diet has to be improved and should include a lot of green vegetables and fruit with the addition of vitamin B-complex supplements for a while. Adequate rest and relaxation are also necessary. Herbs such as *Ginseng, Hops, Jamaican Dogwood, Passion Flower, Pasque Flower, St John's Wort* and *Valerian* are especially useful, and in addition to those used as teas, herbal preparations like

Rosemary and *Lavender* liniments and *St John's Wort* oil, rubbed into the affected part, can ease the pain.

In any nervous condition, the liberal use of *Oats* – in the diet and perhaps as an infusion in the bath – is also strongly recommended. If it occurs in association with shingles, then take *Echinacea* and *Marigold* over a period of at least three months as well. This could be as a tea or as tinctures.

Humulus lupulus Hops are very effective as a relaxant; they strongly affect the central nervous system and so may help to relieve the pain of neuralgia.

• **Multiple Sclerosis** is a chronic degenerative disease of the nerve sheaths. Medicine has not clearly identified the cause; it has been suggested that viral or immuno-logical actions play a part.

From the viewpoint of holistic healing, multiple sclerosis is clearly a disease arising when the inner harmony is out of balance, causing the degenerative changes. As such, the holistic approach will aim at restoring a balance. It is possible to improve multiple sclerosis consid-erably with the aid of appropriate

herbs and with careful digestive control.

Detailed dietary advice can be found in any good cookbook on holistic nutrition; the main factors are the total elimination of dairy products and possibly of foods which contain gluten. Further, saturated fats have to be kept to a minimum and need to be replaced by poly-unsatu-rated ones, from vegetables.

With a disease such as multiple sclerosis, a holistic herbal treatment has to aim at strength-ening and rebuilding the system. Thus, the treatment will vary with each individual and should be centred around the use of nervine tonics and stimulants and digestive tonics. The only herbal remedy to be recommended in all cases is the oil of *Evening Primrose,* which is rich in poly-unsaturated fats and should be taken in capsules over a long period in order to enable the nerve sheaths to be rebuilt.

As multiple sclerosis is a very complex condition, professional help should always be sought.

• **Shingles** are caused by a viral infection of the nerve ganglia which can be extremely painful and longlasting if not treated properly. The infection is usually accompanied by vesicles on the skin.

In the treatment of shingles it is necessary to strengthen the nerve cells with the aid of nervine tonics. Anti-microbials have to be used to aid the body in overcoming the infection, and anodynes in the form of nervine relaxants should

be included to reduce the pain. A useful mixture would be:

Echinacea	2 parts
Jamaican Dogwood	1 part
Oats	1 part
Passion Flower	1 part
St John's Wort	1 part
Valerian	1 part

This tea should be drunk three times a day.

For a local treatment of the symptoms, regular herbal baths with the above herbs are

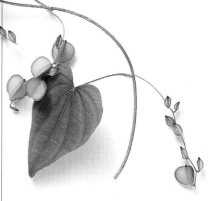

Dioscorea villosa Wild Yam *has many properties, one of which is to act as a normalizer on female hormones.*

recommended. The treatment has to be applied over a period of time. You should also pay attention to good nutrition, following a diet rich in vitamin B-complex supplements.

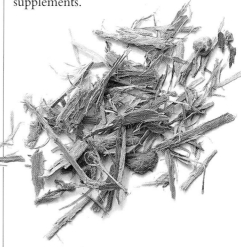

Piscidia piscipula Jamaican Dogwood *is excellent for calming extremely painful conditions such as migraine and dysmenorrhea.*

THE SKIN

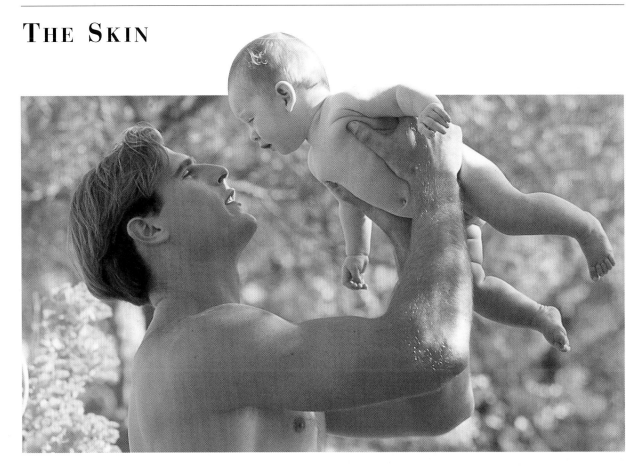

Our skin has numerous functions. It is the primary protective organ of our body; without a complete and coherent skin we would soon die of massive infection or of allergic shock, for the skin protects the body from injury, from light and chemicals, from extremes of temperature and from invasion by micro-organisms. Some of the protective functions are maintained through complex ecological processes, like protection against infections. Not only does the skin itself secrete anti-microbial substances, it also harbours a friendly natural community of bacteria. These resident bacteria protect the skin against the invasion of unfriendly micro-organisms by maintaining an environment unfavourable to them.

One of the potential problems of antibiotic therapy is the disruption of this friendly community, which opens the way for infections via the skin. Similarly, chemical deodorants and anti-perspirants work partly by destroying the natural skin bacteria and thus disrupt this delicate balance.

As the skin is responsible for the excretion of approximately a quarter of the body's waste products, any dysfunction of the skin in this field will put stress on the other three eliminative organs, namely, the kidneys, the lungs and the bowels, as they will have to deal with the extra burden. Thus a problem in the eliminative capacity of the skin can lead to secondary

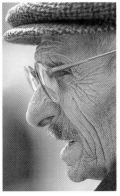

The skin is the largest organ in the body. Elastic, waterproof, lightproof and self-mending, it renews itself constantly and adapts to fit us perfectly, from babyhood and adulthood (above) to venerable old age (left).

problems in the other organs and difficulties with the skin. The skin also plays a part in temperature control, as its sweat glands can regulate the excretion of water. It is through the skin that we have physical contact with our environment, as the whole area of the skin is rich in sensory nerve endings. In fact it is worth noting that in the growing embryo the skin develops from the same source as the nervous tissue. This common origin points to the close relationship between skin and nervous system, a relationship which can be seen as a physical manifestation of the close connection between our inner being and the way it is reflected into the world. Thus, skin diseases will often be an outer reflection of internal problems and must be treated as such. Only rarely, as in bruises and wounds, can the skin be related to in isolation.

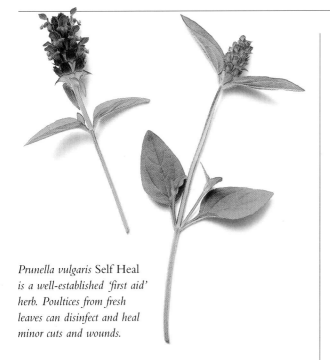

Prunella vulgaris Self Heal *is a well-established 'first aid' herb. Poultices from fresh leaves can disinfect and heal minor cuts and wounds.*

Herbs for the Skin

Even though skin problems may reflect a variety of internal conditions and all groups of herbs may play a role in its treatment, some groups are especially indicated. In particular the vulneraries, the alteratives, the diaphoretics, the anti-microbials and the nervines will be discussed.

VULNERARIES

Nature is rich in plants which promote the healing of fresh cuts and wounds, and this is to be expected if herbs are truly part of an ecological support system, integrated into and created by Gaia. As injuries of one sort or another are perhaps the most common physical problems, we find that every natural habitat is rich in those healing plants. The traditional knowledge of their use is reflected in their common names such as Woundwort, Knitbone and Self-Heal.

Along with its pain-relieving qualities, Stachys palustris Woundwort *is an excellent vulnerary when applied directly to wounds.*

Some of these herbs are astringents, and part of their efficiency is based upon their ability to arrest bleeding and to condense the tissue. The most common and useful vulneraries are *Aloe, American Cranesbill, Chickweed, Comfrey, Elder*

Flower and *Berries, Golden Seal, Horsetail, Irish Moss, Marigold Flowers, Marshmallow Root, Self-Heal, Slippery Elm, Witch Hazel* and *Woundwort*. Some are applied externally, whilst others are used both externally and internally. Study them in The Herbal section to get to know them.

ALTERATIVES

Alteratives gradually alter and correct a 'polluted' condition of the bloodstream and restore a healthier functioning. The way the alteratives operate is poorly understood, but they certainly work and they are perhaps the herbs most often used in the context of skin conditions, the roots of which lie deep within the metabolism of the individual. They cleanse the whole of the body, but their activity is focused in different areas, some in the kidneys, some in the liver, for example, and they have to be chosen according to their specific indications.

Alteratives include *Blue Flag, Burdock, Cleavers, Figwort, Fumitory, Golden Seal, Mountain Grape, Nettles, Red Clover, Sarsaparilla, Sassafras, Thuja* and *Yellow Dock*.

Urtica dioica Nettle *is an astringent particularly suitable for child eczema.*

ANTI-MICROBIALS

For some skin conditions anti-microbials have to be used to rid the body of micro-organisms that have invaded it or act on the skin. Herbs that help here include *Chickweed, Echinacea, Garlic, Marigold, Myrrh, Pasque Flower, Thuja, Thyme* and *Wild Indigo*.

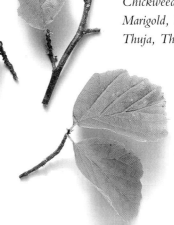

Hamamelis virginiana Witch Hazel *is a very useful healing astringent, an excellent soother of bruises.*

Patterns of Skin Disease

Skin problems can be manifestations of internal problems and should be treated as such and not as local phenomena. Three areas can usefully be identified. There are internal causes, where the origins of a skin disease lie purely in internal disharmony, as in psoriasis or some eczema; and internal reactions to external factors, where the skin problem is due to the body's inability to cope with an external factor, such as an allergen; and external causes, where the skin problem is the direct result of external influences, as with wounds, bruises or sunburn.

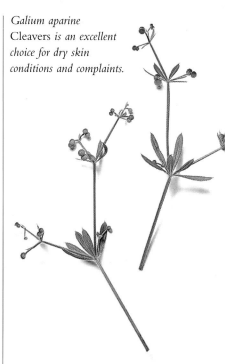

Galium aparine
Cleavers *is an excellent choice for dry skin conditions and complaints.*

INTERNAL CAUSES

Most of the intransigent and chronic skin conditions that affect humanity are the result of internal processes. As our skin is our interface with the world it is often the site where disharmony in our life is manifested.

• **Psoriasis** can be caused by a wide range of factors, often working together; therefore the treatment will have to vary according to individual needs. The root of the problem has to be identified, whether it is physical, psychological or spiritual.

While certain herbs are traditionally indicated for psoriasis, correct diagnosis and awareness of individual needs is important. Most of the herbs are alteratives. They include *Burdock Root, Cleavers, Dandelion, Figwort, Mountain Grape,*

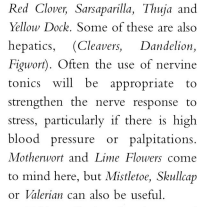

Scrophularia nodosa
Figwort, *a useful external skin remedy*

Red Clover, Sarsaparilla, Thuja and *Yellow Dock.* Some of these are also hepatics, (*Cleavers, Dandelion, Figwort*). Often the use of nervine tonics will be appropriate to strengthen the nerve response to stress, particularly if there is high blood pressure or palpitations. *Motherwort* and *Lime Flowers* come to mind here, but *Mistletoe, Skullcap* or *Valerian* can also be useful.

Taking all that has been said into account, a basic herbal approach that can be added to and modified includes:

Burdock	1 part	
Sarsaparilla	1 part	
Cleavers	1 part	
Yellow Dock	1 part	

This tea should be drunk three times daily. The treatment has to be continued over a long period of time, while attention should be given to a wholesome diet and to enough physical exercise.

External remedies will ease irritations or help with the removal of scales, but will not give permanent relief. Ointments for this purpose can be made from *Comfrey, Chickweed* or *Marshmallow.*

• **Eczema** With eczema, as with psoriasis, it is necessary to search for the roots within. If an allergic reaction is involved, the allergen has to be identified and removed, as otherwise the body has no chance to heal itself or to take advantage of the herbal support that is given.

The herbal remedies will be selected according to individual needs, but the digestive process should be examined and the use of bitters, carminatives or laxatives considered. If the liver is suspected of impaired function, cholagogues or hepatics may be needed, and if the kidneys do not fulfil their vital responsibilities, then diuretics will be indicated. Nervines may also be appropriate.

Traditionally, herbs such as *Burdock Root, Figwort, Fumitory, Mountain Grape, Nettle, Pansy* and *Red Clover* have a good reputation in the treatment of eczema, as internal remedies. A useful basic mixture can be made from the following.

Figwort	1 part	
Nettles	1 part	
Red Clover	1 part	

This tea should be drunk three times daily and is especially good for infantile eczema.

Herbs such as *Burdock, Chickweed, Comfrey, Golden Seal, Marigold, Pansy* or *Witch Hazel* can all be used successfully for compresses or ointments.

• **Acne** If there is any metabolic problem or a preponderance of fatty or carbohydrate food in the diet, acne may result or be aggravated.

The herbal approach aims at supporting the metabolism of these foods and at helping lymphatic drainage and bodily elimination. Alteratives such as *Figwort, Cleavers, Red Clover, Mountain Grape* and *Yellow Dock* are especially useful, but lymphatics such as *Poke Root* and *Echinacea* and hepatics such as *Blue Flag* and *Dandelion* should also be considered.

A mixture such as the following can be taken for a while.

Blue Flag	1 part	
Cleavers	1 part	✒
Echinacea	1 part	📦
Figwort	1 part	🕐
Poke Root	1 part	

This tea should be drunk three times daily.

Externally, a lotion of equal parts or an infusion of *Marigold, Chickweed* and distilled *Witch Hazel* may be useful, as may frequent washing with a pure soap.

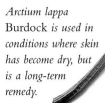

Arctium lappa Burdock *is used in conditions where skin has become dry, but is a long-term remedy.*

INTERNAL REACTIONS TO EXTERNAL FORCES

Sometimes the skin will show reactions to external factors, such as bacteria, that have led to internal processes, which reflect on the skin instead of manifesting internally. While symptoms on the skin should be attended to, the real problem lies in the weakened defence system, which should be toned and strengthened so that the body will rid itself of infection.

The general guidelines for the treatment of infections also hold true here. If antibiotics have been used recently, at least 1g of vitamin C should be taken daily.

• **Boils** The staphylococcus aureus become a problem when the body is weakened and can then lead to boils. To effectively rid the body of boils, herbs have to be used both internally and externally. This can best be achieved with a combination of anti-microbials and alteratives, and possibly bitters. Three remedies which are considered specifics for boils are *Echinacea, Pasque Flower* and *Wild Indigo*. They are best used in combinations that will aid the lymphatic system. A typical mixture would be:

Echinacea	1 part	
Wild Indigo	2 parts	✒
Pasque Flower	1 part	📦
Poke Root	1 part	🕐

This tea should be drunk three times daily.

Externally, an ointment or a poultice should be used to draw pus from the boil. A poultice can be made from *Marshmallow Leaf* or *Cabbage Leaf*, while *Echinacea* or *Myrrh* can control the infection.

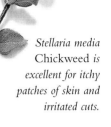

Stellaria media Chickweed *is excellent for itchy patches of skin and irritated cuts.*

• **Impetigo** is a highly contagious infection that commonly occurs in children. Scrupulous hygiene is vital in its treatment, in conjunction with a diet rich in fruits, fresh green vegetables and extra doses of vitamin C of about 2g daily, together with raw garlic as part of the diet. Herbally, the defence of the body has to be aided by the use of anti-microbials and supported by alteratives and tonics. Externally, a lotion of one or more herbs such as *Echinacea, Marigold, Myrrh* or *Wild Indigo* can be used to combat the infection. This will only be truly effective in conjunction with an internal treatment *(see Boils)*.

Chelidonium majus
Greater Celandine *can
be used externally on
fungal skin infections.*

• **Warts** are
caused by viral
infections, which can
only occur if the 'soil' is
right, so a herbal environment aims
at creating a clean and sound inner
environment. Diet and lifestyle
should be wholesome and life-
affirming and herbs like *Cleavers,
Garlic, Poke Root, Prickly Ash* or
Wormwood, which are lymphatic
cleansers and tonics, should be
taken internally. Also take some
vitamin C, about 2g daily. For an
external treatment and a quick
removal of warts, *Greater Celandine*
and *Thuja* are considered to be
specifics. *Greater Celandine* is used
by expressing the latex from fresh

Thuja occidentalis Thuja *can be used
externally as an effective treatment
for warts.*

stems and applying it directly
to the wart, whereas *Thuja* is
made into a lotion or a
tincture, which should
be used often.

• **Herpes Simplex**
This very common
virus infection, which
is also known as cold
sores, is a secondary
manifestation of an
initial infection
with the herpes
virus that usually
occurs early in life. The
infection often remains
unnoticed, as the virus can reside
latent within the body for the rest
of the person's life, unless the
resistance of the
body is lowered.
The treatment
aims primarily at
improving bodily
health through a good
diet, a high level of vitamin C
(3–5g daily) and by supporting the
body's eliminative processes. The
treatment should be supported by a
herbal mixture, which has to be
taken for a period of time, such as:

Cleavers	2 parts	
Echinacea	2 parts	
Oats	1 part	
Poke Root	1 part	

Drink this tea twice daily.
    Externally, a lotion of *Echinacea*
with or without *Myrrh* will prove
very useful.

• **Ringworm** is caused by a
fungal infection of the skin,
which can occur on various parts
of the body and give rise to
symptoms like athlete's foot. It
commonly occurs between the
toes, around the groin or in
circular patches anywhere on the
body. It is made worse by sweating

and by poor hygiene. The key to its
effective removal lies in scrupulous
hygiene and in making sure that
some air can reach the affected
parts. The herbal approach consists
of internal and external remedies.
Internally, a mixture that raises the
body's resistance and increases
lymphatic drainage should be used.

Echinacea	2 parts	
Cleavers	1 part	
Poke Root	1 part	
Wild Indigo	1 part	
Yellow Dock	1 part	

This tea should be drunk three
times daily.

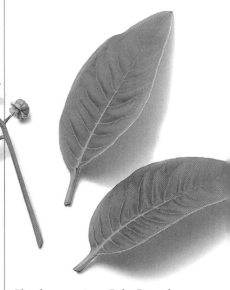

Phytolacca americana Poke Root *has a
useful supporting role in viral skin infections
such as cold sores.*

Externally, anti-fungal herbs like
*Echinacea, Garlic, Golden Seal,
Marigold, Myrrh* or *Thuja* can be
directly applied as lotions or as
tinctures. *Marigold* is by far the
most effective, especially used in a
proportion of 50:50 with *Myrrh* as
tincture and applied undiluted to
the site three times a day.

EXTERNAL CAUSES
The value of *Marigold* cannot be
exaggerated when it comes to
treating skin problems like wounds,

bruises or burns. Its properties make it a healing plant that reduces soreness and inflammation whilst also acting as an anti-microbial, which makes it a primary first aid herb for any problem.

• **Wounds** Of the multitude of vulnerary herbs, *Comfrey, Elder Flower, Golden Seal, Plantain* and *St John's Wort* are the most important, but in addition to the vulneraries it must be remembered that the first stage of wound healing lies in the clotting of blood, where the astringents

Aloe vera Aloe *is an external remedy for minor burns. The gel inside the leaf can be used straight from the plant.*

TO MAKE AN ARNICA COMPRESS

It is very effective to use Arnica tincture: if using dried Arnica flowers, one part flowers should be mixed with ten parts 70% alcohol. If fresh flowers are available, equal amounts of Arnica and alcohol can be used. Put the mixture in a tightly sealed glass container for two weeks, leave it in a warm place and shake it every day. After two weeks strain it through a muslin cloth and press out as much liquid as possible. This can be left for another two days to settle, when it can be filtered to obtain a clear liquid. To make a compress, mix one tablespoonful of tincture with 500ml/1pt of water.

can be extremely useful. Of all these herbs, *Comfrey* has a deserved reputation as a potent healer of wounds, which is in part due to its content of allantoin in roots and leaves. This chemical stimulates cell division and so speeds up scar formation and total healing. As with the other herbs mentioned, it may be used in the form of a poultice, a compress or as an ointment. If there is danger of an infection, an anti-microbial like *Echinacea* should also be added.

• **Bruises** To help the body deal with bruises, sprains and concussion, herbs such as *Arnica, Daisy, Marigold, Witch Hazel* or *Yarrow,* used as compresses, will be exceptionally effective. Of these, *Arnica* is the best and can produce astounding improvements in a very short time. You can also make lotions, tinctures, compresses or ointments from any of the other herbs mentioned above to help in home first aid.

If bruising is a recurring problem without obvious external causes, increase the vitamin C foods in the diet. It may be necessary to investigate why the blood vessels rupture so readily. An infusion of *Horsechestnut* and *Yarrow* drunk regularly for quite a while will help strengthen the blood vessel walls. Rutin and other bioflavonoids will help, either as dietary supplements or in buckwheat.

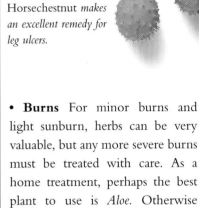

Aesculus hippocastanum Horsechestnut *makes an excellent remedy for leg ulcers.*

• **Burns** For minor burns and light sunburn, herbs can be very valuable, but any more severe burns must be treated with care. As a home treatment, perhaps the best plant to use is *Aloe.* Otherwise *Marigold* or *St John's Wort* will help *(page 224).* This is nature's answer for bad sunburn and it will leave the skin in better shape than when it started.

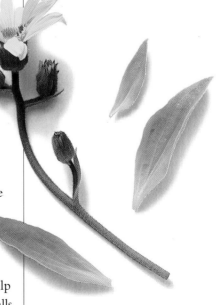

Arnica montana Arnica *is the best herbal help for bruising, both external and internal.*

THE MUSCULO/SKELETAL SYSTEM

Our skeleton, the connective tissue, our muscles and our joints hold us together, enable us to stand and to move, and give us our form. They are used – and misused – a lot and are the site of much physical wear and tear. But the health of these tissues depends not only on the use to which they are put or the structure they are part of, but also to a large extent on our inner environment, the state of our metabolism, and our diet and lifestyle.

Of course genetically-based weaknesses can play a very important part as well, but if they are recognized, much can be done to keep them from manifesting as problems. If problems are due to structural mis-alignments, a great deal can be done with the help of manipulation therapies such as osteopathy or chiropractic. Sometimes the skeleton is so far out of normal alignment that proper neurological functions are impaired and the function of the organs is disturbed or the harmony of the whole body is affected. Osteopathic or chiropractic techniques can help to realign the body, as can methods of psycho-physical adjustments such as Rolfing, the Alexander Technique or Feldenkrais.

JOINTS

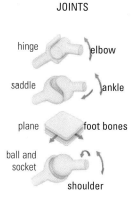

hinge — elbow

saddle — ankle

plane — foot bones

ball and socket — shoulder

There are several types of movable joint, allowing different kinds of movement to the various bones they connect. Hinge joints allow great movement; saddle joints restrict movement to a certain radius; plane joints allow bones to slide over each other; ball and socket joints give flexibility.

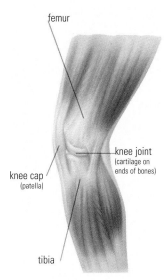

femur

knee joint (cartilage on ends of bones)

knee cap (patella)

tibia

The knee joint allows the femur and tibia to move freely in relation to each other. Strong leg muscles connect the two bones, ligaments keep the joint in place and the knee cap protects the joint.

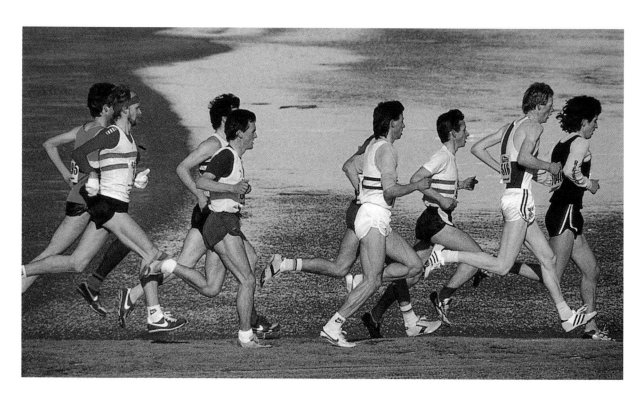

A healthy body in motion is an engine of joy. Using all our bones and muscles to the full in the way they were designed to be used is to experience life holistically. The bones and muscles of your body are strong and hard-wearing. Exercised properly and supported by diet and gentle remedies, they should serve you well throughout life.

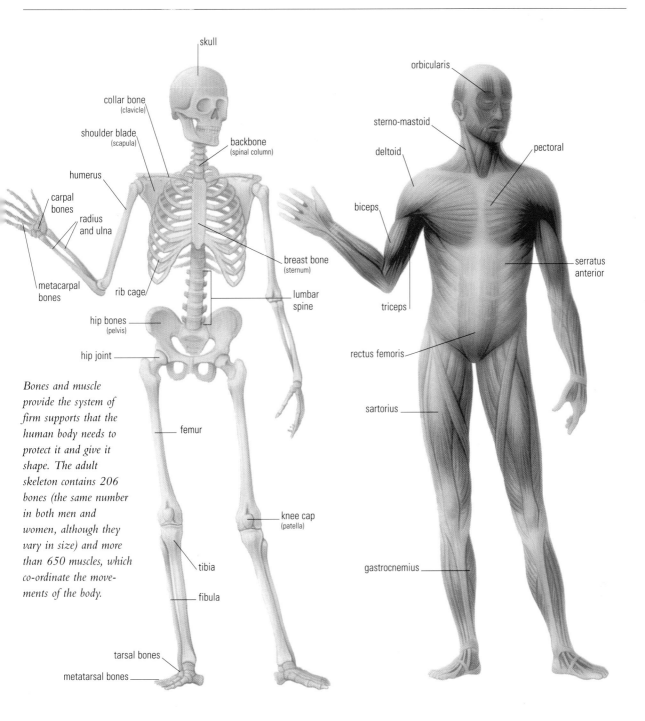

skull

collar bone
(clavicle)

shoulder blade
(scapula)

humerus

carpal
bones

radius
and ulna

metacarpal
bones

rib cage

hip bones
(pelvis)

hip joint

backbone
(spinal column)

breast bone
(sternum)

lumbar
spine

*Bones and muscle
provide the system of
firm supports that the
human body needs to
protect it and give it
shape. The adult
skeleton contains 206
bones (the same number
in both men and
women, although they
vary in size) and more
than 650 muscles, which
co-ordinate the move-
ments of the body.*

femur

knee cap
(patella)

tibia

fibula

tarsal bones

metatarsal bones

orbicularis

sterno-mastoid

deltoid

biceps

pectoral

serratus
anterior

triceps

rectus femoris

sartorius

gastrocnemius

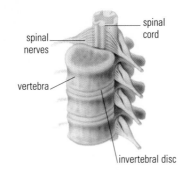

spinal
cord

spinal
nerves

vertebra

invertebral disc

*Spinal nerves carry impulses between
the spinal cord and the body's trunk
and limbs, leaving the backbone by
the gaps between the vertebrae.*

But a major source of conditions that plague this system is the systemic health of the body as a whole. Only as long as the inner environment and metabolism are in harmony is health and wholeness maintained. If our bio-chemical and metabolic processes are out of tune, one of the effects is that the body will be under much strain to remove waste and toxins. If this condition lasts for some years –

which it often does, unnoticed – toxins can build up in the connective tissue of the joints and sow the seeds for the development of rheumatism and arthritis, particularly if there is a genetic disposition in that direction.

Of all the problems that can affect this system, it is in this area of chronic and degenerative ailments of the bones and joints that herbal medicine has most to offer.

219

Herbs for the Musculo/Skeletal System

In this system, particularly in disease such as rheumatism or arthritis, the body has to be led back to a state of health and balance.

To treat problems that manifest in the bones or muscles effectively, digestion and assimilation have to work well, as do the various aspects of elimination. This should be kept in mind when choosing different kinds of herbs for particular needs.

ANTI-RHEUMATICS

A vast array of herbs has the reputation of preventing, relieving or curing rheumatic problems. I will give you a long – though far from complete – list of anti-rheumatics, including a variety of herbs with different primary actions.

They can be chosen according to the needs of the whole body, as they include alteratives, anti-inflammatories, rubifacients, diuretics, stimulants and digestives: *Angelica, Bearberry, Black Cohosh, Black Willow, Bladderwrack, Blue Flag, Bogbean, Boneset, Burdock, Cayenne, Celery Seed, Couchgrass, Dandelion, Devil's Claw, Guaiacum, Ginger, Juniper, Mountain Grape, Mustard, Nettles, Poke Root, Prickly Ash, Ragwort, Sarsaparilla, White Poplar, Wild Yam, Wintergreen, Wormwood, Yarrow* and *Yellow Dock.*

Eupatorium perfoliatum Boneset *is well known in folk-medicine as a support remedy to be taken while broken bones heal.*

ALTERATIVES

Alteratives gradually cleanse and correct a 'polluted' condition of the bloodstream and restore healthier functioning.

Fucus vesiculosus Bladderwrack *is very helpful used externally on inflamed joints.*

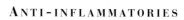
Menyanthes Trifoliata Bogbean *is recommended for rheumatism, arthritis and rheumatoid arthritis.*

The herbs work through different mechanisms, many of which are not yet fully understood, and they work in a wide range of conditions, including rheumatism.

While most alteratives will help in problems of this section, *Black Cohosh, Bogbean, Celery Seed, Devil's Claw, Guaiacum* and *Sarsaparilla* are most widely used. Most rheumatic and arthritic conditions are improved through the general revitalization and cleansing brought about by these herbs.

ANTI-INFLAMMATORIES

It is perhaps misleading to call these herbs anti-inflammatories, as in a holistic treatment we are not aiming at suppressing inflammation, which is usually part of a healthy body-response. Rather, these herbs reduce inflammations by helping the body to overcome the problem. These herbs can be helpful, particularly in rheumatic and arthritic conditions, where long-standing inflammations of joints and other tissues become self-defeating.

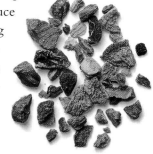
Harpagophytum procumbens Devil's Claw *is particularly effective in cases of arthritis.*

A good example is *Meadowsweet;* it is rich in natural aspirin-like substances that reduce swelling and pain, while it is also a diuretic and hepatic, thus aiding the body in cleaning and elimination and in time clearing the roots of the inflammation, which lie in an accumulation of waste and toxins.

The most effective anti-inflammatories are *Black Willow, Devil's Claw, Guaiacum, Meadowsweet, White Poplar* and *Wild Yam.* Unlike drug anti-inflammatories, these herbs are safe in large doses, since they are in the dilute and balanced form designed by nature. A safe and effective dose of *Black Willow* could be 250ml/^{1}/2pt of tincture a week.

Mentha x piperita Peppermint *is excellent as a liniment to relieve painful joints.*

RUBEFACIENTS

Rubefacients, when applied to the skin, stimulate circulation in that area. This increases the blood supply, which in turn relieves congestion and inflammation, thus making rubefacients particularly useful as the basis for liniments used in muscular rheumatism and similar conditions.

Most rubefacients are too strong to be used internally. Even on sensitive skin they should be used with care, and not at all when the skin is damaged. The particular way to use them is described on pages 223–4: the most useful ones are *Cayenne, Ginger, Horseradish, Mustard, Peppermint* (as oil), *Ragwort, Rosemary* (as oil), and *Wintergreen.*

DIURETICS

Diuretics help the work of the kidney and thus the elimination of metabolic waste and toxins, or the products of inflammation, which is essential, as these can lie at the root of many problems such as arthritis or rheumatism. If there is any kidney problem, it must also be treated. To support the work of this vital organ generally, herbs such as *Boneset, Celery, Juniper Berries* or *Yarrow* can be used, and *Celery Seeds* are often considered specific for rheumatism.

Rosmarinus officinalis Rosemary *stimulates circulation and so encourages toxins to leave the body.*

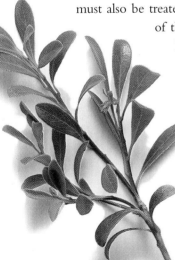

Arctostaphylos uva-ursi Bearberry *is a diuretic which also helps the body to pass toxins quickly.*

CIRCULATORY STIMULANTS

Another way to cleanse the body of toxins is to stimulate the circulation which increases blood flow to muscles and joints. This can be done without straining the heart by using herbs that stimulate the peripheral circulation, such as *Cayenne, Ginger, Poke Root, Prickly Ash* or *Rosemary.* Of course, if there is any circulatory or heart problem, this must be seen to as well.

PAIN RELIEVERS

While the purist will never treat symptoms, the healer's art aims at relieving suffering. It may be necessary to use herbs that will reduce the often severe pain of conditions such as rheumatism, which of course should only be given as part of a whole treatment of the cause. The anti-inflammatories will reduce pain to some degree, but the only effective way to reduce and eliminate pain is to clear the underlying problem. While this is being done, herbs such as *Guaiacum, Jamaican Dogwood, St John's Wort* or *Valerian* can help to relieve the pain. They will be less effective if no other steps are taken.

DIGESTIVE TONICS

The digestive process needs to be in good working order; otherwise nutrients will not be properly absorbed and the musculo/skeletal system will be impaired. The use of bitter tonics like *Gentian, Golden Seal, Wormwood* or *Yarrow* may well be useful.

If there is any appreciable degree of constipation or a build-up of fecal matter, the use of evacuants is called for, especially those that act by stimulating the liver, like *Boldo, Rhubarb Root* or *Yellow Dock.*

Rumex crispus Yellow Dock *helps digestion and re-establishes the body's ability to absorb and use food efficiently.*

Patterns of Muscle and Bone Disease

Most diseases that afflict the bones and muscles are degenerative and associated with old age: rheumatism, arthritis, osteoporosis, osteoarthritis. However, they are not an inevitable adjunct of a long life; many problems can be minimized or even avoided by paying attention to diet and exercise early in life. Occupational hazards such as bursitis or repetitive strain injury are not so easy to avoid, but may be counteracted by specific exercises or better monitoring at work. A truly holistic approach, combining diet, exercise and support from relevant herbs can be very effective in the treatment of everyday bone and joint problems.

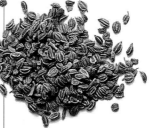

Apium graveolens Celery Seed *is an excellent remedy for gout, arthritis and rheumatism.*

RHEUMATISM AND ARTHRITIS

We will not look into the differences between the various sorts of rheumatism and arthritis. It is arguable whether a differential diagnosis is necessary for a holistic treatment. What is necessary is to recognize the general and individual causes and the influences of the genetic framework. These conditions are a result of the body's inability to deal with pressures from wrong diet and lifestyle or from other stresses.

The aim of the treatment will be to bring the individual to a state of health and vitality where the body can take care of the symptom, instead of attacking the symptom to attain the vitality.

An important insight into approaching these conditions is the idea of friction. The changes in the joints that occur in cases of arthritis cause a rubbing together of bones in such a way as to cause friction, but there is often a long history of friction leading up to this physical change.

It could be due to a particular physical job, as when farmers develop osteoarthritis in the shoulder on which they have carried hay bales for years, or it could be muscle tension

binding joints too tightly together, which is usually due to a history of friction in life. A dictionary definition of friction is 'a resistance encountered when one body moves relative to another body with which it is in contact; ... disagreement or conflict.' When looking at the roots of rheumatic and arthritic problems this definition covers it all, whether the two bodies are bones, people or differing emotions and beliefs.

Conflicts, and the friction that ensues, can take many forms but the experience is fundamentally an inner one. For some, conflict is a state of mind, an attitude with which to relate to the world. Such conflict is really between inner aspects of the individual, a manifestation of psychological disharmony. This will externalize as conflict in relationships or lifestyle, but the roots are often buried deep in the psyche.

When trying to create the right environment within the body for healing to occur, as much attention has to go into emotional and mental

Smilax regelii Sarsaparilla *can be used in combination with other herbs in cases of chronic rheumatism.*

harmony as into diet and herbal medicine.

If an individual has an outlook on life that is tight, defensive and lacking in vulnerability and openness, the rheumatism will be fed. If an inner process of relaxation is initiated that reduces emotional friction, allows a free interaction with people, and an opening up of emotions and beliefs, the stage will be set for the miracle of self-healing to occur, facilitated by the use of herbs.

• **Toxic Build-up** One of the causes of rheumatism and arthritis is an accumulation of toxins or waste products in the affected tissue. A major contributing factor in the development of this condition is an inappropriate diet, either using foods that are wrong for your body or foods that are so devitalized and adulterated that they are detrimental anyway.

As a general guideline, foods that cause the body to have an acidic reaction should be avoided, as should those that cause digestive problems or other adverse conditions, such as subtle allergic reactions.

Instead of eating processed foods full of additives and preservatives, try to make sure that your diet contains food that is as fresh and untreated as possible.

Overt allergic reactions, or subtle ones like the minor digestive upsets of heartburn or wind, are often caused by gluten (mainly from wheat products) and by dairy products, which should both then be avoided. Acidic reactions are caused by meat (especially red meat), eggs and dairy products; by refined carbohydrates and refined sugar; and by most spices.

Foods rich in oxalic acid, such as rhubarb, gooseberries, black and red currants, should also be shunned. Coffee, black tea, alcohol, anything made from black grapes, sugar and salt should also be avoided for various reasons, as they all contribute to the accumulation of toxins and are detrimental to a cleansing process.

Cimicifuga racemosa Black Cohosh *is an excellent pain reliever in cases of rheumatism, osteoarthritis and general muscular pain.*

Instead, fruits (including citrus which, in spite of their citric acid, appear to have an alkaline action on the metabolism) and vegetables should be eaten in abundance, particularly green and root vegetables, and at least 1.5l/3pt of fluid should be drunk daily to help flush the body. The fluid should preferably be water (but water low in mineral content), or water mixed with a little apple cider vinegar or apple juice. A vitamin C supplement of at least 500mg daily is recommended. Fish and white meat may also be eaten.

• **A Cleansing Regime** Through the use of appropriate herbs and in combination with other techniques to support and aid the whole body, it is possible to cleanse the whole system and to remove the source of the rheumatic or arthritic development. Such a treatment takes time, as a degenerative process that took a long time to develop is not reversed in four weeks. But when the right treatment is used, it is not uncommon to hear comments like 'I already feel better within myself' long before the actual symptoms of pain or stiffness are gone.

In addition to the general need for cleansing, each person has to be approached as a unique being.

Does the digestive system need help in any way? Are the kidneys working well? Is there much stress in the person's life? Is the endocrine system working harmoniously? How is the diet?

With rheumatic and arthritic problems, more than with any others, it is essential to treat the whole being, otherwise healing will only be slight or temporary.

But when the unique picture of the individual is taken into account, it is possible to open the gates for a quite miraculous healing to occur.

Having made that point quite clearly, here is a basic mixture for rheumatic and arthritic conditions.

Bogbean	2 parts	
Black Cohosh	1 part	✓
Celery Seed	1 part	▣
Meadowsweet	1 part	◉
Yarrow	1 part	

This tea should be drunk three times a day for a long period of time.

This is just one possibility. The specifics should be selected in view of the particular individual, according to the suggestions given on pages 220–1.

If, for instance, a lot of inflammation or pain is involved, consider the anti-inflammatories and maybe the pain relievers, and you might want to use *Black Willow, Guaiacum* or *Wild Yam.*

If the person lacks sleep due to pain, it is necessary to do something about this, as much healing happens during sleep. A useful herbal combination to aid sleep and to reduce pain is:

Jamaican Dogwood	1 part	✓
Valerian	1 part	▣
Passion Flower	1 part	◉

Drink this tea half an hour before going to bed. It is a safe mixture and may be used in stronger dosage than the normal one or two teaspoonfuls, if required.

• **External Help** In addition, external remedies can be used to ease pain and reduce inflammation, while at the same time stimulating circulation to the affected area to help in the elimination of toxins. Whilst such treatment will not lead to a fundamental change by itself, it will help the whole process and ease discomfort.

A very warming and stimulating liniment can be made by mixing equal parts of tincture of *Cayenne* and glycerine, which should be rubbed into the affected joints or muscles. Care must be taken not to use it on broken skin or to get it on the sensitive skin of the face.

Capsicum annuum Cayenne *is excellent for stimulating circulation in the extremities, and preventing chilblains.*

TO MAKE A LINIMENT USING ST JOHN'S WORT

If there is pain in the muscle tissue or any nerve pain, a liniment based on *St John's Wort* oil can be most effective. You can prepare the oil yourself in late summer by picking fresh blossoms and putting them into oil.

1 *Pick 120g/ 4oz of fresh, just-opened blossoms and crush them into a table-spoonful of olive or sunflower oil.*

2 *Pour 500ml/ 1pt of the same oil over the whole, mix it well and put it into a clear glass container.*

3 *Leave the container open in a warm place to ferment for three to five days, then seal the container well and place it in sunshine or put it in another warm place for three to six weeks, shaking it daily, until the oil has become bright red.*

4 *After this time, press the mixture through a cloth and let the oil stand for a day to separate the oily from the watery part. Use the oily part only, which should be carefully poured off and stored in an airtight opaque container.*

It won't do any harm but it may appear to 'burn' until the volatile oil fades or is washed away. It is the same heat that relieves pain in cold, aching joints and stiff muscles.

St John's Wort oil may be rubbed on areas of rheumatic pain, and it can also be used for neuralgic or sciatic pains or on light burns.

You can also make other oils, either by making the base for them yourself or by using a base with essential oils. If you use essential oils, add 2–3ml of the oil to 30ml of a base such as *Almond, Olive* or *Sunflower* oil. Suitable oils are *Lavender, Marjoram, Peppermint* and *Rosemary,* and they can also be mixed with each other.

Another simple but effective way of relieving pain and swelling is to alternate hot and cold fomentations of water. This first-aid technique can be used when oils and herbs are not at hand.

FIBROSITIS

The advice given for rheumatism and arthritis should be followed.

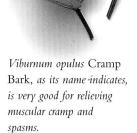

Viburnum opulus Cramp Bark, *as its name indicates, is very good for relieving muscular cramp and spasms.*

CRAMP

We have all experienced muscular cramps at one time or another, which are painful but nothing much to worry about. However, if it becomes an intransigent condition it should be treated, not only to avoid the stressful symptoms, but also because it suggests circulatory problems since it is a symptom of a lack of oxygen.

It is quite an easy matter to remove the problem herbally, if the treatment is continued for a period of time. A mixture of *Cramp Bark, Prickly Ash* and *Ginger* may be used.

Cramp Bark	6 parts	
Prickly Ash	2 parts	
Ginger	1 part	

Drink this decoction three times a day for a number of months.

BURSITIS

The bursae around the knee and elbow joints act as small water-filled cushions between the larger tendons and bones. Inflammation of these sacs is called bursitis.

When it occurs in the knees it is often called housemaid's knee, in the elbow, it is called tennis elbow.

The condition may be due to a hard knock or accident or to a slow change. When it is part of the gradual development of rheumatic tendencies it should be treated as described in the section on rheumatism. When of short-term duration it is best to help the tissues by using a compress on the affected area, or a stimulating liniment *(see box above)*. Both will help reduce the inflammation and ease pain. However, if the problem continues, internal treatment as for rheumatism and arthritis should be started.

Achillea millefolium
Yarrow, *used as a diuretic, can help relieve the symptoms of gout.*

GOUT

This is a specific variety of joint problems due to a build-up of uric acid in the body, which causes extremely painful inflammations. The body needs aid in elimination, especially from the kidneys. The use of diuretics as well as anti-rheumatic herbs will help. Herbs such as *Celery, Boneset, Wild Carrot* and *Yarrow* are especially useful out of all the diuretics available. The following mixture may prove useful.

Burdock Root	1 part	
Celery Seed	1 part	
Yarrow	1 part	

Drink this infusion three times daily over a period of time. If there is much pain, *Thuja* might be included in the mixture.

Diet is paramount in treating and preventing recurrence of gout. A low acid diet provides the basis with a strict avoidance of foods rich in purines that are metabolized in the body to uric acid. These foods include fish such as sardines, anchovies, fish roe, shellfish and crab, liver, kidney, sweetbreads, and beans. Coffee and tea should be left alone and any over-indulgence in general is out. Alcohol has to be totally avoided.

Thymus vulgaris Thyme
makes an excellent herbal bath to soothe and relieve sprains.

LUMBAGO

Lumbago is a general name for pain in the lower back and can be caused by a variety of conditions, ranging from kidney and reproductive system problems to rheumatism and back lesions. The root of the pain must be sought and the appropriate treatment used, whether it be herbs or osteopathy. A warming and stimulating liniment, as described for rheumatism and arthritis, will help. Hot compresses may also be considered for quick symptomatic relief while the cause is being investigated properly.

SCIATICA

This is strictly speaking a form of neuralgia characterized by intense pain and tenderness felt along the length of the sciatic nerve, the longest in the body, extending from the back of the thigh to the lower calf. The term is often used to describe pain that radiates from the hips to the thighs, which can have many causes. There is often a misalignment of spine and hips involved, which in turn presses on the nerve and causes the pain to occur. If this is the case, osteopathic or chiropractic therapy will be most appropriate. Where there is nerve pain or neuralgia, relaxing nervines and tonics will help *(see the section on The Nervous System, pages 202–11)*. However, it is often found that abdominal congestion lies at the root of this painful problem. It is essential to ensure that the bowels are free of constipation, and that the kidneys are working well. In the first place a herb such as *Yellow Dock* is appropriate, but for the kidneys *Bearberry* or *Dandelion* should be used. The general advice given for rheumatism and arthritis *(see pages 222–4)* is appropriate for sciatica. Massage of the lower back and legs may help.

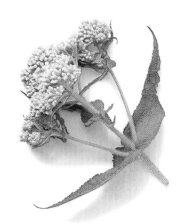

Eupatorium perfoliatum Boneset *helps relieve the symptoms of muscular rheumatism.*

SPRAINS

Muscles can be pulled, and ligaments and tendons sprained through accidents. Hot baths with a stimulating herb added can increase the circulation to the area involved and so speed healing. *Rosemary* or *Thyme* make an excellent addition to a bath, either for the whole body or just the feet.

Add 30–60g/1–2oz of the dried herb to 500ml/1pt of water and either soak the affected part in the hot solution for 15 minutes or soak a bandage or gauze in the solution and apply to the part. This should be repeated every four hours. When there has been a marked reduction in swelling and pain, the affected part should be bandaged and the bandage moistened with distilled *Witch Hazel.*

225

THE GLANDULAR SYSTEM

The body's wisdom is demonstrated by the way in which it maintains a steady internal state and regulates itself. Pervading every activity is the influence of the brain, the master control, with its servants the endocrine and nervous systems.

The endocrine glands are situated in various parts of the body and are characterized by the fact that they release their hormones (chemical messengers) directly into the bloodstream. The hormones then travel to cells in all parts of the body. The membrane of each cell has receptors for one or more hormones, and the binding of a hormone to its specific receptor site starts particular changes in the internal metabolism of this 'target' cell. To gain an overview it will be helpful to examine the roles of the pituitary and hypothalamus glands in this introduction. The activity of these glands is constantly regulated by the

nervous, hormonal and chemical information being fed to them. Hormone production is controlled in many cases by a negative feedback system in which overproduction of a hormone leads to a compensatory decrease in subsequent production until balance is restored. The pituitary gland has a central role in this process of maintaining harmony.

In a small area of the forebrain, just above the pituitary, is the hypothalamus, which is the main co-ordinating centre between the endocrine and nervous system. It functions as a monitor and regulator of the autonomic nervous system, as well as the body's metabolism through eating, drinking and temperature control, and also monitors the menstrual cycle. The anterior pituitary responds to hormones secreted by the hypothalamus, which either stimulate or inhibit the secretion of its own hormones.

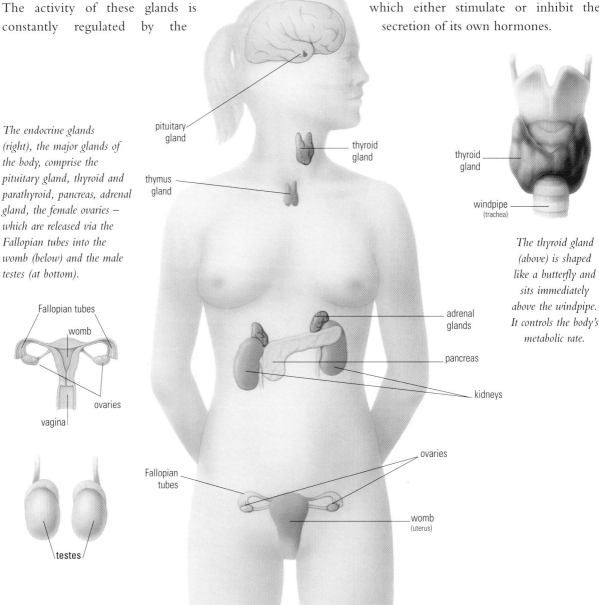

The endocrine glands (right), the major glands of the body, comprise the pituitary gland, thyroid and parathyroid, pancreas, adrenal gland, the female ovaries – which are released via the Fallopian tubes into the womb (below) and the male testes (at bottom).

pituitary gland

thyroid gland

thymus gland

Fallopian tubes

womb

ovaries

vagina

thyroid gland

windpipe
(trachea)

The thyroid gland (above) is shaped like a butterfly and sits immediately above the windpipe. It controls the body's metabolic rate.

adrenal glands

pancreas

kidneys

ovaries

Fallopian tubes

womb
(uterus)

testes

THE PITUITARY GLAND

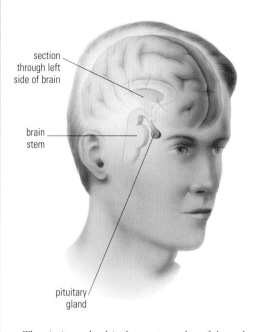

section through left side of brain

brain stem

pituitary gland

The pituitary gland is the most complex of the endocrine glands. A reddish-grey bundle of cells, it is situated just behind the cavity of the nose and secretes eight hormones. It controls the activity of other glands by means of a feedback mechanism; if a particular hormone is lacking in the body, it releases the relevant stimulating hormone, which travels through the blood to the appropriate gland, where more of the necessary hormone is then made.

HEALTH AND THE GLANDS

To be healthy is to have an integrated and smoothly functioning endocrine system. To ensure such health means living a truly whole lifestyle, with appropriate diet, life-affirming emotions and thinking, and a vital spiritual life. The endocrine system is a focus for such techniques as polarity therapy and energy balancing, for through this system the whole body can be healed, and if there is an endocrine imbalance, these therapies can be most effective in regaining harmony.

Herbs for the Glands

The group of herbs best indicated for endocrine treatment are the bitters. Their role in the glandular system is through a generalized reflex stimulation of the whole system. A stimulating action of this sort will promote right homeostatic function, reducing over-activity and increasing underactivity. Some specific agents have powerful effects, but most herbs help the whole body to heal and balance where appropriate.

In addition to the bitters, the alteratives are most useful in their action of cleansing and promoting proper blood functions. The best bitters for the glandular system include *Golden Seal, Mugwort, Rue, Wormwood* and *Yarrow*. Useful alteratives are *Burdock, Cleavers, Echinacea, Dandelion, Red Clover, Sarsaparilla, Violet Leaves* and *Yellow Dock*. There are also specific glandular agents such as *Bladderwrack, Borage, Bugleweed, Ginseng, Goat's Rue, Licorice* and *Wild Yam*. Since endocrine problems are so complex, herbs that are specific to another area, the kidney or liver for instance, may well be the ideal help to regain inner harmony. We must remember to view everything within the context of the whole.

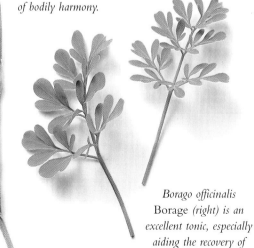

Galega officinalis Goat's Rue *(left) may help stimulate the development of mammary glands.*

Ruta graveolens Rue *(below) has long been used in the restoration of bodily harmony.*

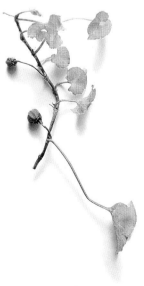

Viola odorata Sweet Violet *(right) may be used in the treatment of urinary infections.*

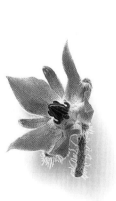

Borago officinalis Borage *(right) is an excellent tonic, especially aiding the recovery of adrenal glands following medical treatment.*

Patterns of Glandular Disease

Endocrine problems have many causes, from external ones like stressful situations to internal ones like genetic disorders. The herbal approach is therefore broad, ensuring that the body becomes strong and vital, and at the same time using specific remedies for different glands.

Even in the absence of overt glandular illness, the endocrine system plays such a fundamental role in health and wholeness that any minor functional problem may lead to a general state of imbalance.

Chionanthus virginicus Fringetree is specific in the treatment of pancreatic problems.

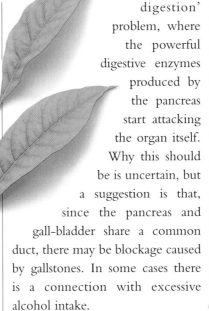

THE PANCREAS

Scattered throughout the tissue of the pancreas are groups of endocrine cells called Islets of Langerhans, which produce two major hormones to control the handling of both glucose and fatty acids in the body.

When blood sugar rises, after a meal for instance, insulin is released which reduces glucose production by the liver and also encourages its usage by the tissues of the body.

The other hormone produced, glucagon, has the opposite effect in the liver and increases glucose production.

• **Pancreatitis** is a very painful inflammation of the pancreas and can show itself in acute or chronic attacks. There appears to be an 'auto-

Lycopus europaeus Bugleweed is very useful in the treatment of over-active thyroid glands, especially where symptoms include shaking and palpitations.

digestion' problem, where the powerful digestive enzymes produced by the pancreas start attacking the organ itself. Why this should be is uncertain, but a suggestion is that, since the pancreas and gall-bladder share a common duct, there may be blockage caused by gallstones. In some cases there is a connection with excessive alcohol intake.

The herbal and dietary indications given in the section on the gall-bladder should be observed. A herb that can be of specific help with this kind of pancreatic problem is *Fringetree Bark*.

• **Diabetes Mellitus** is the most common of the endocrine disorders, affecting over 1% of all people living in the Western world.

The basic problem in diabetes is that the level of glucose in the blood is higher than normal, whilst inside the cell it is low. The causes of this condition are complex and it can result in a range of complications that occur primarily in the arteries and the capillaries.

Diet is a major consideration in the treatment and control of diabetes. It is not simply a matter of avoiding foods rich in carbohydrate, but setting up an eating regime that avoids peaks of glucose entering the blood. Each diet must be tailor-made to suit the individual concerned.

The roots of diabetes are complex and treatment must get to these roots. Professional advice is definitely recommended. Herbs such as *Garlic, Ginseng, Goat's Rue, Jambul, Nettles, Sweet Sumach* and *Fringetree Bark* can be considered for diabetes, although treatment will vary with different conditions.

THE THYROID

The thyroid gland has an important role to play in the regulation of body metabolism. The two main thyroid hormones ensure that the appropriate metabolic rate of body biochemical activity is maintained.

Allium sativum Garlic, along with all its other uses, can be considered for the treatment of diabetes.

• **Over-active Thyroid** When the gland is producing too much of these hormones, the body will burn up food much faster than normal and appetite will increase, but weight will be lost. To treat this effectively involves the use of nervine relaxants to reduce excitability, digestive bitters and a specific herb for this problem, which is *Bugleweed*.

These can relieve the symptoms quite effectively, but a longer-term use of *Bugleweed* and other hormonal tonics is essential. A useful mixture would be:

Bugleweed	2 parts
Nettles	1 part
Valerian	1 part
Yarrow	1 part

This should be drunk three times a day over a period of time.

• **Under-active Thyroid** In this condition the opposite is occurring. The body's basic rate of activity lowers, weight is put on, lethargy and apathy are common, and there is a tendency to deep depression. The herbs that benefit here are the bitters, nervine tonics and the specific thyroid agent, which in this case is *Bladderwrack*. An appropriate mixture is:

Bladderwrack	2 parts
Damiana (or Kola)	1 part
Nettles	1 part
Oats	1 part
Wormwood	1 part

This should be drunk three times a day.

Panax ginseng Ginseng *can alleviate depression brought on by exhaustion.*

• **Goitre** This is a condition where there is an enlargement of the thyroid gland, causing swelling around the front of the neck. It may be due to a variety of medical causes, the most common being either over- or under-active thyroid glands, but it can also simply be due to a deficiency of the trace element iodine in the diet.

By far the richest plant source of iodine is seaweed, and especially *Bladderwrack*.

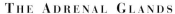

Fucus vesiculosus Bladderwrack *is an exceptional remedy for under-active thyroid glands and the obesity this condition causes.*

THE ADRENAL GLANDS

The adrenal glands are found just above each of the kidneys. They consist of two distinct parts, the outer cortex and inner medulla. The adrenal medulla acts quite separately from the cortex, being the site of the production of adrenalin and nor-adrenalin. These hormones are responsible for the rapid bodily response to extreme stress, the so-called 'fight or flight' effect. It is essential that when this response to a situation occurs, the energy released is used. If the response is inhibited, as it often is when triggered by emotional reactions, the body cannot simply forget the adrenalin. It reacts internally, as external expression is suppressed. Over a period of time this can lead to exhaustion and possibly lay the foundations for chronic disease to present itself anywhere in the body.

With herbal medicine there is the possibility of feeding and renewing the adrenal glands, promoting activity and reintegration in body function. In any case where there has been overexposure to stress, leading to nervous exhaustion and debility, the herbs that aid adrenal function should be considered.

A number of plants are known to contain the natural precursors of the adrenal hormones *(see the section on the Chemistry of Herbs, pages 32–5, for more details).*

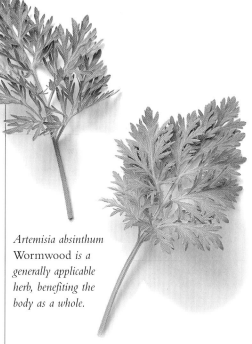

Artemisia absinthum Wormwood *is a generally applicable herb, benefiting the body as a whole.*

The most important of these herbs are *Borage, Ginseng, Licorice* and *Wild Yam*. The long-term use of these herbs can be highly beneficial for anyone in very stressful conditions, especially through regular drinking of *Borage* tea and taking *Ginseng*. If a person has been on steroid drug therapy, *Licorice* is indicated for the revitalization of the adrenals.

THE REPRODUCTIVE SYSTEM

The focus of this section is primarily on the reproductive system of women, as this system is prone to some specific problems. By the nature of human anatomy, there is not the same degree of complexity of structure or function in the male reproductive system. The main physical problem that arises in men is associated with the prostate gland and this is discussed in the section on the urinary system. Infections of the male reproductive system should be approached in the same way as described for infections of the female system.

For the reproductive system to be whole and functioning in a well-balanced and integrated way, body and spirit must be well and thriving as a whole. If the diet is deficient, menstrual problems or vaginal discharges may be generated. If your way of living is not life-affirming, the system

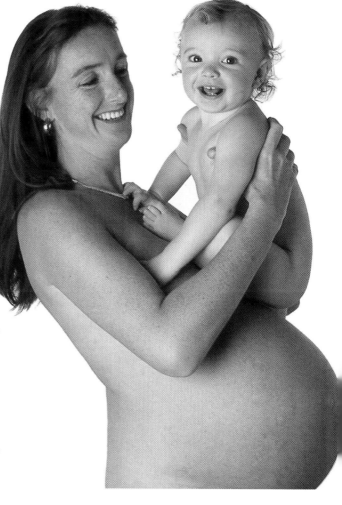

The female reproductive organs (below) are situated in the lower abdomen between the backbone and the pubic bone. The pelvic girdle (below right) protects the ovaries, the Fallopian tubes and the uterus.

The mother's environment and the care she takes of her body (right) before and during pregnancy will affect the health of her baby.

PELVIC GIRDLE

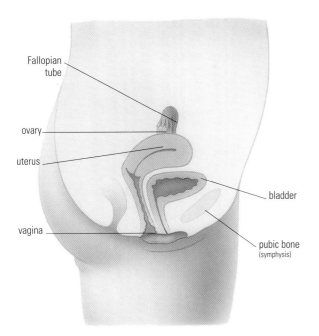

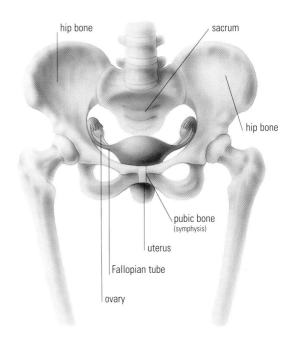

THE MENSTRUAL CYCLE

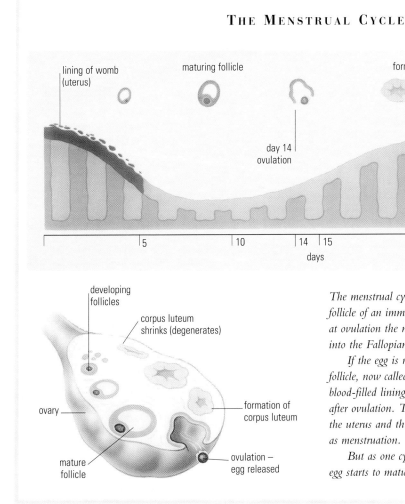

lining of womb (uterus)

maturing follicle

formation of corpus luteum

degenerates

day 14 ovulation

days
5   10   14   15   20   25   28

developing follicles

corpus luteum shrinks (degenerates)

ovary

mature follicle

formation of corpus luteum

ovulation – egg released

The menstrual cycle centres around the life of an egg. The follicle of an immature egg develops in the ovary (left) and at ovulation the mature follicle bursts and releases the egg into the Fallopian tube.

If the egg is not fertilized within seven days the empty follicle, now called the corpus luteum, degenerates and the blood-filled lining of the womb is shed about fourteen days after ovulation. The unfertilized egg is flushed out of the uterus and through the vagina in the process known as menstruation.

But as one cycle ends another is beginning, as a new egg starts to mature.

dedicated to the creation of new life will be adversely affected. For children to be born healthy and happy, and for them to grow well, your lifestyle during pregnancy has to be as good as you can make it. So it is best to check your health in general, but also check your relationships to the world – go for loving and nurturing emotional support. Check your thought life – do you think positively? What sort of books do you read, what films do you watch, what kind of politics are you involved in? The energy within your body is affected by the energy around you and – more importantly – by the way you relate to it. Be at peace with your world and your relationships with it.

Hydrangea arborescens
Hydrangea is extremely useful to the male reproductive system; it is a specific for the treatment of an inflamed or enlarged prostate gland.

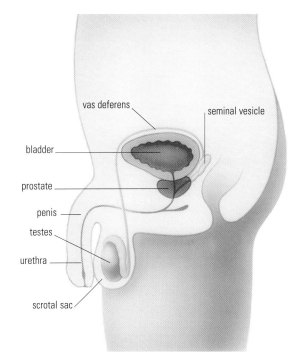

vas deferens

seminal vesicle

bladder

prostate

penis

testes

urethra

scrotal sac

The male reproductive organs are partly external and partly internal. Sperm from the testes move along

the vas deferens to the urethra. Fluid is added and the semen is then ejaculated through the penis.

Herbs for the Female Reproductive System

A great number of herbs benefit the female reproductive system. To help understand the herbal approach we will, as usual, group them according to their actions.

Remarkably, many herbs for the female reproductive system which cannot be duplicated by European remedies have come to us from the cultures of the Native North Americans. We can speculate that this may be due to the deep resonance that existed between these people and the Earth Mother, a resonance that manifested itself in physical terms, of deep healing and aid for women and for the birthing process.

UTERINE TONICS

The uterine tonics have a specifically toning and strengthening action upon the whole system, both on the tissue of the organs and on their functioning. Whilst each has its unique associated actions – which should be checked out to find the most appropriate ones – they all aid the whole reproductive system. Remedies such as *Black Cohosh, Blue Cohosh,* *Chaste Tree, False Unicorn Root, Life Root, Motherwort, Raspberry* and *Squaw Vine* are used as healers in a holistic sense. They are often indicated when there is no obvious acute disease but where a weakness of the sexual organs has a detrimental affect on the whole body.

EMMENAGOGUES

The emmenagogues stimulate and promote a normal menstrual flow. While most of the uterine tonics are also emmenagogues, which act through normalizing the system, there are many other emmenagogues which are not especially healing to the system as a whole. There are even emmenagogues that work by a stimulation that verges on irritation, which can be of benefit in some cases, but it is also the action of herbal abortifacients. A list of those herbs that have to be avoided during pregnancy is given later.

The most useful emmenagogues, out of a potentially endless list, are *Blue Cohosh, False Unicorn Root, Life Root, Motherwort, Parsley, Pennyroyal, Rue, Southernwood, Squaw Vine* and *Yarrow.* The most appropriate one of these for specific treatment should be determined by considering their associated actions.

Cimicifuga racemosa Black Cohosh *is a versatile relaxing nervine, which can be used to normalize the female reproductive system and to aid uterine activity in labour.*

Caulophyllum thalictrioides Blue Cohosh *is a good uterine tonic, which eases false labour pains and helps ensure an easy delivery.*

Petroselinum crispum Parsley *is an effective emmenagogue but should not be used in medicinal dosage during pregnancy, as it may stimulate the womb excessively.*

Rubus idaeus Raspberry *is taken to tone womb tissue, assist contractions and check hemorrhage during labour.*

Artemisia abrotanum Southernwood *can be used to initiate delayed menstruation. It is also known as Lad's Love.*

HORMONAL NORMALIZERS

The hormonal normalizers are an important group. They balance and normalize the functioning of the endocrine glands and so aid the proper functioning of the reproductive system. As they are discussed in detail in the section on the glandular system, I will only mention the most important one, *Chaste Tree*.

This valuable remedy normalizes estrogen and progesterone activity and thus finds a use in all aspects of menstrual dysfunction and especially in conditions associated with menopause.

ASTRINGENTS

Astringents will often be used in the context of this system, and the following have a special affinity to it; *American Cranesbill, Beth Root, Burr-Marigold, Lady's Mantle, Periwinkle* and *Shepherd's Purse.*

DEMULCENTS

Demulcents are often used to provide a soothing and healing action on the system's mucous membranes. The urinary demulcents are often appropriate. A list of these would include *Bearberry, Blue Cohosh, Corn Silk, Golden Seal, Irish Moss* and *Marshmallow.*

ANTISEPTICS

When a condition calls for the use of antiseptics, either one of the general ones or one of the urinary antiseptics can be used: *Bearberry, Couchgrass, Echinacea, Garlic, Juniper, Wild Indigo* and *Yarrow.*

ALTERATIVES AND LYMPHATIC TONICS

As conditions of the reproductive system will affect the whole body, it is often appropriate to use alteratives and lymphatic tonics such as *Blue Flag, Burdock, Cleavers, Echinacea, Poke Root* or *Sarsaparilla.*

NERVINES

The proper and healthy activity of the nerves is vital for the reproductive system to work correctly. Many of the emmenagogues have nervine activity, but in addition it is worth considering the relaxing herbs *Cramp Bark, Skullcap* and *Valerian.* Nervine tonics such as *Damiana* and *Oats* will also be useful.

OTHERS

As there is often a build-up of water associated with conditions of the reproductive system, diuretics may need to be used.

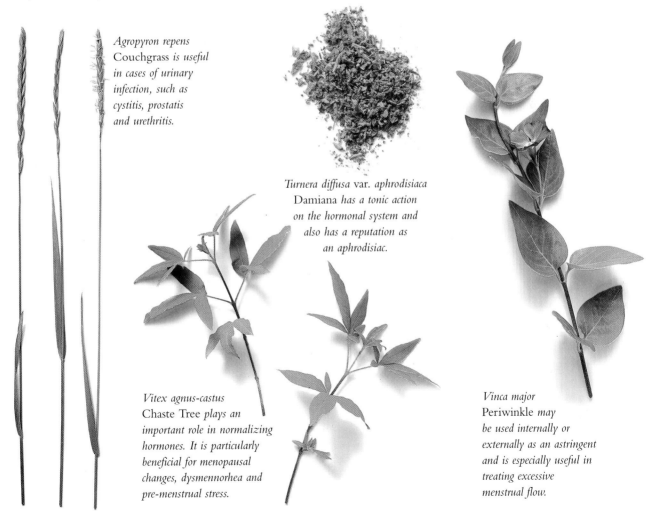

Agropyron repens
Couchgrass *is useful in cases of urinary infection, such as cystitis, prostatis and urethritis.*

Turnera diffusa var. *aphrodisiaca*
Damiana *has a tonic action on the hormonal system and also has a reputation as an aphrodisiac.*

Vitex agnus-castus
Chaste Tree *plays an important role in normalizing hormones. It is particularly beneficial for menopausal changes, dysmennorhea and pre-menstrual stress.*

Vinca major
Periwinkle *may be used internally or externally as an astringent and is especially useful in treating excessive menstrual flow.*

Patterns of Reproductive Disease

We will consider the diseases of the reproductive system in four groups: those associated with the menstrual cycle, those with pregnancy and childbirth, those with menopause and those associated with infections.

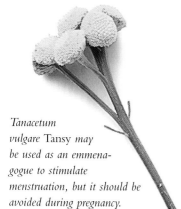

Tanacetum vulgare Tansy may be used as an emmena-gogue to stimulate menstruation, but it should be avoided during pregnancy.

THE MENSTRUAL CYCLE

To ensure a normal and easy menstrual cycle, any of the uterine tonics may be used regularly or perhaps just for the time leading up to the expected onset of the period. 'Normal' is used here recognizing that normalcy is relative and that each individual will have her own norm.

If problems like amenorrhea, menorrhagia, metrorrhagia, dysmenorrhea or pre-menstrual syndrome occur, they can be treated herbally.

• **Amenorrhea** is a condition where there is an absence of menstruation. In adolescents, the first period cycle can be apparently delayed for various reasons, in which case the uterine tonics may help the body to establish its natural rhythm. Perhaps the best herbs are *Blue Cohosh, Chaste Tree Berry, False Unicorn Root, Rue* and *Southernwood*.

If menstruation is delayed or obstructed in adults, the uterine tonics will also help, especially where the cause lies primarily in a withdrawal from the contraceptive pill, with the need for the body to find its way back into its natural rhythm. A mixture of *Blue Cohosh, Chaste Tree Berry, False Unicorn Root* and *Rue* will be very beneficial:

Chaste Tree Berry	2 parts	
False Unicorn Root	2 parts	
Blue Cohosh	1 part	
Rue	1 part	

This tea should be drunk three times a day.

An excellent old remedy for delayed periods is an infusion of equal parts of *Pennyroyal* and *Tansy*, which should be drunk three times a day until the period begins.

PREGNANCY

A word or two about pregnancy. Menstruation may be delayed because of conception. Check first whether the delay is due to a pregnancy, otherwise these herbs might act as abortifacients. The present Western herbal tradition does not have a safe and effective herbal abortifacient. Other traditions may. The emmenagogues are potentially dangerous if used to induce abortion. If you are pregnant and unhappy about it, go to a Family Planning Clinic. If you are not pregnant, these herbs are safe and healing when used as directed.

• **Menorrhagia** Occasionally, period flow will be stronger than normal, a condition called menorrhagia. This excessive flow can be normalized with the use of astringents, which will regulate it without inhibiting the natural process. If the excessive flow continues over a number of periods, it is advisable to consult a gynecologist to make sure that it does not indicate a more severe problem.

While most astringents will help, those with a special affinity for the uterus and associated tissues are certainly the best *(see page 233)*. They should be studied to find the most applicable one, but a treatment could be based on:

American Cranesbill	1 part	
Beth Root	1 part	
Periwinkle	1 part	

This tea should be drunk three times a day in the week leading up to a period and during the flow itself. If it is an ongoing problem, the tea should be drunk once or twice a day throughout the cycle.

• **Metrorrhagia** Where bleeding occurs in the middle of the cycle – or for that matter at any unexpected time – the herbs recommended for menorrhagia will prove useful.

However, it is important to establish the cause, which will often suggest the use of uterine tonics to help in a more fundamental way. Also, the use of *Chaste Tree Berry* is often indicated.

To balance the loss of additional blood during this time, a diet rich in natural iron is essential.

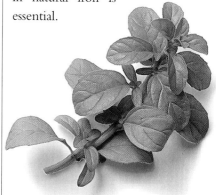

Mentha pulegium Pennyroyal is taken principally to strengthen uterine contractions and as an emmenagogue. It too should be avoided during pregnancy.

• **Dysmenorrhea** is a condition where the period is accompanied by cramping pains, which can be incapacitating in their intensity.

Herbs like uterine tonics, anti-spasmodics and nervines have a lot to offer in the relief of these pains. A mixture of *Black Haw Bark, Cramp Bark* and *Pasque Flower* may be tried:

Black Haw Bark	2 parts	
Cramp Bark	2 parts	
Pasque Flower	1 part	

This tea should be drunk three times daily when needed.

Herbs such as *Black Cohosh, False Unicorn Root* and *Wild Yam* should be considered as well, depending on the condition. Consult The Herbal section to choose the most appropriate herb or combination of herbs for the individual case.

• **Pre-menstrual Syndrome** In the days leading up to the onset of menstruation, tension and anxiety, agitation and depression can occasionally develop, sometimes together with a build-up of water in the body, a heightened sensitivity of the breasts and a range of other symptoms.

All of these are caused by the body's response to the hormonal changes at that time. An important question arises as to whether this is a 'normal' response for that individual or compounded by psychological factors. Which comes first, the psychological condition or the hormone problem?

Deep insights into the inner nature of a culture and its relationship to life can be found in examining whether it relates to menstruation as a magical time that is honoured or an unclean time

Pulsatilla vulgaris Pasque Flower *is a relaxing nervine, useful for the relief of dysmenorrhea, ovarian pain and painful conditions of the testes.*

that is to be hidden. How a woman relates to the whole process of menstruation will deeply affect her body's response to it. Factors that may play a role in compounding pre-menstrual tension can be her relationship to sexuality, the attitudes of relatives, childhood experiences, expectation of tension, or expectation of its interference with work and other activities. If the inner attitude to menstruation is blocked and congested, the experience of the period will reflect this. If the attitude – consciously or not – is clear, at ease and flowing, the experience of menstruation will be the same.

Taking all the above into account, herbs can do a lot to ease pre-menstrual tension. An infusion of equal parts of *Skullcap* and *Valerian* can be taken when and as often as needed. If there is associated cramping, *Cramp Bark* and *Pasque Flower* might be used and if water retention also occurs, then *Dandelion* can be added to the mixture.

• **The Contraceptive Pill** While the need for effective contraception in our over-crowded world is undeniable, the extensive use of contraceptive pills – which are based on hormones – has also created its own problems in our society.

On the physical level, the systemic impact of the pill poses important questions about the effect of its long-term use. The pill is a good example of the two-edged sword of technology, where the solution of one problem raises at least one new problem.

When you stop using the pill, the body – especially its hormonal balance – takes a while to regain its natural harmonic functions. Herbal remedies that act as endocrine balancers and uterine tonics can speed up the process.

Black Cohosh	1 part	
Chaste Tree Berry	1 part	
Licorice	1 part	
Motherwort	1 part	

Drink this tea three times a day for the first two weeks after coming off the pill, twice daily for the third week and once a day for the fourth week.

In this mixture, *Licorice* will aid the adrenal glands, *Black Cohosh* and *Chaste Tree Berry* will tone the uterus and support the glands involved in the production of sex hormones, and *Motherwort,* while augmenting these actions, will also support the nervous system and allow an emotional balance to be regained.

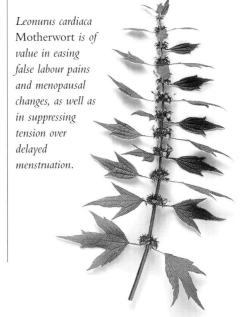

Leonurus cardiaca Motherwort *is of value in easing false labour pains and menopausal changes, as well as in suppressing tension over delayed menstruation.*

235

PREGNANCY AND CHILDBIRTH

Pregnancy is a most special time, for mother and father as much as for the baby coming into life, a time to be treated with great respect and awe. For the baby, this time of peace and still-ness, of security and wholeness, is dependent on the mother's lifestyle and that of those around her.

What she eats and drinks will construct the child's body. The energies of her thoughts and feelings, and of the people around her, will colour and influence the child. Be aware and take care!

Whilst it is the mother who carries the child and directly experiences the miracle of ges-tation, we have all started our lives within the womb. Everybody involved should be wholly present in the process, with willingness, understanding and love – all essential to the wellbeing of the child. Loving consciousness is the key, and the willingness to manifest that which is appropriate. This attitude is basic to all matters of wholeness. Herbal remedies or attention to diet are just parts of the process and will not alone be sufficient to ensure a natural birth and a healthy child.

Whilst nature ensures that the placenta and other physical pro-cesses of mother and child will do the very best that can be done for the new being, much special care can be taken and herbs can be used to assist the process. Many excellent books on natural child-birth are now available and should be studied.

Nature offers an abundance of plants for all stages of the birthing process. Some may be used at specific times, and some

Rubus idaeus Raspberry *leaves have long been used to strengthen and tone the tissue of the womb during pregnancy and to help check the threat of hemorrhage during the birth.*

throughout pregnancy, to ease, aid and tone the tissue and to facilitate the birth itself. By far the best of these are *Raspberry Leaves* and *Squaw Vine,* which may be taken individually or together. A cup per day should be taken for at least the last three months and better for the whole of the nine months – or at least as soon as you know you are pregnant. Apart from these two

HERBS TO BE AVOIDED DURING PREGNANCY

A number of herbs markedly stimulate the uterus; this is the basis of the action of some emmenagogues. Under most conditions this is of no consequence, but during preg-nancy it is important that no externally produced stimula-tion or spasm occurs in the uterus, as this may trigger a miscarriage.

The most common of these stimulating herbs are Autumn Crocus, *Barberry, Golden Seal, Juniper, Male Fern,* Mandrake, *Pennyroyal, Poke Root, Rue, Sage, Southernwood, Tansy, Thuja* and *Wormwood.* Whilst these will not always act as abortifacients, it is well worth avoiding the risk of taking them, as their desired actions can equally be attained by other herbs.

toners, it may be appropriate to use other herbs to augment health in general, ensuring that both nu-trition and bodily function are at their peak.

A typical and usually appro-priate example would be the use of *Nettles* as a source of iron.

• Threatened Miscarriage

Occasionally miscarriage is the body's natural response to certain situations. In such circumstances no herbal remedy will oppose the body's purpose. However, miscarriage can also be threatened in cases of inadequate diet, stress or trauma, and then herbs can provide that extra strength or vitality to avoid an unnecessary miscarriage.

The body can use herbal aid to ensure that the baby thrives. While specific herbs may be appropriate, general uterine tonics such as *Black Haw Bark, Blue Cohosh, Cramp Bark, False Unicorn Root* or *True Unicorn Root* are indicated to protect against a threatened mis-carriage. While all of these may be useful, a combination of toning, anti-spasmodic and nervine relaxant actions can be especially effective.

Blue Cohosh	2 parts	✓
False Unicorn Root	2 parts	▣
Cramp Bark	1 part	◷

Drink this tea three times daily.

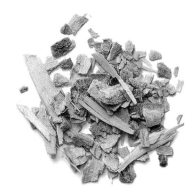

Viburnum opulus Cramp Bark *relaxes the uterus, thus relieving the painful cramp associated with periods and protecting the body from miscarriage.*

If there is a considerable amount of stress involved, stronger nervines like *Skullcap* or *Valerian* may be considered as well.

• **Morning Sickness**
A common occurrence in the first few months of pregnancy is morning sickness, coming most frequently in the morning when the stomach is empty, although it can happen at other times. It seems to be the result of a number of factors acting together. Most important is the massive change in hormone levels that is going on, combined with low blood sugar and possibly low blood pressure. In more naturopathic terms it can be seen as a cleansing of toxins from the system in preparation for pregnancy.

Whilst it is best to avoid any medication during pregnancy, there are some specific and safe remedies that can be used if needed, such as *Black Horehound*, *Irish Moss* and *Meadowsweet*. Gentle nervines that will help as well are *Chamomile*, *Hops* and *Peppermint*. A useful mixture is:

Meadowsweet	2 parts	
Black Horehound	1 part	
Chamomile	1 part	

This tea should be drunk three times a day or as needed. It will be needed less if the diet is nurturing, stress is avoided and the woman respects her body and spirit, herself and her child.

• **Labour** If you drink a tea of *Raspberry Leaves* and *Squaw Vine* through at least the last three months of pregnancy, labour will probably be easy and not too prolonged. However, if labour should be protracted and if the strength of the uterus seems to be

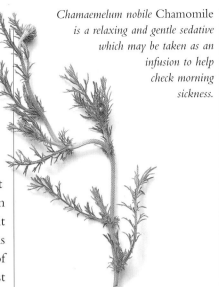

Chamaemelum nobile Chamomile *is a relaxing and gentle sedative which may be taken as an infusion to help check morning sickness.*

waning, herbs may be usefully employed to stimulate the uterus into contraction. By far the most useful and safe oxytocic herb in this case is *Golden Seal*. Whilst it should *not* be used in pregnancy, during labour it may be used to both support and strengthen the body's endeavours.

Cnicus benedictus Blessed Thistle *is an astringent which not only benefits appetite loss and indigestion but also helps to stimulate the flow of breast milk.*

• **Milk Production**
Some mothers find it difficult to either commence milk production or to maintain a high enough level of production when breastfeeding.

Since it is best for the child to be on breast milk for as long as it is feasible, herbs that will help can be invaluable. For this, herbs such as *Aniseed, Blessed Thistle, Caraway Seeds, Fennel Seeds, Fenugreek Seeds, Goat's Rue* and *Vervain* are available, with *Goat's Rue* being perhaps the most powerful. It can safely be drunk three times a day as an

infusion made from one or two tablespoonfuls per cup of water.

The seeds mentioned, which are rich in volatile oils, are also very effective and can be combined to make a very pleasant tea.

Caraway	2 parts
Fennel	1 part
Aniseed	1 part
OR: Fenugreek	2 parts
Aniseed	1 part

To make either of these teas, crush two tablespoonfuls of the seeds and put them in a cup of cold water. Bring it to simmering point and then remove it from the heat. Leave it to stand for 10 minutes, covered to reduce the loss of the volatile oils. Drink a cup of this tea three times a day.

If for some reason the milk flow needs to be stopped, the most effective herb is *Red Sage,* or – if not available – ordinary *Garden Sage,* made into an infusion and drunk three times daily until the desired result is obtained.

THE MENOPAUSE
In our 'civilized' society, the menopause is approached with dread by many women, as it is feared as a time when their role as women becomes devalued. They feel they are no longer sex objects, and that their role as mothers or potential mothers is reduced. The children have left home, and their role as support for the husband in his struggle to earn money and establish himself has often been accomplished. As we tend to draw our identity from socially-defined roles, indeed tend

Hydrastis canadensis Golden Seal *is a tonic and an astringent useful for uterine conditions such as hemorrhage and menorrhagia, but it may also be taken in combination with other herbs to help balance the body during the menopause.*

to become those identities, there seems to be not much left when these roles are gone. But we are not just socially-defined roles! The menopause can be a great gift in a woman's life, a liberation, an initiation. It presents an opportunity to re-evaluate her purpose in life, perhaps to change her life, to see change not as something to fear but as something to embrace as a friend and thus to move onward to greater fulfilment.

Apart from the psychological changes associated with the menopause, there are also hormonal changes which manifest in a physical way and may lead to distressing symptoms.

The most notable of these are the 'hot flushes', brought about by rushes of hormones into the blood as the gland system adjusts to the new situation. As a combined effect of the physiological changes and the psychological impact of the new situation, there may be associated symptoms of 'neurosis' or 'depression'. Disruptions due to the hormonal changes, problems related to the change in self-image and the resistance to that change, can all interact and lead to such psychological symptoms.

As this is a book about herbs, I shall limit my advice to herbal remedies. However, remember that there is much more going on than hormonal change, and that a number of psychotherapeutic

techniques are available to help during this time of change.

The following mixture will help the body to balance and to adapt to the changes, reducing the severity of hot flushes and their frequency, quite quickly too. It should be taken for a few months until all symptoms are gone and the change is completed.

Chaste Tree Berry	2 parts	
Wild Yam	2 parts	
Black Cohosh	1 part	✒
Golden Seal	1 part	▣
Life Root	1 part	◉
Oats	1 part	
St John's Wort	1 part	

Drink this tea three times daily. Use *Motherwort* in place of *St John's Wort,* however, if heart palpitations, high blood pressure or tension are present.

This mixture will ease most of the associated problems and enable the body to establish a new level of hormonal function and integration. Remember that the body knows best. However, in cases of associated anxiety or depression, *Skullcap* or *Valerian* may also be added to the mixture.

INFECTIONS

The whole reproductive system is as susceptible to infections as any other part of the body and because it opens to the outside world it also has distinct problems

Cimicifuga racemosa Black Cohosh *has a normalizing action on the balance of female sex hormones. It may safely be used to regain normal hormonal activity.*

due to infections through contact. In some respects the problems are similar to those of the ear, nose and throat, for here as well it is the mucous membranes that are open to the infection. Discharges of mucus are also common as responses to infections, or are due to the body's effort to get rid of excessive mucus accumulating elsewhere in the body.

To truly heal an infection of the vagina or of any other part of the system, remedies must be used that aid and clear the whole body. Douches or other local applications will at best only get rid of the symptoms for a while.

An appropriate treatment for vaginal infections involves the use of anti-microbials in association with herbs that clear the lymphatics, usually alteratives. To aid the healing of infected tissue, astringents will usually be indicated, especially in cases with mucus discharge. In addition, the whole picture has to be taken into account and the state of general health augmented with the addition of appropriate remedies.

One common cause to bear in mind is the use of the pill or a recent withdrawal from it, for its use will often affect the ecology of the vaginal region. The anti-microbials to use here include *Echinacea, Garlic* or *Wild Indigo,* the lymphatics for this area should be *Cleavers* or *Poke Root,* and of the many astringents that can be applied, *American Cranesbill, Beth Root, False Unicorn Root, Life Root, Oak* and *Periwinkle* are the most frequently used. Most astringents will also prove effective as external applications in combination with a tea. A useful internal mixture would be:

American Cranesbill	2 parts	
Beth Root	2 parts	↗
Echinacea	2 parts	▣
Periwinkle	2 parts	◉
Cleavers	1 part	

This tea should be drunk three times daily.

The mixture may also be used as a douche, made in the same way as an infusion. It should be used three times a day also, to support the internal treatment, and has to be continued for a few days after the infection has cleared. In a similar way yoghurt may be used both internally and externally. This re-establishes the natural bacterial flora so that the regained ecology can look after itself. This is especially good when a problem follows the use of antibiotic drugs.

Humulus lupulus Hops *have a noticeably relaxing effect on the central nervous system and may be used to reduce sexual over-excitability in men.*

The general guidelines on combating infection of course apply here. The diet should be rich in natural vitamins and minerals, especially from fruit and vegetable sources. Perhaps a vitamin C supplement is indicated, especially after antibiotic therapy. Abundant garlic in the diet is advisable, preferably raw.

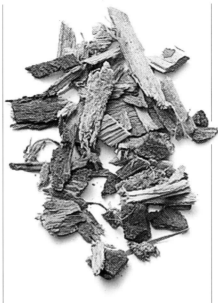

Quercus robur Oak *is an effective astringent in combating diarrhea, dysentery and hemorrhoids, but is also of value in combating vaginal infections.*

HERBS AND SEXUALITY

Almost all cultural traditions in the world have favourite herbs that have the reputation of increasing libido and of reversing impotence. For one of them, *Damiana*, such a reputation was even carried into its botanical name, *Turnera diffusa* var. *aphrodisiaca*. Whether the aphrodisiacs work by directly stimulating a sexual urge is highly debatable. In my opinion such an action does not exist. However, it is possible to enhance sexuality by using herbs if we look at it in holistic terms. If the body is full of vitality, is at ease and the mind is poised and at peace, sex can be a powerful expression of that vitality. From this angle, herbs that will help us to be in such a space of ease and wholeness, will act in a roundabout way as aphrodisiacs. A few herbs such as *Damiana, Ginseng* and *Saw Palmetto*

have a reputation as tonics for the reproductive glands and especially for the male system. They not only undoubtedly strengthen the system itself, but can also help to move a person into a state of greater embodiment of their innate wholeness and vitality.

If sexual problems arise in connection with stress and tension, nervine relaxants and tonics such as *Lime Blossom, Oats* or *Skullcap* may be indicated.

If the general state of health is in any way below par, it should be aided by the appropriate remedies, with the bitter tonics often being very helpful.

The old herbals are also rich in remedies that will reduce the sexual drive. Cures for nymphomania and masturbation abound! If it is appropriate to reduce the experience or expression of sexual energy, the combined used of nervine relaxants (to take off some of the energy) and nervine tonics (to strengthen and support the system) can be indicated, with good herbs being *Passion Flower, Valerian* or *Wild Lettuce. Hops* are especially good for men if there is a need to reduce sexual over-excitability.

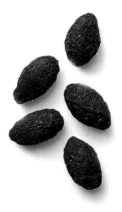

Seronoa repens Saw Palmetto Berries *are valuable in toning and strengthening the male reproductive system. They are particularly effective for enlarged prostate glands.*

THE URINARY SYSTEM

Much that can be said about the relationship of the kidneys to the body can also be said about the role of any individual or group within an ecosystem, about an ecosystem within the biosphere, about planets within our solar system, and so on outward. If we go inward, into our body and into the cell structure, we find similar patterns of relationships.

The kidney is primarily dedicated to the maintenance of a constant and healthy internal environment in the body. It is an organ of homeostasis. The inner architecture of the kidney and the way its amazing structure fulfils its complex functions is beyond the scope of this book. However, we should at least look at some of the things the kidney can do, and how it works.

Its most important function is the regulation of the body's water content. Although the kidney is often described as excreting water, its duty is really more one of conserving it, for much of

the water that passes through the kidneys is reabsorbed. Only a comparatively small amount, which acts as a solvent for the waste materials, is actually passed on into the bladder. The kidney also regulates the relative salt balance in the body, excreting excess amounts. Another important function of the kidney is the role it plays in the maintenance of the acid/alkali balance of the blood.

It is also responsible for separating waste from useful substances. As the blood filters through the kidneys, many vital molecules, such as glucose and amino-acids, leave the blood and enter the urine fraction. These important molecules are later reabsorbed, while waste products are excreted. The complexity of the kidney reflects its function of differentiating between waste products and vital substances. The kidney is also involved in the production of the hormone renin, which is involved in the regulation of blood pressure.

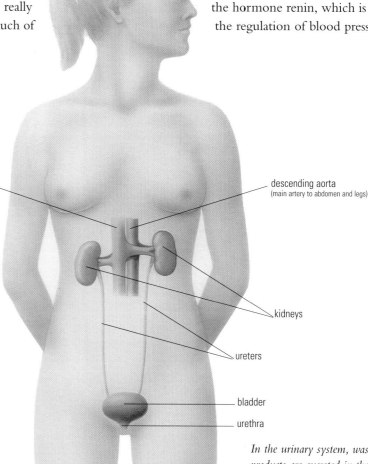

inferior vena cava
(main vein of abdomen)

descending aorta
(main artery to abdomen and legs)

kidneys

ureters

bladder

urethra

Inflammation of the male prostate gland, which is situated immediately below the bladder, causes pain on urination and also restricts the flow of urine.

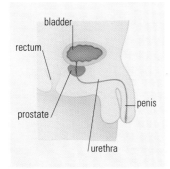

bladder

rectum

prostate

penis

urethra

In the urinary system, waste products are excreted in the urine, which is carried from the kidneys down the ureters, through the bladder and out of the body via the urethra.

Herbs for the Urinary System

Considering the importance of the kidneys, it is not surprising that nature is abundant in herbs that can aid their functions. Looking at the role of the kidneys in a holistic context, it is obvious that the proper function of any part of the body is dependent on the effective elimination of waste products and toxins. As our diet tends to include unnatural and harmful chemicals, and as our lifestyle is largely out of harmony with our outer environment and the needs of the inner environment, the role of the kidneys becomes even more important.

Herbs that aid the kidneys are not only useful for urinary problems but may be relevant to aid the body's cleansing mechanism in treating the whole body, no matter what the problem.

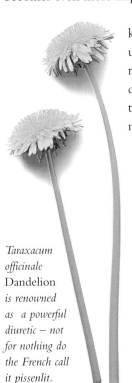

Taraxacum officinale Dandelion *is renowned as a powerful diuretic – not for nothing do the French call it pissenlit.*

DIURETICS

In a strict sense, a diuretic is a plant that increases the excretion and flow of urine. However, the term tends to be used more generally for any herb that acts on the kidneys or the bladder. The list of diuretics is enormous but perhaps the most effective and valuable diuretic recommended for general use is *Dandelion*. Not only is it as effective as synthetic diuretics, *Dandelion* also contains a high percentage of potassium, an element that is often washed out of the body by the use of such synthetic diuretics.

All the plants described throughout this section have diuretic properties associated with other specific actions related to the urinary system. One more general diuretic worth mentioning here is *Cleavers*. Its simple diuretic action combined with alterative properties can safely benefit most conditions.

URINARY ANTISEPTICS

The antiseptic action of some diuretic herbs is usually due to a content of volatile oils or glycosides which are excreted through the kidney tubules, thus

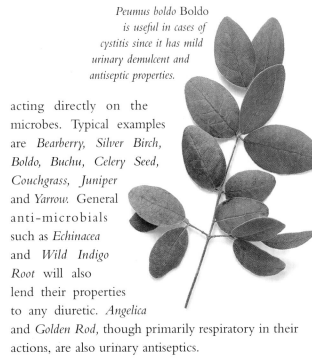

Peumus boldo Boldo *is useful in cases of cystitis since it has mild urinary demulcent and antiseptic properties.*

acting directly on the microbes. Typical examples are *Bearberry, Silver Birch, Boldo, Buchu, Celery Seed, Couchgrass, Juniper* and *Yarrow*. General anti-microbials such as *Echinacea* and *Wild Indigo Root* will also lend their properties to any diuretic. *Angelica* and *Golden Rod,* though primarily respiratory in their actions, are also urinary antiseptics.

URINARY DEMULCENTS

In some conditions, the tissue of the urinary membranes needs to be soothed if it is irritated because of an infection or friction, as from a kidney stone. Herbs such as *Corn Silk, Couchgrass* or *Marshmallow Leaf* supply a demulcent action and can be used together with other urinary remedies.

URINARY ASTRINGENTS

Whilst blood in the urine is a symptom that needs professional attention and diagnosis, it can be treated with the aid of astringents if it turns out to be caused by a minor problem. Astringents will stop hemorrhaging in the kidneys, bladder, urethra or ureter and will also aid the healing of lesions. The best urinary astringents are *Beth Root, Burr-Marigold, Horsetail* and *Plantain*. *Tormentil* is another good astringent which is mildly antiseptic and vulnerary at the same time.

ANTI-LITHICS

Another important property of some diuretics is their ability to prevent the formation, or aid in the removal, of calculi (stones or gravel) in the urinary system. There are many herbs with the reputation of being anti-lithics, but *Gravel Root, Hydrangea, Parsley Piert, Pellitory of the Wall* and *Stone Root* are perhaps the most effective ones.

Juniperus communis Juniper Berries *also act as an effective* antiseptic in urinary conditions such as cystitis.

Patterns of Urinary Disease

The urinary system, kidney and bladder are prone to a range of problems that reflect those developing in the body as a whole. It is best to view urinary conditions as manifestations of systemic problems, which is really the way all specific diseases should be approached.

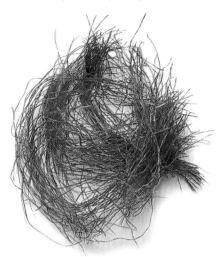

Zea mays Corn Silk *is a soothing diuretic that will help relieve any urinary irritation. It is frequently used for renal problems in children.*

INFECTIONS

The urinary system is subject to a variety of infections. Low resistance may be caused by such things as inadequate diet or chronic constipation; another common cause is the use of antibiotics.

When antibiotics are used they inflict a physiological shock upon the system and disturb our inner ecology. After their use it is vital to help the body re-strengthen its defence system, which may be done by eating live yoghurt to renew the beneficial bacterial flora of the intestines and by taking additional vitamin C.

• **Cystitis** This infection of the bladder is characterized by a scalding pain experienced on passing water as well as by pain in the groin before, during and just after urination.

Cystitis may also be accompanied by an intense desire to pass water even though the bladder is empty. Herbs such as *Bearberry, Buchu, Couchgrass, Juniper Berries* and *Yarrow* may be used. Do not use *Juniper Berries* if there is a tendency for an inflamed condition of the kidneys. While a hot tea of *Yarrow*, taken often, might solve the problem by itself, this mixture can also be used.

Bearberry	1 part	
Couchgrass	1 part	
Yarrow	1 part	

This tea should be drunk hot every two hours as long as the cystitis is acute, then three times a day for a while to totally cure it. If the burning is very strong or if there is blood in the urine, a demulcent such as *Corn Silk* may be added.

The diet has to be low in acid-forming foods as well as in sugar and artificial additives.

As a precaution, and particularly in acute cases, the use of deodorant douches is to be avoided as they disrupt the area's ecology.

• **Urethritis** This infection of the urethra can be treated in the same way as cystitis, but it may be beneficial to increase the proportion of demulcent herbs in the mixture.

• **Prostatitis** In an infection of the prostate gland, the symptoms may not be as localized as in the case of cystitis. Therefore, in addition to the urinary antiseptics used in cystitis, the systemic antimicrobial *Echinacea* can be added and the masculine gonad gland tonic *Saw Palmetto Berries* should also be considered.

This is also used in the case of a swollen prostate gland. A useful mixture consists of:

Bearberry	1 part	
Couchgrass	1 part	
Echinacea	1 part	
Horsetail	1 part	
Hydrangea	1 part	

This tea should be drunk three times daily.

• **Pyelonephritis** is an infection located in the pelvis or the kidney. It may also affect other kidney tissue and can be accompanied by intense and incapacitating pain. It is advisable to seek professional help with this problem.

The herbal approach is to treat the sufferer for systemic infection and fever, giving prominence to the urinary antiseptics such as *Bearberry, Buchu* and *Pellitory of the Wall*, which is sometimes considered to be a specific remedy for this problem.

KIDNEY PROBLEMS

Herbal remedies have much to offer in the treatment of kidney problems, whether minor or major in nature. However, as this organ is so fundamental to health and life, any treatment of kidney disease should be undertaken by qualified and trained practitioners.

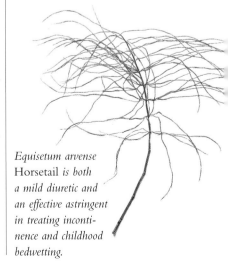

Equisetum arvense Horsetail *is both a mild diuretic and an effective astringent in treating incontinence and childhood bedwetting.*

Eupatorium purpureum Gravel Root *is an anti-lithic and diuretic, which is used particularly in cases of kidney stones and gravel and, to a lesser extent, in infections such as cystitis and urethritis.*

• **Water Retention**

When kidneys do not eliminate enough water, some of it collects in the body and is often retained, due to gravity, in the feet and lower legs. The cause for the retention must be sought, and it usually lies in the kidneys themselves or in the circulatory system. The basis of water retention can vary from pre-menstrual tension, through pregnancy to heart failure. It is impossible to give guidelines for differential diagnosis. Please get skilled advice before embarking on using herbs to remove the water. If the use of herbal diuretics produces little or no change within ten days, then you should definitely seek professional advice.

Only when the basic cause is identified and treated can the water retention be truly stopped, but there are herbs that will remove the retained water. All of the diuretic herbs may be used, but the most effective ones are *Bearberry, Dandelion Leaf* and *Yarrow.*

• **Kidney Stones** The formation of mineral deposits – stones or gravel – is a process that responds well to herbal treatment.

A low acid diet is indicated, totally avoiding foods high in oxalic acid such as rhubarb and spinach. It is important that anyone with stones or a tendency for their formation should drink a lot of water to ensure that the system is being flushed. At least three litres (six pints) of water a day is recommended, preferably water low in mineral content. If there is a lot of sweating, it must also be compensated for. To treat kidney stones herbally, anti-lithics are called for to dissolve the stones or aid their passing and to guard against further deposits. Diuretic action is also needed to increase the amount of fluid going through the kidneys and thus to flush out deposits. Fortunately most anti-lithics are also diuretics. Herbs such as *Gravel Root, Hydrangea, Parsley Piert, Pellitory of the Wall, Stone Root* and *Wild Carrot* fall into this category. Urinary demulcents such as *Corn Silk, Couchgrass* and *Marshmallow Leaf* should also be considered to soothe the mucous membranes and to guard against any abrasion through friction. If there is any hint of an infection or even if there is only a tendency for one to develop, anti-microbials such as *Bearberry, Echinacea* or *Yarrow* should be used.

For a good general treatment of stones and gravel the following mixture can be used.

Corn Silk	1 part	
Gravel Root	1 part	
Hydrangea	1 part	
Stone Root	1 part	

This tea should be drunk three times daily.

If you have a tendency to form kidney stones, you can also use this tea regularly once a day as a preventative measure.

• **Renal Colic** If a small stone moves into the ureter and gets stuck there, it may obstruct the flow of urine and cause renal colic, which can be extremely painful. The use of anti-spasmodic herbs like *Cramp Bark, Sea Holly* or *Valerian* may help, but the attack will be relieved completely only when the blockage either moves or is passed altogether.

• **Incontinence** can be caused by a number of physical and psychological factors. As long as there is no organic defect or illness involved, it can be brought under control herbally, even where it is due to a loss of tone of the sphincter muscle of the bladder or to a general muscle or nervous debility. A good herbal mixture would be:

Horsetail	2 parts	
Agrimony	1 part	
Sweet Sumach	1 part	

Drink this tea three times a day.

Night incontinence in children is often due to psychological factors that should be recognized and worked with if the herbs are not effective.

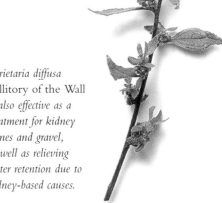

Parietaria diffusa Pellitory of the Wall *is also effective as a treatment for kidney stones and gravel, as well as relieving water retention due to kidney-based causes.*

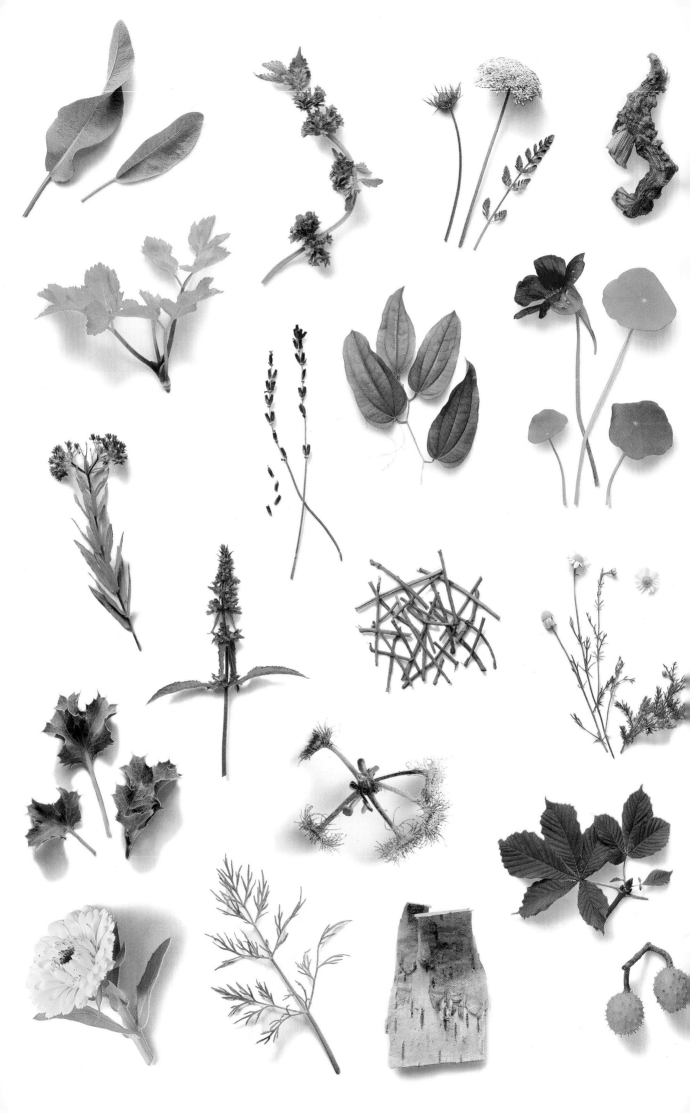

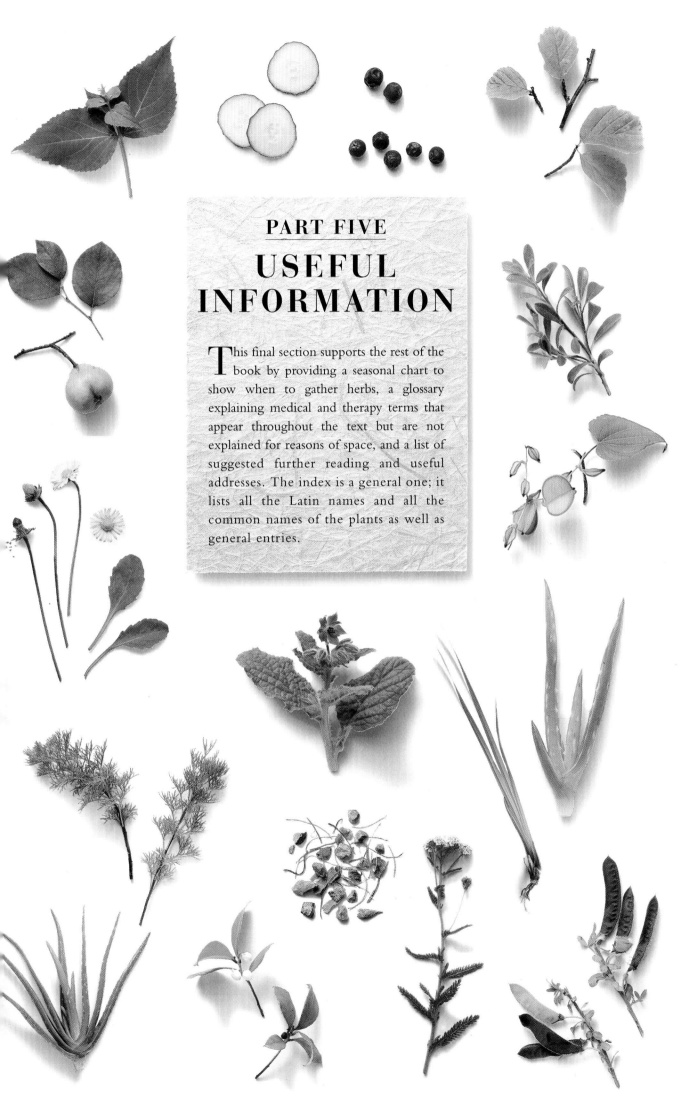

PART FIVE

USEFUL INFORMATION

This final section supports the rest of the book by providing a seasonal chart to show when to gather herbs, a glossary explaining medical and therapy terms that appear throughout the text but are not explained for reasons of space, and a list of suggested further reading and useful addresses. The index is a general one; it lists all the Latin names and all the common names of the plants as well as general entries.

WHEN TO GATHER HERBS

In every season nature offers herbs, but naturally not everything is available at all times. To find out when a herb can be collected, refer to the chart below. When different parts of a herb are collected at different times, they are listed separately. The information is a general guide; obviously local conditions will vary.

Name	Spring	Summer	Fall	Winter
Agrimony	-	●	-	-
Angelica, leaves	-	●	-	-
Angelica, root	-	-	●	-
Aniseed	-	●	●	-
Avens, aerial parts	-	●	-	-
Avens, root	●	-	-	-
Balm	-	●	●	-
Balmony	-	●	●	-
Barberry	●	-	●	-
Bayberry	●	-	●	-
Bearberry	●	●	-	-
Beth Root	-	●	●	-
Birch, Silver	●	●	-	-
Bistort	-	●	●	-
Bittersweet	-	-	●	-
Black Cohosh	-	-	●	-
Black Haw	-	-	●	-
Black Horehound	-	●	-	-
Black Root	-	-	●	-
Black Willow	●	-	-	-
Blessed Thistle, aerial parts	-	●	-	-
Blessed Thistle, seeds	-	-	●	-
Blood Root	●	●	●	-
Blue Cohosh	-	-	●	-
Blue Flag	-	-	●	-
Bogbean	●	●	-	-
Boldo	●	●	●	●
Boneset	-	●	●	-
Borage	●	●	●	-
Broom Tops	●	●	●	-
Buchu	●	●	●	-
Buckthorn	-	-	●	-
Burdock	-	-	●	-
Burr-Marigold	-	●	●	-
Butterbur, leaves	●	●	●	-
Butterbur, rhizome	●	●	-	-

Name	Spring	Summer	Fall	Winter
Calamus	-	-	●	-
Californian Poppy	-	●	●	-
Caraway	-	●	-	-
Carline Thistle	-	-	●	-
Catnip	-	●	●	-
Celery	-	●	●	-
Chamomile	●	●	-	-
Chaste Tree	-	-	●	●
Chickweed	●	●	●	●
Cleavers	●	-	-	-
Coltsfoot, flowers	●	-	-	●
Coltsfoot, leaves	●	●	-	-
Comfrey	●	-	-	-
Coriander	-	●	-	-
Couchgrass	●	●	●	-
Cowslip, flowers	●	-	-	-
Cowslip, root	●	-	-	●
Cramp Bark	●	-	-	-
Cranesbill, American	-	-	●	-
Cudweed	-	●	-	-
Daisy	●	●	●	-
Dandelion, leaves	●	●	●	●
Dandelion, root	-	●	-	-
Dill	-	●	●	-
Echinacea	-	-	●	-
Elder, bark and berries	-	●	●	-
Elder, flowers	●	●	-	-
Elecampane	-	-	●	-
Ephedra	-	-	●	●
Eyebright	-	●	●	-
False Unicorn Root	-	-	●	-
Fennel	-	●	●	-
Figwort	-	●	-	-
Flax	-	-	●	-
Fringetree Bark	●	-	●	-
Fumitory	-	●	●	-
Garlic	-	-	●	-
Gentian	-	-	●	-
Goat's Rue	-	●	-	-
Golden Rod	-	●	●	-
Gravel Root	-	-	●	-
Greater Celandine	-	●	●	●
Ground Ivy	●	●	-	-
Hawthorn Berries	-	-	●	-
Hops	-	●	●	-
Horsechestnut	-	-	●	-

Name	Spring	Summer	Fall	Winter
Horseradish	–	–	●	●
Horsetail	●	●	–	–
Hydrangea	–	–	●	–
Hyssop	–	●	–	–
Iceland Moss	●	●	●	–
Juniper Berries	–	–	●	–
Lady's Mantle	–	●	–	–
Lavender	–	●	●	–
Life Root	–	●	–	–
Lily of the Valley	●	●	–	–
Lime Blossom	–	●	●	–
Lobelia	–	●	●	–
Lungwort Herb	●	●	●	–
Male Fern	–	–	●	–
Mallow	–	●	●	–
Marigold	–	●	●	–
Marjoram, Wild	–	●	●	–
Marshmallow, leaves	●	●	–	–
Marshmallow, root	–	–	●	–
Meadowsweet	–	●	–	–
Mistletoe	●	–	–	–
Motherwort	–	●	●	–
Mountain Grape	–	–	●	–
Mouse Ear	●	●	–	–
Mugwort	–	●	●	–
Mullein, flowers	–	●	–	–
Mullein, leaves	–	●	–	–
Mustard	–	●	●	–
Nasturtium	–	●	●	–
Nettle	●	●	–	–
Oak Bark	●	–	–	–
Oats	–	●	–	–
Pansy	●	●	–	–
Parsley Piert	–	●	–	–
Pasque Flower	●	–	–	–
Passion Flower	●	●	–	–
Peach, bark	●	–	–	–
Peach, leaves	–	●	–	–
Pellitory of the Wall	–	●	●	–
Pennyroyal	–	●	–	–
Periwinkle	●	–	–	–
Pilewort	●	●	–	–
Pine, Scots	●	–	–	●
Plantain	–	●	●	–
Pleurisy Root	●	–	–	–
Poke Root	●	–	–	●

Name	Spring	Summer	Fall	Winter
Prickly Ash Bark	–	–	●	–
Pumpkin	–	●	●	–
Queen's Delight	–	●	–	–
Quince	–	–	●	–
Ragwort	–	●	●	–
Raspberry	●	●	●	–
Red Clover	●	●	●	–
Red Poppy	–	●	–	–
Red Sage	●	●	–	–
Rosehips	–	–	●	–
Rosemary	–	●	●	–
Rue	●	●	–	–
St John's Wort	–	●	●	–
Self-Heal	–	●	–	–
Senega	–	–	●	–
Shepherd's Purse	●	●	●	●
Silverweed	–	●	–	–
Skullcap	–	●	●	–
Soapwort, leaves	–	●	–	–
Soapwort, root and rhizome	–	–	●	–
Squaw Vine	●	●	–	–
Stone Root	–	–	●	–
Sundew	–	●	–	–
Sweet Violet	●	–	–	●
Tansy	–	●	●	–
Thuja	●	●	●	–
Thyme	–	●	–	–
Tormentil	–	–	●	–
True Unicorn Root	–	●	–	–
Valerian	–	–	●	–
Vervain	–	●	–	–
Wahoo	–	–	●	–
White Horehound	–	●	●	–
White Poplar	●	–	–	–
Wild Carrot, aerial parts	–	●	–	–
Wild Carrot, seeds	–	●	●	–
Wild Cherry	–	–	●	–
Wild Indigo	–	–	●	–
Wild Lettuce	–	●	–	–
Wintergreen	●	●	●	–
Witch Hazel	●	●	●	–
Wood Sage	●	●	●	–
Wormwood	–	●	●	–
Woundwort	–	●	–	–
Yarrow	–	●	●	–
Yellow Dock	–	●	●	–

GLOSSARY

For further definitions of the actions of herbs refer to pages 36-9 The Action of Herbs

abortifacient
substance that causes
the early expulsion
of an unborn baby

abscess
a lump of pus caused
by inflammation or
bacteria

acne
common skin
disorder
usually caused
by hormone
imbalance
(especially during
adolescence)

adaptogen
a substance that
modulates hormones

Addison's disease
disease caused by
underactivity of the
adrenal glands

adenitis
inflammation of a gland

adenoids
lymphatic tissue at the back
of the nose

adrenal gland
a two-part gland situated
just above each kidney

adrenaline
substance secreted by part
of the adrenal gland that
increases the heart rate in
response to stress

allergy
abnormal response by the
body to a food or foreign
substance

Alexander Principle
a manipulative
technique based on
improving posture
and encouraging
the practice of
deep
breathing;
established
at the end
of the 19th
century by
F. Matthias
Alexander,
an Australian
Hops actor

alveolus
air pockets in the lung;
they cluster together like
grapes

amebic dysentery
dysentery caused by a
parasitic ameba

amenorrhea
absence of menses
(periods)

anal fissure
a split between the
skin and the mucous
membrane around
the anus

anemia
defiency of hemoglobin in
the blood

angina pectoris
severe pain in the lower
chest, usually on the left
side

anodyne
pain-killing

anorexia nervosa
psychological problem
causing extreme loss
of appetite and drastic
weight loss

anti-allergic
substance that reduces
allergic reactions

anti-bacterial
substance that prevents
bacteria from forming

anti-depressive
substance that relieves
depression

anti-hemorrhagic
substance that halts
bleeding

anti-hidrotic
substance that prevents
perspiration

anti-neoplastic
substance that helps prevent
abnormal growths

anti-pyretic
preventing fever

anti-rheumatic
substance that relieves
rheumatic problems

anti-tussive
substance that prevents
coughing

anti-viral
substance that prevents
viruses attacking
the body

appendicitis
inflammation of the
appendix

arteriosclerosis
hardening of the arteries

arthritis
painful inflammation of
joint tissues

asthma
spasm of the bronchi in
the lungs, narrowing
the airways

astringent
substance able to
contract cell walls
and stop unwanted
discharge

atony
lack of normal tension
in the muscles

bile
thick, oily fluid
excreted by the
liver; bile helps the
body digest fats

biliousness
disorder of bile
production (to
excess)

blepharitis
inflammation of
the eyelids

bronchitis *Pellitory of*
infection of *the Wall*
the bronchi,
the tubes that
take air to the
lungs

brucellosis
bacterial infection caught
from close contact with
animals. Symptoms similar
to flu

bursitis
inflammation of the water-
filled cushions surrounding
the knee (bursae)

carbuncle
collection of boils in the
skin

carcinogenic
substance that can cause
cancer

cardio-active
substance that stimulates
heart activity

caries
decay occuring in teeth

catarrh
excessive excretion of the
phlegm from the air
passage

cathartic
substance that purges the
body, usually the intestine,
and cleanses the system

celiac disease
a condition caused by a
strong allergy to gluten

chiropractic
a manipulative
therapy which places
importance on the
spine, the pivot of the
nervous system,
removing pressure
from the nerves
and allowing
them to function
more efficiently.
Founded by
American
osteopath David
Daniel Palmer
in 1895

colic
abdominal pain
caused by
wind in the
intestines

concussion
loss of conciousness
due to a blow on
the head

conjunctivitis
infection of the mucous
membrane (conjunctiva)
of the eye

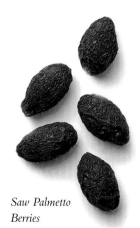

*Saw Palmetto
Berries*

constipation
condition where evacuating the bowels is infrequent and difficult

Crohn's Disease
inflammatory disease of the bowel

croup
inflammation of the larynx affecting young children and babies

cystitis
bladder infection causing infrequent and painful urination

debility
weakness

dermatitis
inflammation of the skin

diabetes mellitus
condition whereby the pancreas produces little or no insulin, resulting in a high blood sugar level that could lead eventually to a hyperglycemic coma

diarrhea
frequent evacuation of loose (watery) stools

diverticulitis
inflammation of weak points in the large intestine (especially in the elderly)

duodenum
the first stretch of the small intestine

dysentery
acute intestinal infection causing severe pain and diarrhea

dysmenorrhea
severe pains accompanying monthly period

dyspepsia
indigestion

eczema
term for a wide range of skin conditions

emphysema
condition caused by air entering the tissues of the air sacs (alveoli) in the lungs and breaking down the thin walls so that gas exchange cannot take place

enteritis
inflammation that can occur in any section of the small intestine

epilepsy
abnormality of brain function causing seizures

Feldenkrais Technique
a manipulative therapy that works on posture, stance and gesture to improve self-awareness of the body image and so change or improve mental patterns. Founded by Russian engineer and physicist Dr Moshe Feldenkrais in the 1940s

Woundwort

fibrositis
inflammation of the body's connective tissue

fistula
abnormal channel linking body cavities

flatulence
excessive amount of gas in stomach or intestines

gall-bladder
organ that stores bile and sends it to the duodenum

gallstones
insoluble stones which occur in the gall-bladder

gas exchange
the exchange of waste carbon dioxide in the blood for fresh oxygen; it takes place in the alveoli of the lungs

gastritis
inflammation of the stomach lining

gingivitis
inflammation of the gums

goitre
condition where there is enlargement of the thyroid gland, causing swelling at the front of the neck

gout
inflammation in joints caused by a build-up of uric acid

hayfever
allergic reaction to pollen causing inflammation of the mucous membranes of the nose and eyes

hemorrhage
loss of blood

hemorrhoids – see piles

impetigo
extremely infectious skin disease

incontinence
partial or complete loss of control of urination

indigestion
condition where digestion is difficult, resulting in abdominal pain

insomnia
condition where falling asleep is difficult or impossible

jaundice
symptom of congestion in the liver where the skin and whites of the eyes turn yellowish in colour

laryngitis
inflammation of the larynx

larynx
section of the top part of the windpipe (trachea) containing vocal cords

Leishmania
parasite which causes skin diseases

leucorrhea
vaginal discharge, often indicating infection

louse
microscopic insect that sucks blood from the skin

lymph glands
tissue masses throughout the body that help protect against infection

malabsorption
condition where the ability of the small intestine to absorb food is diminished

malaria
potentially fatal disease passed on by female mosquitoes from the Anopheles family

mastitis
acute inflammation of the breasts

mastoiditis
ear infection that can often cause a boil on the outer ear

meningitis
inflammation of the membranes that protect the brain

menorrhagia
an excess loss of blood occurring during menstruation

menstrual flow
discharge of blood and tissue debris of monthly period

metrorrhagia
bleeding which occurs in the middle of the menstrual cycle

mucous colitis
irritation of the colon resulting in mucus secretion

nutritive
substance that promotes nutrition

orexigenic
stimulating to the appetite

osteo-arthritis
most common form of arthritis, affecting mainly hips, knees and shoulders

osteopathy
a manipulative technique used on the joints and now accepted in orthodox medicine. Like chiropractic, it concentrates on the spine. Founded in the 1870s by American orthodox medical practitioner Dr Andrew Taylor Still

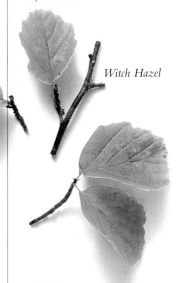

Witch Hazel

palpitations
erratic/fast beating of the heart

pancreatitis
inflammation of the pancreas (one of the endocrine glands that release chemicals into the bloodstream)

parasiticide
parasite killer

Parkinson's Disease
a progressive disease of the nervous system

parturient
encouraging onset of
labour

peptic ulcer
an ulcer occurring on
the internal membranes
of the digestive tract

**peripheral
vasoconstrictor**
substance that constricts
the blood vessel walls
on the surface of the
body

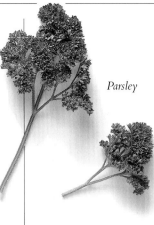

Parsley

peristalsis
rhythmic movement of the
gut to push food along the
intestinal tract

peritonitis
infection in the abdomen

pharyngitis
inflammation of the
pharynx, the airway from
the back of the nose to the
trachea (windpipe)

phlebitis
inflammation of the veins
closest to the skin

piles
swollen veins in the anus
wall

pityriasis
skin disorder resulting in a
scaly rash

pleurisy
inflammation of the
membrane which
surrounds the lungs
(pleura)

pneumonia
a lung infection usually
caused by bacteria
or viruses

polyp
swollen mass of inflamed
mucous membrane,
usually in the nasal
cavity

prostate gland
male gland surrounding
neck of bladder and
urethra

prostatitis
inflamed or enlarged
prostate gland

protozoal infection
parasitic infection

psoriasis
skin disorder causing skin
to become dry and itchy

pulmonary
of the lungs

purgative – see laxative

pyelitis
infection of the pelvis of
the kidney, the bowl-
shaped part into which
urine drains from special
tubules

pyelonephritis
inflammation of the pelvis
of the kidney

pyeorrhea
chronic degenerative
disease of the gums

quinsy
inflammation/abscesses
around the tonsils

refrigerant
substance that reduces fever

relaxant
substance that promotes
relaxation (either muscular
or psychological)

rheumatism
any painful disorder of the
joint tissues

rhinitis – see hayfever

ringworm
skin disease caused by
fungal infection

Rolfing
a manipulative deep
massage technique which
works on the connective
tissues of the body to
correct structural imbalance
after emotional trauma or
physical injury; founded
by American biochemist
Dr Ida Rolf in the 1940s

scabies
a skin disease caused by the
mite *Sarcoptes scabei*

sciatica
pain in the lower back,
usually a sign of some
other problem, like a
slipped disc

septicemia
spread of infection through
the bloodstream by the
circulation of bacteria

shingles
viral infection of the nerve
ganglia

sinusitis
inflammation of mucous
membranes lining the
sinuses (especially nasal)

smooth muscles
muscles with two nerve
supplies which surround
organs and cause both
contraction and relaxation

spasmolytic
able to relieve spasms or
convulsions

spleen
organ that filters dead
blood cells from the blood

stomachic
substance that stimulates
functions of the stomach

stomatitis
inflammation of any natural
opening of the body

stye
a painless swelling on the
eyelid that may become
uncomfortable in time and
need removing surgically

tapeworm
long, flat worm that lives as
a parasite in human
digestive tracts

thrombosis
formation of a blood clot
in a blood vessel

thrush
fungal infection of throat
or vagina

thyrocine antagonist
substance that inhibits
production of the hormone
thyrocine in the thyroid
gland

thyroid gland
gland that
regulates the
body's metabolic
rate, situated in
front of the
windpipe (trachea)

tinea – see
ringworm

tinnitus
a condition where
sounds (ringing) appear
in the ear for no apparent
reason

tonsillitis
inflammation of the tonsils

tonsils
lymph tissue at the back of
the throat

topical irritant
a substance that irritates
the skin

tracheitis
inflammation of the
windpipe (trachea)

tuberculosis
infectious disease caused
by bacteria entering the
body through the digestive
tract, affecting the
lungs first

tumour
abnormal growth of
the cells anywhere in
the body

ulcer
slow-healing sore
occurring internally
or externally

urethritis
inflammation of the tube
from the bladder (urethra)

uric acid
waste product produced by
metabolism

uterine tonic
substance that has a toning
effect on the whole
reproductive system

vasodilator
substance that dilates
the blood vessels and
so improves circulation

vermifuge
anthelmintic; remedy
that eliminates worms
from the body

visceral pain
pain in intestines and
abdominal cavity

whooping cough
infectious childhood
disease of the upper
respiratory tract

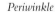

Periwinkle

FURTHER READING

There are generally two types of books about herbs. One type lists plants that are medicinally used and gives their properties. In order to use this type the reader must have prior knowledge about the appropriate plant for a particular condition. The other type focuses on conditions and symptoms, giving herbs that will help to heal. Though neither type is ideal, they can help a lot in the exploration of this fascinating field.

The list that follows is only a small selection of what is currently available.

Beinfield and Korngold
**Between Heaven and Earth:
A Guide to Chinese Medicine**
(Ballantine, 1992)

Bensky and Gamble
**Chinese Herbal Medicine –
Materia Medica**
(Eastland Press, 1986)

British Herbal Pharmacopoeia
*(British Herbal Medicine Association,
1990)*

Christopher, Dr John R
School of Natural Healing
(Dr Christopher's Publications, 1991)

De Smet, Keller, Hansel and
Chandler
**Adverse Effects of Herbal
Drugs, Vol 1**
(Springer-Verlag, 1992)

Frawley, David
**Ayurvedic Healing:
A Comprehensive Guide**
(Morson Publishing, 1990)

Gladstar, Rosemary
**Herbal Healing
for Women**
(Fireside, 1993)

Green, James
Male Herbal
(Crossings Press, 1991)

Grieve, Mrs M
**A Modern Herbal,
Vols 1 and 1**
(Dover Publications, 1971)

Griggs, Barbara
Green Pharmacy
*(Inner Traditions
International Ltd, 1991)*

Harborne and Baxter (eds)
**Phytochemical Dictionary:
A Handbook of Bioactive
Compounds from Plants**
(Taylor & Francis, 1993)

Hoffmann, David
An Elder's Herbal
(Inner Traditions, 1992)

Hoffmann, David
Successful Stress Control
(Healing Arts Press, 1986)

McIntyre, Anne
**The Complete Woman's
Herbal**
(Gaia Books, 1994)

Mills, Simon
**Dictionary of Modern
Herbalism**
(Inner Traditions, 1985)

Mills, Simon
**Out of the Earth:
The Science and
Practice of
Herbal Medicine**
(Viking Penguin, 1992)

Murray, Michael
**Healing Power
of Herbs**
(Prima Publications, 1992)

Priest and Priest
Herbal Medications
(L N Fowler & Co Ltd, 1982)

Ross and Brain
**An Introduction to
Phytopharmacy**
*(Pitman Medical Publishing,
1977)*

Trease and Evans
**Pharmacognosy,
13th edn**
(Baillere Tindall, 1989)

Wess, Rudolf
Herbal Medicine
(Medicina Biologica, 1988)

Wren, R C
**Potter's New
Cyclopaedia of
Botanical Drugs
and Preparations**
(C W Daniel, 1988)

USEFUL ADDRESSES

*Selected organizations and suppliers in the UK, USA, Canada
and Australasia*

HERBAL ORGANIZATIONS UK

**National Institute of
Medicinal Herbalists**
56 Longbrook Street
Exeter EX4 6AH

**Council for Complementary
and Alternative Medicine**
206-8 Latimer Road
London W10 6RE

**The School of
Phytotherapy**
Bucksteep Manor
Bodle Street Green
nr Hailsham,
East Sussex BN277 4RJ

HERBAL ORGANIZATIONS
USA AND CANADA

The American Herbalist Guild
PO Box 1688, Soquel
OA 995703, USA

Herb Research Foundation
1007 Pearl St
Suite 200, Boulder
CO 80802, USA

**The American Herb
Association**
Box 1673, Nevada City
CA 95949, USA

**The Ontario Herbalists
Association**
181 Brookdale Avenue
Toronto, Ontario M5M 1P4
Canada

HERBAL ORGANIZATIONS
IN AUSTRALASIA

**The College of
Naturopathic Medicine**
Box 4529, Christchurch
New Zealand

**National Herbalists
Association of Australia**
Box 65, Kingsgrove, NSW 2208
Australia

HERBAL SUPPLIERS UK

Neal's Yard Apothecary
15 Neal's Yard, Covent Garden
London WC2 9DP

Baldwins
171-173 Walworth Road
London SE17 1RW

Potter Limited
Leyland Mill Lane
Wigan, Lancashire WN1 2SB

Brome & Schimmer Ltd
Unit 42, Romsey Industrial Estate
Romsey,
Hampshire SO51 0HR

Peirce A Arnold & Son
12 Park Road, Hackbridge
Surrey SM6 7ES

Barwinnock Herbs
Barwinnock, Barrhill
Girvan, Ayrshire
KA26 ORB

HERBAL SUPPLIERS USA

Avena Botanicals
Box 365, West Rockport
MA 04865

Blessed Herbs
109 Barre Plains Road
Oakham, MA 01063

Frontier Co-operative Herbs
Box 299, Norway, IA 52318

Gaia Herbs
62 Old Littleton Road, Harvard
MA 011451

Green Terrestrial
PO Box 41, Route 9W
Milton, NY 12547

Herb-Pharm
347 East Fork Road, Williams
OR 97444

Herbalist & Alchemist Inc
PO Box 553, Broadway
NJ 08809

Island Herbs
c/o Ryan Drum, Waldron Island
WA 98297

Mountain Rose
PO Box 2000, Redway
CA 95560

Pacific Botanicals
4350 Fish Hatchery Road
Grants Pass, OR 97527

Sage Mountain Herb Products
PO Box 420, East Barre
VT 05649

Simpler's Botanical,
PO Box 39, Forestville
CA 95436

Wind River
PO Box 3876, Jackson
WY 93001

INDEX

References in **bold** *refer to entries of plants in* The Herbal, *pages 51–166.*

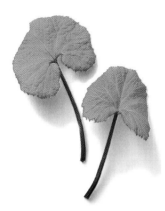

A

abcesses *194*
Acacia catechu (Black Catechu) **53**
Acerola berries *186*
Achillea millefolium (Yarrow) **53**, *173-4,
  186, 217, 223, 225, 229, 242-3*
acne *215*
Acorus calamus (Calamus) **54**, *196, 199*
adaptogens *206*
adrenal glands *229*
Aesculus hippocastanum (Horsechestnut)
  54, *174, 217*
Agathosma betulina (Buchu) **55**, *242*
Agrimonia eupatoria (Agrimony) **55**, *187,
  198-200, 243*
Agrimony *(Agrimonia eupatoria)* **55**, *187,
  198-200, 243*
Agropyron repens (Couchgrass) **56**, *242-3*
Alchemilla mollis (Lady's Mantle) **56**, *193*
alcoholic tincture *23*
alcohols *32*
Aletris farinosa (True Unicorn Root) **57**, *236*
Alfalfa *194*
alkaloids *35*
allergies *181, 199, 210*
Allium sativum (Garlic) **57**, *173, 180, 184-6,
  199, 216, 228, 238*
Allspice *(Pimento dioica)* **123**
Almond *184*
Aloe *(Aloe vera)* **58**, *217*
Aloe vera (Aloe) **58**, *217*
Alpina officinarum (Galangal) **58**
Althaea officinalis (Marshmallow) **59**, *174, 186,
  193-4, 196-9, 201, 214-15, 243*
amenorrhea *234*
American Cranesbill *(Geranium maculatum)* **97**,
  193, 197, 199, 234, 238-9
Anethum graveolens (Dill) **59**
Angelica *(Angelica archangelica)* **60**, *180*
Angelica archangelica (Angelica) **60**, *180*
angina pectoris *172*
Aniseed *(Pimpinella anisum)*
  123, *179-81, 195, 237*
anorexia nervosa *193*
anthaquinones *34*
anti-inflammatories
  220
anti-microbials *42,
  213*
anti-rheumatics *220*
antibiotics *41*
antiseptics *42, 233,
  241*
anxiety *195, 206-7*

Aphanes arvensis (Parsley Piert) **60**, *243*
Apium graveolens (Celery) **61**, *223, 225*
appendicitis *200*
appetite loss *193*
Arctium lappa (Burdock) **61**, *214-15, 225*
Arctostaphylos uva-ursi (Bearberry) **62**, *225,
  242-3*
Aristolochia serpentaria (Virginia Snakeroot) **62**
Armoracia rusticana (Horseradish) **63**, *194*
Arnica *(Arnica montana)* **63**, *173, 217*
Arnica montana (Arnica) **63**, *173, 217*
Artemisia abrotanum (Southernwood) **64**, *234*
Artemisia absinthum (Wormwood) **64**, *193, 195,
  201, 208, 210, 216, 229*
Artemisia cina (Santonica) **65**
Artemisia vulgaris (Mugwort) **65**
arteriosclerosis *173*
arthritis *222-4*
Asclepias tuberosa (Pleurisy Root) **66**, *180*
asthma *181*
Avena sativa (Oats) **66**, *206-7, 210-11, 216,
  229, 238-9*
Avens *(Geum urbanum)* **98**

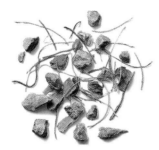

B

Bach Flower Remedies *203*
Ballota nigra (Black Horehound) **67**, *209, 237*
Balm of Gilead *(Populus x gileadensis)* **126**, *187*
Balm *(Melissa officinalis)* **113**, *172, 189, 195,
  198, 208-9*
Balmony *(Chelone glabra)* **76**, *200-1, 210*
Balsam of Tolu *(Myroxylon balsamum)* **116**
Baptisia tinctoria (Wild Indigo) **67**, *184-5,
  215-16, 238*
Barberry *(Berberis vulgaris)* **68**, *192, 200-1*
baths *28, 180, 208*
Bayberry *(Myrica cerifera)* **115**, *193, 198-9*
Bearberry *(Arctostaphylos uva-ursi)* **62**, *225, 242-3*
Bellis perennis (Daisy) **68**, *217*
Berberis vulgaris (Barberry) **68**, *192, 200-1*
Beth Root *(Trillium erectum)* **155**, *234, 238-9*
Betula pendula (Silver Birch) **69**
Bidens tripartita (Burr-marigold) **69**
Birch, Silver *(Betula pendula)* **69**
Bistort *(Polygonum bistorta)* **126**
bitter principles *35*
Bittersweet *(Solanum dulcamara)* **145**
Black Catechu *(Acacia catechu)* **53**
Black Cohosh *(Cimifuga racemosa)* **78**, *185, 210,
  223, 235, 238*
Black Haw *(Viburnu prunifolium)* **161**, *235-6*
  Black Horehound *(Ballota
    nigra)* **67**, *209, 237*
  Black Mustard *(Brassica
    nigra)* **70**
  Black Root *(Veronicastrum
    virginicum)* **160**, *200-1*
  Black Willow *(Salix nigra)*
    138, *209, 223*

Bladderwrack *(Fucus vesiculosus)* **94**, *229*
Blessed Thistle *(Cnicus benedictus)* **79**, *237*
blood pressure *172-3*
Blood Root *(Sanguinaria canadensis)* **140**, *180-1,
  187, 201*
Blue Cohosh *(Caulophyllum thalictriodes)* **7**, *234,
  236*
Blue Flag *(Iris versicolor)* **105**, *184, 187, 194,
  200, 215*
Bogbean *(Menyanthes trifoliata)* **114**, *223*
boils *215*
Boldo *(Peumus boldo)* **121**, *192, 200-1*
Boneset *(Eupatorium perfoliatum)* **91**, *180, 186,
  225*
Borage *(Borago officinalis)* **70**, *229*
Borago officinalis (Borage) **70**, *229*
Brassica nigra (Black Mustard) **70**
bronchitis *179-80*
Broom Tops *(Cytisus scoparius)* **85**, *171-2*
bruises *217*
Buchu *(Agathosma betulina)* **55**, *242*
Buckthorn *(Rhamnus catharticus)* **133**
Buckwheat *173-4*
Bugleweed *(Lycopus europaeus)* **110**, *171-2,
  228-9*
Burdock *(Arctium lappa)* **61**, *214-15, 225*
burns *217*
Burr-marigold *(Bidens tripartita)* **69**
bursitis *224*
Butterbur *(Petasites hybridus)* **120**

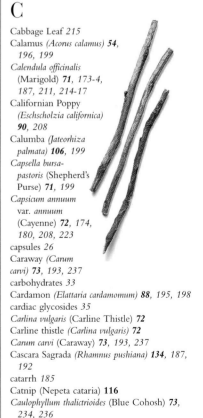

C

Cabbage Leaf *215*
Calamus *(Acorus calamus)* **54**,
  196, 199
Calendula officinalis
  (Marigold) **71**, *173-4,
  187, 211, 214-17*
Californian Poppy
  (Eschscholzia californica)
  90, *208*
Calumba *(Jateorhiza
  palmata)* **106**, *199*
*Capsella bursa-
  pastoris* (Shepherd's
  Purse) **71**, *199*
Capsicum annuum
  var. *annuum*
  (Cayenne) **72**, *174,
  180, 208, 223*
capsules *26*
Caraway *(Carum
  carvi)* **73**, *193, 237*
carbohydrates *33*
Cardamon *(Elattaria cardamomum)* **88**, *195, 198*
cardiac glycosides *35*
Carlina vulgaris (Carline Thistle) **72**
Carline thistle *(Carlina vulgaris)* **72**
Carum carvi (Caraway) **73**, *193, 237*
Cascara Sagrada *(Rhamnus pushiana)* **134**, *187,
  192*
catarrh *185*
Catnip *(Nepeta cataria)* **116**
Caulophyllum thalictrioides (Blue Cohosh) **73**,
  234, 236
Cayenne *(Capsicum annuum* var. *annuum)* **72**,
  174, 180, 208, 223
Celandine, Greater *(Chelidonium majus)* **76**, *216*
Celery *(Apium graveolens)* **61**, *223, 225*
Centaurium erythraea (Centaury) **74**, *207*
Centaury *(Centaurium erythraea)* **74**, *207*

Cetraria islandica (Iceland Moss) **74**

Chamaelirium luteum (False Unicorn Root) **75**, *210, 234-6, 238*

Chamaemelum nobile (Garden Chamomile) **75**, *184-5, 193, 195, 198, 200, 208-9, 237*

Chamomile, Garden *(Chamaemelum nobile)* **75**, *184-5, 193, 195, 198, 200, 208-9, 237*

Chamomile, German *(Matricaria recutita)* **75**, *199*

Chaste Tree *(Vitex agnus-castus)* **164**, *210, 234-5, 238*

Chelidonium majus (Greater Celandine) **76**, *216*

Chelone glabra (Balmony) **76**, *200-1, 210*

Chickweed *(Stellaria media)* **147**, *214-15*

chilblains *174*

childbirth *236-7*

Chionanthus virginicus (Fringetree) **77**, *200-1, 228*

Chondrus crispus (Irish Moss) **77**, *195, 237*

Cimicifuga racemosa (Black Cohosh) **78**, *185, 210, 223, 235, 238*

Cinchona officinalis (Peruvian Bark) **78**

Cinnamomum zeylandicum (Cinnamon) **121**

Cinnamon *(Cinnamomum zeylandicum)* **121**

circulatory system *168-74, 221*

cleansing *14*

Cleavers *(Galium aparine)* **96**, *175, 180, 184, 187, 194, 214-16, 238-9*

Clover, Red *(Trifolium pratense)* **154**, *207-8, 214-15*

Cloves *(Syzygium aromaticum)* **149**, *194*

Cnicus benedictus (Blessed Thistle) **79**, *237*

Cola nitida (Kola) **80**, *207, 210, 229*

colds *186*

Colic Root *see True Unicorn Root*

colitis *198-9*

Collinsonia canadensis (Stone Root) **80**, *243*

Coltsfoot *(Tussilago farfara)* **156**, *179-81*

Comfrey *(Symphytum officinale)* **148**, *173-4, 180-1, 193, 196-9, 214, 217*

Commiphora molmol (Myrrh) **81**, *187, 194-5, 215-16*

compresses *30, 217*

Condurango *(Marsdenia condurango)* **112**, *193*

congestion *179*

constipation *192*

contraceptive pill *235*

Convallaria majalis (Lily of the Valley) **81**, *170-2*

Coriander *(Coriandrum sativum)* **82**

Coriandrum sativum (Coriander) **82**

Corn Silk *(Zea mays)* **165**, *242-3*

Couchgrass *(Agropyron repens)* **56**, *242-3*

coughs *179*

coumarins *34*

Cowslip *(Primula veris)* **128**

cramp *224*

Cramp Bark *(Viburnum opulus)* **161**, *173, 224, 235-6, 243*

Cranesbill, American *(Geranium maculatum)* **97**, *193, 197, 199, 234, 238-9*

Crataegus laevigata (Hawthorn) **82**, *170-4, 181*

Cucumber *(Cucumis sativus)* **83**

Cucumis sativus (Cucumber) **83**

Cucurbita pepo (Pumpkin) **83**

Cudweed *(Gnaphalium uliginosum)* **99**

Cydonia oblonga (Quince) **84**

Cypripedium calceolus var. *pubescens* (Lady's Slipper) **84**, *206-8*

cystitis *242*

Cytisus scoparius (Broom Tops) **85**, *171-2*

D

Daisy *(Bellis perennis)* **68**, *217*

Damiana *(Turnera diffusa* var. *aphrodisiaca)* **156**, *207, 210, 229, 239*

Dandelion *(Taraxacum officinale)* **151**, *171-2, 174, 192, 200-1, 207, 214-15, 225, 235, 243*

dandelion wine *24*

Daucus carota (Wild Carrot) **85**, *225, 243*

deafness *184-5*

decoctions *23*

depression *207-8*

Devil's Claw *(Harpagophytum procumbens)* **102**

diabetes mellitus *228*

diaphoretics *42-3*

diarrhea *192-3*

diet *168-9, 175, 189, 201, 210*

digestive system *188-201, 221*

Digitalis purpurea (Foxglove) **170**

Dill *(Anethum graveolens)* **59**

Dioscorea villosa (Wild Yam) **86**, *193, 198-200, 210, 223, 229, 235, 238*

diuretics *171, 221, 241*

diverticulitis *199*

Dock, Yellow *(Rumex crispus)* **137**, *200, 214-16, 225*

douches *28*

Drosera rotundifolia (Sundew) **86**, *180-1*

drying herbs *20-1*

Dryopteris filix-mas (Male Fern) **87**

dysmenorrhea *235*

E

earache *184*

ears *182-5*

Echinacea angustifolia (Echinacea) **87**, *174-5, 180, 184-7, 194, 197-200, 211, 215-17, 238-9, 242-3*

Echinacea *(Echinacea angustifolia)* **87**, *174-5, 180, 184-7, 194, 197-200, 211, 215-17, 238-9, 242-3*

eczema *214*

Elder *(Sambucus nigra)* **139**, *184-6, 208, 217*

Elecampane *(Inula helenium)* **105**, *180-1*

Eleattaria cardamomum (Cardamon) **88**, *195, 198*

Eleutherococcus senticosus (Siberian Ginseng) **88**, *206*

enteritis *198*

Ephedra *(Ephedra sinica)* **89**, *181, 186*

Ephedra sinica (Ephedra) **89**, *181, 186*

Equisetum arvense (Horsetail) **89**, *242-3*

Eryngium maritimum (Sea Holly) **90**, *243*

Eschscholzia california (Californian Poppy) **90**, *208*

Eucalyptus *180, 185, 194, 216*

Euonymus atropurpureus (Wahoo) **91**, *200-1*

Eupatorium perfoliatum (Boneset) **91**, *180, 186, 225*

Eupatorium purpureum (Gravel Root) **92**, *243*

Euphorbia hirta (Pill-bearing Spurge) **92**, *181*

Euphrasia officinalis (Eyebright) **93**, *185-7*

Evening Primrose *211*

exercise *168-9*

Eyebright *(Euphrasia officinalis)* **93**, *185-7*

eyes *182-3, 187*

F

False Unicorn Root *(Chamaelirium luteum)* **75**, *210, 234-6, 238*

Fennel *(Foeniculum vulgare)* **94**, *192, 195, 237*

Fenugreek *(Trigonella foenum-graecum)* **154**, *237*

Fern, Male *(Dryopteris filix-mas)* **87**

Feverfew *(Tanacetum parthenium)* **150**, *209*

fibrositis *224*

Figwort *(Scrophularia nodosa)* **141**, *171, 214-15*

Filipendula ulmaria (Meadowsweet) **93**, *193, 195-6, 198, 201, 209-10, 223, 237*

flavones *34*

flavonoid glycosides *34*

Flax *(Linum usitatissimum)* **109**, *180-1*

fleas *45*

Foeniculum vulgare (Fennel) **94**, *192, 195, 237*

Foxglove *(Digitalis purpurea)* **170**

Fringetree *(Chionanthus virginicus)* **77**, *200-1, 228*

Fucus vesiculosus (Bladderwrack) **94**, *229*

Fumaria officinalis (Fumitory) **95**, *214*

Fumitory *(Fumaria officinalis)* **95**, *214*

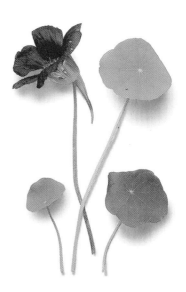

G

Galangal *(Alpina officinarum)* **58**

Galega officinalis (Goat's Rue) **95**, *228, 237*

Galium aparine (Cleavers) **96**, *175, 180, 184, 187, 194, 214-16, 238-9*

gallstones *201*

gall-bladder *200-1*

Garden Chamomile *(Chamaemelum nobile)* **75**, *184-5, 193, 195, 198, 200, 208-9, 237*

Garlic *(Allium sativum)* **57**, *173, 180, 184-6, 199, 216, 228, 238*

gastritis *195-6*

gathering herbs *20-1*

Gaultheria procumbens (Wintergreen) **96**

Gentian *(Gentiana lutea)* **97**, *193, 195, 201*

Gentiana lutea (Gentian) **97**, *193, 195, 201*

Geranium maculatum (American Cranesbill) **97**, *193, 197, 199, 234, 238-9*

German Chamomile *(Matricaria recutita)* **75**, *199*

Geum urbanum (Avens) **98**

Ginger *(Zingiber officinale)* **165**, *174, 192-3, 199, 224*

gingivitis *194*

Ginseng *(Panax ginseng)* **118**, *206-7, 210, 228-9, 239*

Ginseng, Siberian *(Eleutherococcus senticosus)* **88**, *206*

glands *175*

glandular system *226-9*
Glechoma hederacea (Ground Ivy) **98**, *208*
Glycyrrhiza glabra (Licorice) **99**, *179, 181, 186, 192, 194, 229, 235*
glycerine-based tinctures *25*
Gnaphalium uliginosum (Cudweed) **99**
Goat's Rue *(Galega officinale)* **95**, *228, 237*
goitre *229*
Golden Rod *(Solidago virgauria)* **146**, *184-6*
Golden Seal *(Hydrastis canadensis)* **103**, *175, 184-7, 195-8, 200-1, 209-10, 214, 216-17, 237-8*
gout *225*
Gravel Root *(Eupatorium purpureum)* **92**, *243*
Greater Celandine *(Chelidonium majus)* **76**, *216*
Greater Plantain *(Plantago major)* **125**, *217*
Grindelia camporum (Grindelia) **100**, *181*
Grindelia *(Grindelia camporum)* **100**, *181*
Ground Ivy *(Glechoma hederacea)* **98**, *208*
Guaiacum *(Guaiacum officinale)* **100**, *223*
Guaiacum officinale (Guaiacum) **100**, *223*

H

Hagenia abyssinica (Kousso) **101**
Hamamelis virginiana (Witch Hazel) **101**, *174, 187, 194, 200, 214-15, 217, 225*
Harpagophytum procumbens (Devil's Claw) **102**
Hawthorn *(Crataegus laevigata)* **82**, *170-4, 181*
hayfever *186*
headaches *208-9*
hearing problems *184-5*
heart *168-74*
hemorrhoids *200*
herpes simplex *216*
Hops *(Humulus lupulus)* **102**, *181, 195, 197-8, 208, 210, 237, 239*
hormonal problems *210*
Horsechestnut *(Aesculus hippocastanum)* **54**, *174, 217*
Horseradish *(Armoracia rusticana)* **63**, *194*
Horsetail *(Equisetum arvense)* **89**, *242-3*
Humulus lupulus (Hops) **102**, *181, 195, 197-8, 208, 210, 237, 239*
Hydrangea aborescens (Hydrangea) **103**, *242-3*
Hydrangea *(Hydrangea aborescens)* **103**, *242-3*
Hydrastis canadensis (Golden Seal) **103**, *175, 184-7, 195-8, 200-1, 209-10, 214, 216-17, 237-8*
hyperactivity *207*
Hypericum perforatum (St John's Wort) **104**, *210-11, 217, 224, 238*
Hyssop *(Hyssopus officinalis)* **104**, *180, 184*
Hyssopus officinalis (Hyssop) **104**, *180, 184*

I

Iceland Moss *(Cetraria islandica)* **74**
immune system *16-17*
impetigo *215*
incontinence *243*
indigestion *195*

infections *40-5, 184, 238-9, 242*
influenza *186*
infusions *22-3*
insomnia *208*
Inula helenium (Elecampane) **105**, *180-1*
Ipecacuanha *(Psychotria ipecacuanha)* **130**
Iris versicolor (Blue Flag) **105**, *184, 187, 194, 200, 215*
Irish Moss *(Chondrus crispus)* **77**, *195, 237*

J

Jamaican Dogwood *(Piscidia piscipula)* **124**, *208-11, 223*
Jambul *(Syzygium cumini)* **150**, *228*
Jateorhiza palmata (Calumba) *106, 199*
jaundice *201*
Juniper *(Juniperus communis)* **106**, *242*
Juniperus communis (Juniper) **106**, *242*

K

Kelp *see Bladderwrack*
kidney stones *243*
kidneys *240-3*
Kola *(Cola nitida)* **80**, *207, 210, 229*
Kousso *(Hagenia abyssinica)* **101**
Krameria triandra (Rhatany) **107**, *187*

L

labour *237*
Lactuca virosa (Wild Lettuce) **107**, *179, 195, 239*
Lady's Mantle *(Alchemilla mollis)* **56**, *193*
Lady's Slipper *(Cypripedium calceolus var. pubescens)* **84**, *206-8*
large intestine *198-200*
laryngitis *187*
Lavandula angustifolia (Lavender) **108**, *195, 198, 207-9, 211*
Lavender *(Lavandula angustifolia)* **108**, *195, 198, 207-9, 211*
laxatives *190*
Leonurus cardiaca (Motherwort) **108**, *171-2, 179, 181, 214, 235, 238*
lice *45*
Licorice *(Glycyrrhiza glabra)* **99**, *179, 181, 186, 192, 194, 229, 235*
Life Root *(Packera aureua)* **117**, *210, 238*
Lily of the Valley *(Convallaria majalis)* **81**, *170-2*
Lime Blossom *(Tilia x vulgaris)* **153**, *172-3, 181, 198-9, 206-8, 239*
liniments *31, 224*
Linum usitatissimum (Flax) **109**, *180-1*
liver *200-1*
Lobaria pulmonaria (Lungwort Moss) **109**
Lobelia inflata (Lobelia) **110**, *180-1, 184*
Lobelia *(Lobelia inflata)* **110**, *180-1, 184*
lozenges *27*
lumbago *225*
lungs *176-81*
Lungwort Herb *(Pulmonaria officinalis)* **131**, *180*
Lungwort Moss *(Lobaria pulmonaria)* **109**
Lycopus europaeus (Bugleweed) **110**, *171-2, 228-9*
lymphatic system *175*

M

Ma Huang *see Ephedra*
Mahonia aquifolium (Mountain grape) **111**, *201, 214-15*
malabsorption *198*
Male Fern *(Dryopteris filix-mas)* **87**
Mallow *(Malva sylvestris)* **111**
Malva sylvestris (Mallow) **111**
Marigold *(Calendula officinalis)* **71**, *173-4, 187, 211, 214-17*

Marjoram, Wild *(Origanum vulgare)* **117**, *208-9*
Marrubium vulgare (White Horehound) **112**, *179-80*
Marsdenia condurango (Condurango) **112**, *193*
Marshmallow *(Althaea officinalis)* **59**, *174, 186, 193-4, 196-9, 201, 214-15, 243*
mastoiditis *184*
Matricaria recutita (German Chamomile) **75**, *199*
Meadowsweet *(Filipendula ulmaria)* **93**, *193, 195-6, 198, 201, 209-10, 223, 237*
Melissa officinalis (Balm) **113**, *172, 189, 195, 198, 208-9*
menopause *237-8*
menorrhagia *234*
menstrual cycle *231, 234*
Mentha pulegium (Pennyroyal) **114**
Mentha x piperita (Peppermint) **113**, *185-6, 194-5, 208-9, 237*
Menyanthes trifoliata (Bogbean) **114**, *223*
metrorrhagia *234*
migraine *209-10*
milk production *237*
Milk Thistle *(Silybum marianum)* **144**
miscarriage, threatened *236-7*
Mistletoe *(Viscum alba)* **163**, *172-3, 206, 210, 214*
Mitchella repens (Squaw Vine) **115**, *236-7*
morning sickness *237*

Motherwort *(Leonurus cardiaca)* **108**, *171-2, 179, 181, 214, 235, 238*
Mountain Grape *(Mahonia aquifolium)* **111**, *201, 214-15*
Mouse Ear *(Pilosella officinarum)* **122**, *180-1*
mouth *193-5*
Mugwort *(Artemisia vulgaris)* **65**
Mullein *(Verbascum thapsus)* **159**, *179-80, 184*
multiple sclerosis *211*
musculo/skeletal system *218-25*
Mustard, Black *(Brassica nigra)* **70**
Myrica cerifera (Bayberry) **115**, *193, 198-9*
Myroxylon balsamum (Tolu Balsam) **116**
Myrrh *(Commiphora molmol)* **81**, *187, 194-5, 215-16*

N

Nasturtium *(Tropaeolum majus)* **155**
Navelwort *see Pennywort*

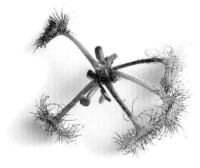

Nepeta cataria (Catnip) **116**
nervous system 202-11
Nettle *(Urtica dioica)* **158**, 214, 228-9, 236
neuralgia 210-11
neurological diseases 208-11
Night Blooming Cereus *(Selenicereus grandiflorus)* **142**, 170
nose 182-3, 185-7
nosebleed 187

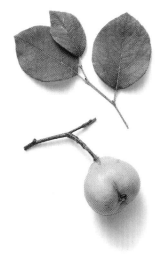

O

Oak *(Quercus robur)* **132**, 193, 199, 238
Oats *(Avena sativa)* **66**, 206-7, 210-11, 216, 229, 238-9
oils 31
ointments 28-30, 215
Origanum vulgare (Wild Marjoram) **117**, 208-9
overeating 195
oxymel 25

P

Packera aurea (Life Root) **117**, 210, 238
pain 193
pain relievers 221
palpitations 172
Panax ginseng (Ginseng) **118**, 206-7, 210, 228-9, 239
pancreas 228
pancreatitis 228
Pansy *(Viola tricolor)* **163**, 214
Papaver rhoeas (Red Poppy) **118**
Parietaria diffusa (Pellitory of the Wall) **119**, 242-3
Parsley *(Petroselinum crispum)* **120**
Parsley Piert *(Aphanes arvensis)* **60**, 243
Pasque Flower *(Pulsatilla vulgaris)* **131**, 210, 215, 235
Passiflora incarnata (Passion Flower) **119**, 172, 208-11, 223, 239
Passion Flower *(Passiflora incarnata)* **119**, 172, 208-11, 223, 239
Peach *(Prunus persica)* **129**
Pellitory of the Wall *(Parietaria diffusa)* **119**, 242-3
Pennyroyal *(Mentha pulegium)* **114**
Pennywort *(Umbilicus rupestris)* **157**, 184
Peppermint *(Mentha x piperata)* **113**, 185-6, 194-5, 208-9, 237
Periwinkle *(Vinca major)* **162**, 199-200, 234, 238-9
Peruvian Bark *(Cinchona officinalis)* **78**
Petasites hybridus (Butterbur) **120**
Petroselinum crispum (Parsley) **120**
Peumus boldo (Boldo) **121**, 192, 200-1
phenolic compounds 33-4

phlebitis 173
Phytolacca americana (Poke Root) **121**, 175, 180, 184-5, 187, 194, 215-16, 238
Picrasma excelsor (Quassia) **122**
Pilewort *(Ranunculus ficaria)* **133**, 200
Pill-bearing Spurge *(Euphorbia hirta)* **92**, 181
pills 26
Pilosella officinarum (Mouse Ear) **122**, 180-1
Pimento dioica (Allspice) **123**
Pimpinella anisum (Aniseed) **123**, 179-81, 195, 237
Pine, Scots *(Pinus sylvestris)* **124**, 185
Pinus sylvestris (Scots Pine) **124**, 185
Piscidia piscipula (Jamaican Dogwood) **124**, 208-11, 223
pituitary gland 227
plant acids 32
Plantago major (Greater Plantain) **125**, 217
Plantain, Greater *(Plantago major)* **125**, 217
pleurisy 180
Pleurisy Root *(Asclepias tuberosa)* **66**, 180
Poke Root *(Phytolacca americana)* **121**, 175, 180, 184-5, 187, 194, 215-16, 238
Polygala senega (Senega) **125**, 180-1
Polygonum bistorta (Bistort) **126**
polyps 187
Pomegranate *(Punica granatum)* **132**
Poppy, Red *(Papaver rhoeas)* **118**
Populus x gileadensis (Balm of Gilead) **126**, 187
Populus tremuloides (White Popular) **127**
Potentilla anserina (Silverweed) **127**
Potentilla erecta (Tormentil) **128**, 200
poultices 31, 180, 215
pregnancy 234, 236-7
pre-menstrual syndrome 235
pre-menstrual tension 207
preparation 22-31
prevention 12
Prickly Ash *(Zanthoxylum americanum)* **164**, 174, 216, 224
Primula veris (Cowslip) **128**
prostatitis 242
Prunella vulgaris (Self-Heal) **129**
Prunus persica (Peach) **129**
Prunus serotina (Wild Cherry) **130**, 181
psoriasis 214
Psychotria ipecacuanha (Ipecacuanha) **130**
Pulmonaria officinalis (Lungwort Herb) **131**, 180
Pulsatilla vulgaris (Pasque Flower) **131**, 210, 215, 235
Pumpkin *(Cucurbita pepo)* **83**
Punica granatum (Pomegranate) **132**
pyelonephritis 242
pyorrhea 194

Q

Quassia *(Picrasma excelsor)* **122**
Queen's Delight *(Stillingia sylvatica)* **148**
Quercus robur (Oak) **132**, 193, 199, 238
Quince *(Cydonia oblonga)* **84**

R

Ragwort *(Senecio jacobaea)* **143**
Ranunculus ficaria (Pilewort) **133**, 200
Raspberry *(Rubus idaeus)* **136**, 187, 236-7
Red Clover *(Trifolium pratense)* **154**, 207-8, 214-15
Red Poppy *(Papaver rhoeas)* **118**
Red Sage *(Salvia officinalis)* **138**, 187, 194, 237
relaxants 178, 191, 203
relaxation 204-5
renal colic 243
reproductive system 230-9
respiratory system 176-81
Rhamnus catharticus (Buckthorn) **133**
Rhamnus pushiana (Cascara Sagrada) **134**, 187, 192
Rhatany *(Krameria triandra)* **107**, 187
Rheum palmatum (Rhubarb Root) **134**, 192, 199
rheumatism 222-4
Rhubarb Root *(Rheum palmatum)* **134**, 192, 199
Rhus aromatica (Sweet Sumach) **135**, 228, 243
ringworm 216
Rosa canina (Rosehips) **135**, 186
Rosehips *(Rosa canina)* **135**, 186
Rosemary *(Rosmarinus officinalis)* **136**, 195, 207-9, 211, 225
Rosmarinus officinalis (Rosemary) **136**, 195, 207-9, 211, 225
Rubus idaeus (Raspberry) **136**, 187, 236-7
Rue *(Ruta graveolens)* **137**, 208, 234
Rumex crispus (Yellow Dock) **137**, 200, 214-16, 225
Ruta graveolens (Rue) **137**, 208, 234

S

Sage, Red *(Salvia officinalis)* **138**, 187, 194, 237
St John's Wort *(Hypericum perforatum)* **104**, 210-11, 217, 224, 238
Salix nigra (Black Willow) **138**, 209, 223
Salvia officinalis (Red Sage) **138**, 187, 194, 237
Sambucus nigra (Elder) **139**, 184-6, 208, 217
Sanguinaria canadensis (Blood Root) **140**, 180-1, 187, 201
Santonica *(Artemisia cina)* **65**
Saponaria officinalis (Soapwort) **140**
saponins 34-5
Sarsaparilla *(Smilax regelii)* **145**, 214
Sassafras albidum (Sassafras) **141**
Sassafras *(Sassafras albidum)* **141**
Saw Palmetto *(Seronoa repens)* **144**, 239, 242
scabies 45
sciatica 225
Scots Pine *(Pinus sylvestris)* **124**, 185
Scrophularia nodosa (Figwort) **141**, 171, 214-15
Scutellaria laterifolia (Skullcap) **142**, 172-3, 181, 186, 193, 198-9, 206-10, 214, 235, 237-9
Sea Holly *(Eryngium maritimum)* **90**, 243

Selenicereus grandiflorus (Night Blooming Cereus) **142**, 170
Self-Heal (Prunella vulgaris) **129**
Senecio jacobaea (Ragwort) **143**
Senega (Polygala senega) **125**, 180-1
Senna alexandrina (Senna) **143**, 199
Senna (Senna alexandrina) **143**, 199
Seronoa repens (Saw Palmetto) **144**, 239, 242
sexuality 239
Shepherd's Purse (Capsella bursa-pastoris) **71**, 199
shingles 211
Siberian Ginseng *(Eleutherococcus senticosus)* **88**, 206
Silver Birch *(Betula pendula)* **69**
Silverweed *(Potentilla anserina)* **127**
Silybum marianum (Milk Thistle) **144**
sinusitis 186
skin 212-17
Skullcap *(Scutellaria laterifolia)* **142**, 172-3, 181, 186, 193, 198-9, 206-10, 214, 235, 237-9
Skunk Cabbage *(Symplocarpus foetidus)* **149**
Slippery Elm *(Ulmus rubra)* **157**, 196-9
small intestine 197-8
Smilax regelii (Sarsaparilla) **145**, 214
Soapwort *(Saponaria officinalis)* **140**
Solanum dulcamara (Bittersweet) **145**
Solidago virgauria (Golden Rod) **146**, 184-6
Southernwood *(Artemisia abrontanum)* **64**, 234
sprains 225
Squaw Root *see* Blue Cohosh
Squaw Vine *(Mitchella repens)* **115**, 236-7
Squill *(Urginea maritima)* **158**
Stachys officinalis (Wood Betony) **146**, 173, 208-9
Stachys palustris (Woundwort) **147**
steam inhalation 185

Stellaria media (Chickweed) **147**, 214-15
Stillingia sylvatica (Queen's Delight) **148**
stimulants 178, 190, 203, 220
stomach 195-7
Stone Root *(Collinsonia canadensis)* **80**, 243
stress 169, 171, 195, 205-6, 210
Sundew *(Drosera rotundifolia)* **86**, 180-1
suppositories 30
Sweet Flag *see* Calamus
Sweet Sumach *(Rhus aromatica)* **135**, 228, 243
Sweet Violet *(Viola odorata)* **162**
Symphytum officinale (Comfrey) **148**, 173-4, 180-1, 193, 196-9, 214, 217
Symplocarpus foetidus (Skunk Cabbage) **149**
syrups 25
Syzygium aromaticum (Cloves) **149**, 194
Syzygium cumini (Jambul) **150**, 228

T

Tanacetum parthenium (Feverfew) **150**, 209
Tanacetum vulgare (Tansy) **151**, 208
tannins 34
Tansy *(Tanacetum vulgare)* **151**, 208
Taraxacum officinale (Dandelion) **151**, 171-2, 174, 192, 200-1, 207, 214-15, 225, 235, 243
teas 23
teeth 193-4
tension 195
Teucrium scorodonia (Wood Sage) **152**
throat 182-3, 187
thrombosis 173
Thuja occidentalis (Thuja) **152**, 187, 214, 216
Thuja *(Thuja occidentalis)* **152**, 187, 214, 216
Thyme *(Thymus vulgaris)* **153**, 180, 208, 225
Thymus vulgaris (Thyme) **153**, 180, 208, 225
thyroid 228-9
Tilia x vulgaris (Lime Blossom) **153**, 172-3, 181, 198-9, 206-8, 239
tinctures 24-5
tinnitus 185
tonic wine 24
tonics 12-13, 170, 203, 221, 232
tonsillitis 187
toothbrush 194
Tormentil *(Potentilla erecta)* **128**, 200
Trifolium pratense (Red Clover) **154**, 207-8, 214-15
Trigonella foenum-graecum (Fenugreek) **154**, 237
Trillium erectum (Beth Root) **155**, 234, 238-9
Tropaeolum majus (Nasturtium) **155**
True Unicorn Root *(Aletris farinosa)* **57**, 236
Turkey Rhubarb Root *see* Rhubarb Root
Turnera diffusa var. aphrodisiaca (Damiana) **156**, 207, 210, 229, 239
Tussilago farfara (Coltsfoot) **156**, 179-81

U

ulcers 174, 194-8
Ulmus rubra (Slippery Elm) **157**, 196-9
Umbilicus rupestris (Pennywort) **157**, 184
urethritis 242
Urginea maritima (Squill) **158**
urinary system 240-3
Urtica dioica (Nettle) **158**, 214, 228-9, 236
Uva Ursi *see* Bearberry

V

Valerian *(Valeriana officinalis)* **159**, 172-3, 181, 193, 195-9, 201, 206-11, 214, 223 229, 235, 237-9, 243
Valeriana officinalis (Valerian) **159**, 172-3, 181, 193, 195-9, 201, 206-11, 214, 223, 229, 235, 237-9, 243
varicose veins 174
Verbascum thapsus (Mullein) **159**, 179-80, 184
Verbena officinalis (Vervain) **160**, 186, 200, 207, 210, 237
Veronicastrum virginicum (Black Root) **160**, 200-1
Vervain *(Verbena officinalis)* **160**, 186, 200, 207, 210, 237
Viburnum opulus (Cramp Bark) **161**, 173, 224, 235-6, 243
Viburnum prunifolium (Black Haw) **161**, 235-6
Vinca major (Periwinkle) **162**, 199-200, 234, 238-9

vinegar-based tinctures 25
Viola odorata (Sweet Violet) **162**
Viola tricolor (Pansy) **163**, 214
Virginia Snakeroot *(Aristolochia serpentaria)* **62**
Viscum alba (Mistletoe) **163**, 172-3, 206, 210, 214
vitamin C 186
Vitex agnus-castus (Chaste Tree) **164**, 210, 234-5, 238
volatile oils 32-3

W

Wahoo *(Euonymus atropurpureus)* **91**, 200-1
warts 216
water retention 243
White Horehound *(Marrubium vulgare)* **112**, 179-80
White Poplar *(Populus tremuloides)* **127**
whooping cough 180-1
Wild Carrot *(Daucus carota)* **85**, 225, 243
Wild Cherry *(Prunus serotina)* **130**, 181
Wild Indigo *(Baptisia tinctoria)* **67**, 184-5, 215-16, 238
Wild Lettuce *(Lactuca virosa)* **107**, 179, 195, 239
Wild Marjoram *(Origanum vulgare)* **117**, 208-9
Wild Yam *(Dioscorea villosa)* **86**, 193, 198-200, 210, 223, 229, 235, 238
Willow, Black *(Salix nigra)* **138**, 209, 223
wines 24-5
Wintergreen *(Gaultheria procumbens)* **96**
Witch Hazel *(Hamamelis virginiana)* **101**, 174, 187, 194, 200, 214-15, 217, 225
Wood Betony *(Stachys officinalis)* **146**, 173, 208-9
Wood Sage *(Teucrium scorodonia)* **152**
worms 45
Wormwood *(Artemisia absinthum)* **64**, 193, 195, 201, 208, 210, 216, 229
wounds 217
Woundwort *(Stachys palustris)* **147**

Y

Yarrow *(Achillea millefolium)* **53**, 173-4, 184, 186, 217, 223, 225, 229, 242-3
Yellow Dock *(Rumex crispus)* **137**, 200, 214-16, 225

Z

Zanthoxylum americanum (Prickly Ash) **164**, 174, 216, 224
Zea mays (Corn Silk) **165**, 242-3
Zingiber officinale (Ginger) **165**, 174, 192-3, 199, 224

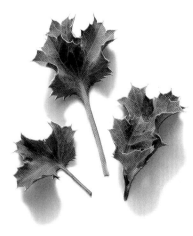